Medication Safety and Pharmacovigilance in Clinical: From the Researcher Bench to the Patient Bedside

Medication Safety and Pharmacovigilance in Clinical: From the Researcher Bench to the Patient Bedside

Editors

Alfredo Vannacci
Niccolò Lombardi
Giada Crescioli

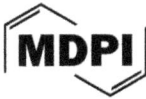

Basel • Beijing • Wuhan • Barcelona • Belgrade • Novi Sad • Cluj • Manchester

Editors

Alfredo Vannacci
University of Florence
Florence
Italy

Niccolò Lombardi
University of Florence
Florence
Italy

Giada Crescioli
University of Florence
Florence
Italy

Editorial Office
MDPI
St. Alban-Anlage 66
4052 Basel, Switzerland

This is a reprint of articles from the Special Issue published online in the open access journal *Journal of Clinical Medicine* (ISSN 2077-0383) (available at: https://www.mdpi.com/journal/jcm/special_issues/medication_pharmacovigilance).

For citation purposes, cite each article independently as indicated on the article page online and as indicated below:

Lastname, A.A.; Lastname, B.B. Article Title. *Journal Name* **Year**, *Volume Number*, Page Range.

ISBN 978-3-7258-0681-2 (Hbk)
ISBN 978-3-7258-0682-9 (PDF)
doi.org/10.3390/books978-3-7258-0682-9

© 2024 by the authors. Articles in this book are Open Access and distributed under the Creative Commons Attribution (CC BY) license. The book as a whole is distributed by MDPI under the terms and conditions of the Creative Commons Attribution-NonCommercial-NoDerivs (CC BY-NC-ND) license.

Contents

Giada Crescioli, Roberto Bonaiuti, Renato Corradetti, Guido Mannaioni, Alfredo Vannacci and Niccolò Lombardi
Pharmacovigilance and Pharmacoepidemiology as a Guarantee of Patient Safety: The Role of the Clinical Pharmacologist
Reprinted from: *J. Clin. Med.* 2022, 11, 3552, doi:10.3390/jcm11123552 1

Silvia Pagani, Niccolò Lombardi, Giada Crescioli, Violetta Giuditta Vighi, Giulia Spada, Paola Andreetta, et al.
Drug-Related Hypersensitivity Reactions Leading to Emergency Department: Original Data and Systematic Review
Reprinted from: *J. Clin. Med.* 2022, 11, 2811, doi:10.3390/jcm11102811 7

Mohammad A. Al-Mamun, Jacob Strock, Yushuf Sharker, Khaled Shawwa, Rebecca Schmidt, Douglas Slain, et al.
Evaluating the Medication Regimen Complexity Score as a Predictor of Clinical Outcomes in the Critically Ill
Reprinted from: *J. Clin. Med.* 2022, 11, 4705, doi:10.3390/jcm11164705 27

Nadir Yalçın, Merve Kaşıkcı, Hasan Tolga Çelik, Karel Allegaert, Kutay Demirkan, Şule Yiğit and Murat Yurdakök
Novel Method for Early Prediction of Clinically Significant Drug–Drug Interactions with a Machine Learning Algorithm Based on Risk Matrix Analysis in the NICU
Reprinted from: *J. Clin. Med.* 2022, 11, 4715, doi:10.3390/jcm11164715 44

Fahad M. Althobaiti, Safaa M. Alsanosi, Alaa H. Falemban, Abdullah R. Alzahrani, Salma A. Fataha, Sara O. Salih, et al.
Efficacy and Safety of Empagliflozin in Type 2 Diabetes Mellitus Saudi Patients as Add-On to Antidiabetic Therapy: A Prospective, Open-Label, Observational Study
Reprinted from: *J. Clin. Med.* 2022, 11, 4769, doi:10.3390/jcm11164769 57

Yoshihiro Noguchi, Shunsuke Yoshizawa, Tomoya Tachi and Hitomi Teramachi
Effect of Dipeptidyl Peptidase-4 Inhibitors vs. Metformin on Major Cardiovascular Events Using Spontaneous Reporting System and Real-World Database Study
Reprinted from: *J. Clin. Med.* 2022, 11, 4988, doi:10.3390/jcm11174988 70

Claudia Rossi, Rosanna Ruggiero, Liberata Sportiello, Ciro Pentella, Mario Gaio, Antonio Pinto and Concetta Rafaniello
Did the COVID-19 Pandemic Affect Contrast Media-Induced Adverse Drug Reaction's Reporting? A Pharmacovigilance Study in Southern Italy
Reprinted from: *J. Clin. Med.* 2022, 11, 5104, doi:10.3390/jcm11175104 80

Carina Amaro, Cristina Monteiro and Ana Paula Duarte
COVID-19 Vaccines Adverse Reactions Reported to the Pharmacovigilance Unit of Beira Interior in Portugal
Reprinted from: *J. Clin. Med.* 2022, 11, 5591, doi:10.3390/jcm11195591 93

Tigist Dires Gebreyesus, Eyasu Makonnen, Tafesse Tadele, Habtamu Gashaw, Workagegnew Degefe, Heran Gerba, et al.
Safety Surveillance of Mass Praziquantel and Albendazole Co-Administration in School Children from Southern Ethiopia: An Active Cohort Event Monitoring
Reprinted from: *J. Clin. Med.* 2022, 11, 6300, doi:10.3390/jcm11216300 114

Giorgia Teresa Maniscalco, Cristina Scavone, Annamaria Mascolo, Valentino Manzo, Elio Prestipino, Gaspare Guglielmi, et al.
The Safety Profile of COVID-19 Vaccines in Patients Diagnosed with Multiple Sclerosis: A Retrospective Observational Study
Reprinted from: *J. Clin. Med.* **2022**, *11*, 6855, doi:10.3390/jcm11226855 128

Ligang Liu, Armando Silva Almodóvar and Milap C. Nahata
Medication Adherence in Medicare-Enrolled Older Adults with Chronic Obstructive Pulmonary Disease before and during the COVID-19 Pandemic
Reprinted from: *J. Clin. Med.* **2022**, *11*, 6985, doi:10.3390/jcm11236985 139

Valentina Brilli, Giada Crescioli, Andrea Missanelli, Cecilia Lanzi, Massimo Trombini, Alessandra Ieri, et al.
Exposures and Suspected Intoxications to Pharmacological and Non-Pharmacological Agents in Children Aged 0–14 Years: Real-World Data from an Italian Reference Poison Control Centre
Reprinted from: *J. Clin. Med.* **2023**, *12*, 352, doi:10.3390/jcm12010352 150

Teresa Gavaruzzi, Marta Caserotti, Roberto Bonaiuti, Paolo Bonanni, Giada Crescioli, Mariarosaria Di Tommaso, et al.
The Interplay of Perceived Risks and Benefits in Deciding to Become Vaccinated against COVID-19 While Pregnant or Breastfeeding: A Cross-Sectional Study in Italy
Reprinted from: *J. Clin. Med.* **2023**, *12*, 3469, doi:10.3390/jcm12103469 162

Giorgia Teresa Maniscalco, Daniele Di Giulio Cesare, Valerio Liguori, Valentino Manzo, Elio Prestipino, Simona Salvatore, et al.
Three Doses of COVID-19 Vaccines: A Retrospective Study Evaluating the Safety and the Immune Response in Patients with Multiple Sclerosis
Reprinted from: *J. Clin. Med.* **2023**, *12*, 4236, doi:10.3390/jcm12134236 175

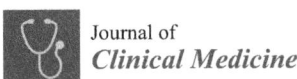 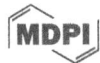

Editorial

Pharmacovigilance and Pharmacoepidemiology as a Guarantee of Patient Safety: The Role of the Clinical Pharmacologist

Giada Crescioli [1,2,*], Roberto Bonaiuti [1,2], Renato Corradetti [1,3], Guido Mannaioni [1,4], Alfredo Vannacci [1,2,*] and Niccolò Lombardi [1,2,*]

1. Pharmacovigilance and Pharmacoepidemiology Research Unit, Section of Pharmacology and Toxicology, Department of Neurosciences, Psychology, Drug Research and Child Health, University of Florence, 50139 Florence, Italy; roberto.bonaiuti@unifi.it (R.B.); renato.corradetti@unifi.it (R.C.); guido.mannaioni@unifi.it (G.M.)
2. Tuscan Regional Centre of Pharmacovigilance, 50122 Florence, Italy
3. Pharmacology Unit, Careggi University Hospital, 50134 Florence, Italy
4. Medical Toxicology Unit and Poison Control Centre, Careggi University Hospital, 50134 Florence, Italy
* Correspondence: giada.crescioli@unifi.it (G.C.); alfredo.vannacci@unifi.it (A.V.); niccolo.lombardi@unifi.it (N.L.)

Citation: Crescioli, G.; Bonaiuti, R.; Corradetti, R.; Mannaioni, G.; Vannacci, A.; Lombardi, N. Pharmacovigilance and Pharmacoepidemiology as a Guarantee of Patient Safety: The Role of the Clinical Pharmacologist. *J. Clin. Med.* **2022**, *11*, 3552. https://doi.org/10.3390/jcm11123552

Received: 16 June 2022
Accepted: 17 June 2022
Published: 20 June 2022

Publisher's Note: MDPI stays neutral with regard to jurisdictional claims in published maps and institutional affiliations.

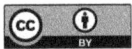

Copyright: © 2022 by the authors. Licensee MDPI, Basel, Switzerland. This article is an open access article distributed under the terms and conditions of the Creative Commons Attribution (CC BY) license (https://creativecommons.org/licenses/by/4.0/).

1. Background

Recent years, particularly the COVID-19 pandemic, can be considered a turning point for pharmacovigilance and pharmacoepidemiology in terms of their role in drug safety and drug utilisation monitoring in clinical practice [1]. Researchers operating in the fields of pharmacovigilance and pharmacoepidemiology have extensive knowledge about approved medications, many of which have been or are currently undergoing clinical trials for repurposing. In this context, clinical pharmacologists' knowledge can be used and translated to optimise dosing and treatment regimens and to assess the relationship between active compound exposure and adverse drug reactions (ADR) or adverse events following immunisation (AEFI), with the crucial aims of optimising drugs or vaccines' efficacy and ensuring patients' safety.

2. Pharmacovigilance

Adverse drug reactions represent a relevant clinical issue, causing each year a significant number of medical consultations, emergency department (ED) visits, and/or patients' hospitalisations [2], including an increase in the length of patients' hospital stay. ADRs are considerable medical occurrence, not only from a clinical point of view, but they also represent an economic burden, since they can be involved in the death of several thousand patients each year, accounting up for a not negligible percentage of a hospital's budget [3]. This scenario is even more complex if we consider that many ADRs are predictable and therefore preventable.

Drug and vaccine safety surveillance is a continuous process, which includes all the phases of the life cycle of a drug/vaccine. Additionally, also surveillance of the safety of products belonging to complementary and alternative medicine (CAM), defined as phytovigilance [4], contributes to guaranteeing the safety of patients.

During the drug development process, safety is investigated in different preclinical and clinical phases. Although drug and vaccine safety evaluation is very rigorous and highly regulated, randomised clinical trials (RCTs) have several limitations, which include limited numbers of patients, strict eligibility criteria, and limited duration. These intrinsic characteristics of RCTs make their results far from representing the real-world population, thus not allowing an exhaustive assessment of the safety profile of drugs and vaccines. Consequently, post-marketing surveillance, also known as pharmacovigilance (during phase IV of drug development), plays a key role in better defining drugs' and vaccines' safety profiles in clinical practice, overcoming the gap of evidence derived from the pre-marketing phases [5,6]. These aspects are even more relevant if we consider that most CAM products (i.e., dietary supplements, herbal supplements, traditional Chinese medicine products, homoeopathic products, etc.) are placed on the market without first being tested on humans, even less in frailer subgroups [6].

In the last decades, spontaneous reporting of suspected ADRs, AEFIs, and adverse events associated with CAM products, has represented the starting point and the milestone to build the modern pharmacovigilance system which is currently operating, although with differences between countries, all over the world under the coordination of the World Health Organisation Uppsala Monitoring Centre. More recently, new methodological approaches have become necessary in the field of pharmacovigilance, to try to overcome the limits of spontaneous reporting, particularly the underreporting [2].

An important example is represented by active pharmacovigilance projects, aimed at estimating the impact of ADRs, AEFIs, and adverse events associated with CAM products through continuous pre-organized activities in specific clinical settings (i.e., ED, hospital ward, nursing home, etc.) [2,5] or through the analysis of local or national administrative healthcare databases (i.e., dispensed drugs, emergency department records, hospital discharge records, exemption codes, etc.) [7].

In the frame of ED, active pharmacovigilance represents a valuable methodology, allowing healthcare professionals and researchers to detect, collect and characterise the clinical burden of ADRs [6], AEFIs [8], and adverse events associated with CAM products [9,10] in outpatients. Furthermore, active pharmacovigilance may help to recognise risk factors associated with adverse reactions among specific patient populations, such as the elderly (age $\geq$ 65 years) [11], women [7], including those in pregnancy or breastfeeding [12,13], children [14], subjects exposed to polypharmacy, or patients affected by substance use disorder [15]. In this framework, an active pharmacovigilance approach can help to early recognise and prevent adverse reactions, minimising their clinical, economic and social impact.

In recent years, new technologies are also making an important contribution to active pharmacovigilance. In particular, machine learning, deep learning, and natural language processing approaches can be used to detect adverse reactions from unconventional data sources, e.g., social media [16,17], and to discover safety signals, underlying some adverse reactions not yet reported [18]. Moreover, safety data collected from healthcare social networks and forums, general social networking, and search logs can be processed by big data sentiment analysis algorithms to provide a more comprehensive picture of the public opinion, experiences, and sentiments about drugs and vaccines [19], and can be used to create effective public health campaigns on drugs/vaccines safety, diseases prevention or to fight vaccine hesitancy [20].

3. Pharmacoepidemiology

Pharmacoepidemiology refers to the study of interactions between drugs, vaccines, or CAM products and populations. In particular, it can be defined as the study of the utilisation, therapeutic effects, and risks of different health products through several epidemiological approaches. Even though RCTs may be preferred for evaluating the efficacy of a drug or a vaccine, the principal aim of the pharmacoepidemiological method is to estimate drug or vaccine effect in real life (effectiveness), avoiding, as much as possible, any modification caused by the study itself (i.e., presence of biases). From a practical point of view, pharmacoepidemiology relates to descriptive methodologies (i.e., describing the use of a drug in a specific demographic or clinical setting) [21], as well as to etiologic methodologies (i.e., estimating the association between drug exposure and a specific clinical outcome) [22]. Researchers operating in the field of pharmacovigilance, first the clinical pharmacologist, can use pharmacoepidemiological studies to identify unexpected or rare safety issues and detect changes in frequency of expected ADRs/AEFIs, making possible a continuous monitoring of the benefit risk ratio of a drug, vaccine or CAM product in the real-world setting [5].

New evidence concerning drug safety obtained through pharmacoepidemiological approaches is relevant for pharmaceutical industries because they can use this information to submit amendments to the approved indications for their products. In fact, pharmacoepidemiology allows industries to demonstrate the safety of their products, especially compared to others (comparative observational studies). Furthermore, it is also fundamental for regulatory agencies, for physicians, and patients using health products. In this context, there is a clear need for high-quality epidemiological research in the post-marketing phase for the timely identification of any significant safety concerns that arise when a drug, vaccine, or CAM product is used in the real-world "uncontrolled" setting. All this is mandatory to protect the health and quality of life of patients.

Over the past decades, more data has become increasingly available due to the constant growth of administrative healthcare databases, in particular those reporting data on prescription drugs. This circumstance has enhanced the improvement of pharmacoepidemiology, a dynamic research field that has undergone a more rapid development than many other research areas of pharmacology and clinical pharmacology. Evidence proliferation in modern society will continue, and population-based observational studies (i.e., cohort and case control studies) aimed at assessing the effectiveness (defined as the extent to which a drug achieves its intended effect in the usual clinical setting) and safety of drugs, vaccines, and CAM products will be increasingly requested by industry, regulatory agencies, payers, healthcare professionals, patients, and caregivers.

The availability of electronic healthcare databases will enable researchers operating in the fields of pharmacovigilance and pharmacoepidemiology to identify a growing number of cases in which effectiveness does not match efficacy. This will challenge the actions of all concerned stakeholders. For these reasons, pharmacoepidemiological studies will also be increasingly requested by reimbursement agencies and other payers to assess the value of health products used in the general population. In conclusion, it is essential that the increasing amount of data collected to monitor the utilisation, effectiveness, and safety of new drugs, vaccines, and CAM products will be used to improve clinical decision-making. In this complex scenario, the clinical pharmacologist will certainly have to play an important role, in concert with the other actors involved in the post-marketing setting.

4. The Role of the Clinical Pharmacologist

In the real-world setting, there are two different actors in the issue of ADRs: the healthcare professional (i.e., medical doctor, pharmacist, nurse, etc.) and the citizen/patient. While they are directly involved, in cooperation with universities, regulatory authorities, and drug manufacturers, the figure of the clinical pharmacologist (with a medicine or pharmacy single-cycle degree background) has also a pivotal role in the management of adverse reactions. However, his/her role is still often underestimated and underused [23].

Generally, the clinical pharmacologist has a dual background, in biomedical science and in pharmacology. Furthermore, a clinical pharmacologist will often be trained in biostatistics and pharmacoepidemiology. For example, in Italy, to become a clinical pharmacologist, a single-cycle master's degree in healthcare (i.e., medicine or pharmacy), followed by a doctorate and/or a specialisation in clinical pharmacology and toxicology is needed. Clinical pharmacologists operate in universities, industry, regulatory authorities, and hospitals. In fact, their activities comprehend teaching in biomedical schools, research in the public or industry fields, regulatory affairs, and hospital activities.

In Italy, the main healthcare professionals that are involved in pharmacovigilance are hospital pharmacists. However, while the hospital pharmacist is directly involved in the management of pharmacovigilance report forms, including all activities related to the proper functioning of the national pharmacovigilance system, clinical pharmacologists have a unique insight into the possible mechanism of the putative adverse reaction, the underlying or concomitant diseases, and the possibility of drug–drug, drug–CAM or drug–disease interactions [1,24]. Thus, more recently, hospital pharmacists have been supported by one or more clinical pharmacologists, and their cooperation at both hospital and territorial level enhance the knowledge of drug safety in the pre- and post-marketing settings. Moreover, the clinical pharmacologist may enhance the quality of information and may help in the interpretation of data collected during adverse events reporting. This could be of utmost importance for modern projects of active pharmacovigilance when the clinical pharmacologist can play the role of a trained monitor.

At the individual patient level, the clinical pharmacologist could be involved in the resolution of several drug-related issues, which can vary from some advice regarding drug administration, to the choice of a drug in specific population subgroups, such as pregnant women. Indications in adverse reactions management can be based on literature evidence or on knowledge of drugs' pharmacokinetics and pharmacodynamics, or they may be part of a more proactive approach. In proactive and preventive approaches, the clinical pharmacologist could take part in the resolution/prevention of adverse reactions, cooperating with other healthcare professionals to improve the appropriateness of use of drugs and CAM products and to increase personalised medicine [25]. Moreover, new technologies for adverse reactions monitoring could be improved by clinical pharmacologists' knowledge. These new applications and tools can be designed taking into account many aspects of pharmacology, pharmacoepidemiology, and pharmacological use in real clinical practice in which the clinical pharmacologist is an expert.

During the SARS-CoV-2 pandemic, great attention was paid to the risk associated with the involuntary intoxication and to the need for correct information concerning the in-home utilisation of several medical and non-medicinal products (i.e., cleaners and disinfectants, medical devices, etc.), thus representing a further field of action in which the clinical pharmacologist can guarantee a fundamental contribution [26]. Actually, the role of clinical pharmacologists, particularly those working in a poison control center, is valuable in the identification and management of exposures and suspected intoxications in the general population or in specific subgroups [27].

5. Future Perspectives

Real-world data are crucial to further establish the safety profile of pharmacological treatments in the general population [28]. As a next step, real-world data from electronic healthcare databases may be used in pharmacovigilance and pharmacoepidemiology to monitor drug utilisation patterns, as well as the effectiveness and safety of drugs in large populations. Big data and machine learning analysis technologies could be used to extract and aggregate pharmacovigilance data from different and unrelated sources (i.e., health insurance companies, academic institutions, healthcare systems, etc.) and associate relevant information on drug safety using artificial intelligence tools [29]. All these approaches will be particularly useful in the near future for the monitoring of COVID-19 vaccines' safety. Moreover, among new technologies, gamification is another promising technology with several potential uses in drug safety. Gamification applications transfer gaming dynamics to the "serious context" of pharmacological therapies, for example, to educate health professionals [30] and patients [31] on the correct management of chronic diseases or to improve adherence to drug treatments thus reducing adverse events [32]. In this context, "digital therapeutics" (algorithms and software) can represent an innovative approach through which the clinical pharmacologist can improve the management and safety of pharmacological and/or integrative treatments [33].

As the amount of data available from randomised controlled trials and pharmacoepidemiological studies will increase over the coming years, the characteristics of adverse events related to medicines, vaccines or CAMs will become clearer and the central role of the clinical pharmacologist should become even more relevant. Managing adverse events should be a routine activity for clinical pharmacologists. This management takes advantage of all the skills of the clinical pharmacologist to explore individual cases and the mechanisms of adverse events. With their knowledge in pharmacovigilance and pharmacoepidemiology, clinical pharmacologists may play a key role by bringing various healthcare professionals together in a proactive discussion/collaboration aimed at improving the safety of pharmacological and/or integrative treatments in clinical practice.

Author Contributions: Conceptualization, G.C. and N.L.; writing—original draft preparation, G.C. and N.L.; writing—review and editing, R.B., R.C., G.M. and A.V. All authors have read and agreed to the published version of the manuscript.

Funding: This research received no external funding.

Conflicts of Interest: The authors declare no conflict of interest.

References

1. Crescioli, G.; Brilli, V.; Lanzi, C.; Burgalassi, A.; Ieri, A.; Bonaiuti, R.; Romano, E.; Innocenti, R.; Mannaioni, G.; Vannacci, A.; et al. Adverse Drug Reactions in SARS-CoV-2 Hospitalised Patients: A Case-Series with a Focus on Drug-Drug Interactions. *Intern. Emerg. Med.* **2021**, *16*, 697–710. [CrossRef] [PubMed]
2. Lombardi, N.; Crescioli, G.; Bettiol, A.; Tuccori, M.; Capuano, A.; Bonaiuti, R.; Mugelli, A.; Venegoni, M.; Vighi, G.D.; Vannacci, A.; et al. Italian Emergency Department Visits and Hospitalizations for Outpatients' Adverse Drug Events: 12-Year Active Pharmacovigilance Surveillance (The MEREAFaPS Study). *Front. Pharmacol.* **2020**, *11*, 412. [CrossRef] [PubMed]
3. Perrone, V.; Conti, V.; Venegoni, M.; Scotto, S.; Esposti, L.D.; Sangiorgi, D.; Prestini, L.; Radice, S.; Clementi, E.; Vighi, G. Seriousness, Preventability, and Burden Impact of Reported Adverse Drug Reactions in Lombardy Emergency Departments: A Retrospective 2-Year Characterization. *Clin. Outcomes Res.* **2014**, *6*, 505–514. [CrossRef]
4. Lombardi, N.; Crescioli, G.; Bettiol, A.; Menniti-Ippolito, F.; Maggini, V.; Gallo, E.; Mugelli, A.; Vannacci, A.; Firenzuoli, F. Safety of Complementary and Alternative Medicine in Children: A 16-Years Retrospective Analysis of the Italian Phytovigilance System Database. *Phytomedicine* **2019**, *61*, 152856. [CrossRef] [PubMed]
5. Marconi, E.; Crescioli, G.; Bonaiuti, R.; Pugliese, L.; Santi, R.; Nesi, G.; Cerbai, E.; Vannacci, A.; Lombardi, N. Acute Appendicitis in a Patient Immunised with COVID-19 Vaccine: A Case Report with Morphological Analysis. *Br. J. Clin. Pharmacol.* **2022**. [CrossRef] [PubMed]
6. Pagani, S.; Lombardi, N.; Crescioli, G.; Giuditta Vighi, V.; Spada, G.; Andreetta, P.; Capuano, A.; Vannacci, A.; Venegoni, M.; Vighi, G.D. Clinical Medicine Drug-Related Hypersensitivity Reactions Leading to Emergency Department: Original Data and Systematic Review. *J. Clin. Med* **2022**, *11*, 2811. [CrossRef]
7. Spini, A.; Crescioli, G.; Donnini, S.; Ziche, M.; Collini, F.; Gemmi, F.; Virgili, G.; Vannacci, A.; Lucenteforte, E.; Gini, R.; et al. Sex Differences in the Utilization of Drugs for COVID-19 Treatment among Elderly Residents in a Sample of Italian Nursing Homes. *Pharmacoepidemiol. Drug Saf.* **2022**, *31*, 489–494. [CrossRef]
8. Luxi, N.; Giovanazzi, A.; Capuano, A.; Crisafulli, S.; Cutroneo, P.M.; Fantini, M.P.; Ferrajolo, C.; Moretti, U.; Poluzzi, E.; Raschi, E.; et al. COVID-19 Vaccination in Pregnancy, Paediatrics, Immunocompromised Patients, and Persons with History of Allergy or Prior SARS-CoV-2 Infection: Overview of Current Recommendations and Pre- and Post-Marketing Evidence for Vaccine Efficacy and Safety. *Drug Saf.* **2021**, *44*, 1247–1269. [CrossRef]
9. Crescioli, G.; Lombardi, N.; Bettiol, A.; Menniti-Ippolito, F.; Roberto, I.; Da Cas, R.; Parrilli, M.; Del Lungo, M.; Gallo, E.; Mugelli, A.; et al. Adverse Events Following Cannabis for Medical Use in Tuscany: An Analysis of the Italian Phytovigilance Database. *Br. J. Clin. Pharmacol.* **2019**, *86*, 106–120. [CrossRef]
10. Lombardi, N.; Crescioli, G.; Maggini, V.; Ippoliti, I.; Menniti-Ippolito, F.; Gallo, E.; Brilli, V.; Lanzi, C.; Guido Mannaioni, G.; Firenzuoli, F.; et al. Acute Liver Injury Following Turmeric Use in Tuscany: An Analysis of the Italian Phytovigilance Database and Systematic Review of Case Reports. *Br. J. Clin. Pharmacol.* **2021**, *87*, 741–753. [CrossRef]
11. Crescioli, G.; Bettiol, A.; Bonaiuti, R.; Tuccori, M.; Rossi, M.; Capuano, A.; Pagani, S.; Spada, G.; Venegoni, M.; Vighi, G.D.; et al. Risk of Hospitalization Associated with Cardiovascular Medications in the Elderly Italian Population: A Nationwide Multicenter Study in Emergency Departments. *Front. Pharmacol.* **2021**, *11*, 611102. [CrossRef] [PubMed]
12. Vannacci, A.; Bettiol, A.; Lombardi, N.; Marconi, E.; Crescioli, G.; Bonaiuti, R.; Maggini, V.; Gallo, E.; Mugelli, A.; Firenzuoli, F.; et al. The Use of Complementary and Alternative Medicines during Breastfeeding: Results from the Herbal Supplements in Breastfeeding InvesTigation (HaBIT) Study. *Br. J. Clin. Pharmacol.* **2018**, *84*, 2040. [CrossRef]
13. Bettiol, A.; Lombardi, N.; Marconi, E.; Crescioli, G.; Bonaiuti, R.; Maggini, V.; Gallo, E.; Mugelli, A.; Firenzuoli, F.; Ravaldi, C.; et al. The Impact of Previous Pregnancy Loss on Lactating Behaviors and Use of Herbal Medicines during Breastfeeding: A Post Hoc Analysis of the Herbal Supplements in Breastfeeding InvesTigation (HaBIT). *Evid. Based Complement. Altern. Med.* **2018**, *2018*, 1035875. [CrossRef] [PubMed]
14. Lombardi, N.; Crescioli, G.; Bettiol, A.; Tuccori, M.; Rossi, M.; Bonaiuti, R.; Ravaldi, C.; Levi, M.; Mugelli, A.; Ricci, S.; et al. Vaccines Safety in Children and in General Population: A Pharmacovigilance Study on Adverse Events Following Anti-Infective Vaccination in Italy. *Front. Pharmacol.* **2019**, *10*, 948. [CrossRef]
15. Sartori, S.; Crescioli, G.; Brilli, V.; Traversoni, S.; Lanzi, C.; Vannacci, A.; Mannaioni, G.; Lombardi, N. Phenobarbital Use in Benzodiazepine and Z-Drug Detoxification: A Single-Centre 15-Year Observational Retrospective Study in Clinical Practice. *Intern. Emerg. Med.* **2022**, *12*, 1–10. [CrossRef] [PubMed]

16. Maggini, V.; Lombardi, N.; Crescioli, G.; Gallo, E.; Sivelli, F.; Gensini, G.F.; Vannacci, A.; Firenzuoli, F. Chelidonium Majus: Relevant Safety Aspects of a Hepatotoxic Plant, Trawling the Web. *Phyther. Res.* **2019**, *33*, 2465–2469. [CrossRef]
17. Soysal, E.; Wang, J.; Jiang, M.; Wu, Y.; Pakhomov, S.; Liu, H.; Xu, H. CLAMP—A Toolkit for Efficiently Building Customized Clinical Natural Language Processing Pipelines. *J. Am. Med. Informatics Assoc.* **2018**, *25*, 331–336. [CrossRef]
18. Lian, A.; Du, J.; Tang, L. Using a Machine Learning Approach to Monitor COVID-19 Vaccine Adverse Events (VAE) from Twitter Data. *Vaccines* **2022**, *10*, 103. [CrossRef]
19. Du, J.; Tang, L.; Xiang, Y.; Zhi, D.; Xu, J.; Song, H.Y.; Tao, C. Public Perception Analysis of Tweets during the 2015 Measles Outbreak: Comparative Study Using Convolutional Neural Network Models. *J. Med. Internet Res.* **2018**, *20*, e236. [CrossRef]
20. Chou, W.Y.S.; Budenz, A. Considering Emotion in COVID-19 Vaccine Communication: Addressing Vaccine Hesitancy and Fostering Vaccine Confidence. *Health Commun.* **2020**, *35*, 1718–1722. [CrossRef]
21. Lombardi, G.; Lombardi, N.; Bettiol, A.; Crescioli, G.; Ferrari, C.; Lucidi, G.; Polito, C.; Berti, V.; Bessi, V.; Bagnoli, S.; et al. Long-Term Use of Pharmacological Treatment in Alzheimer's Disease: A Retrospective Cohort Study in Real-World Clinical Practice. *Eur. J. Clin. Pharmacol.* **2022**, *1*, 3. [CrossRef] [PubMed]
22. Lombardi, N.; Brilli, V.; Crescioli, G.; Bettiol, A.; Ippazio, C.; Mazzaglia, G.; Fumagalli, S.; Mannaioni, G.; Vannacci, A.; Gini, R. Patterns and Trends of Idarucizumab Use in an Italian Region: A Probabilistic Record-Linkage Approach in a Real-Life Setting. *Eur. Heart J.* **2020**, *41*, ehaa946-3364. [CrossRef]
23. van der Graaf, P.H.; Giacomini, K.M. COVID-19: A Defining Moment for Clinical Pharmacology? *Clin. Pharmacol. Ther.* **2020**, *108*, 11–15. [CrossRef] [PubMed]
24. Crescioli, G.; Lanzi, C.; Mannaioni, G.; Vannacci, A.; Lombardi, N. Adverse Drug Reactions in SARS-CoV-2 Hospitalised Patients: A Case-Series with a Focus on Drug-Drug Interactions-Reply. *Intern. Emerg. Med.* **2021**, *16*, 799–800. [CrossRef]
25. Sobiak, J.; Resztak, M.; Crescioli, G.; Lombardi, N.; Vagnoli, L.; Bettiol, A.; Giunti, L.; Cetica, V.; Coniglio, M.L.; Provenzano, A.; et al. STOP Pain Project-Opioid Response in Pediatric Cancer Patients and Gene Polymorphisms of Cytokine Pathways. *Pharmaceutics* **2022**, *14*, 619. [CrossRef]
26. Crescioli, G.; Lanzi, C.; Gambassi, F.; Ieri, A.; Ercolini, A.; Borgioli, G.; Bettiol, A.; Vannacci, A.; Mannaioni, G.; Lombardi, N. Exposures and Suspected Intoxications during SARS-CoV-2 Pandemic: Preliminary Results from an Italian Poison Control Centre. *Intern. Emerg. Med.* **2021**, *17*, 535–540. [CrossRef]
27. Missanelli, A.; Lombardi, N.; Bettiol, A.; Lanzi, C.; Rossi, F.; Pacileo, I.; Donvito, L.; Garofalo, V.; Ravaldi, C.; Vannacci, A.; et al. Birth Outcomes in Women Exposed to Diagnostic Radiology Procedures during First Trimester of Pregnancy: A Prospective Cohort Study. *Clin. Toxicol.* **2022**, *60*, 175–183. [CrossRef]
28. Crescioli, G.; Boscia, E.; Bettiol, A.; Pagani, S.; Spada, G.; Vighi, G.V.; Bonaiuti, R.; Venegoni, M.; Vighi, G.D.; Vannacci, A.; et al. Risk of Hospitalization for Adverse Drug Events in Women and Men: A Post Hoc Analysis of an Active Pharmacovigilance Study in Italian Emergency Departments. *Pharmaceuticals* **2021**, *14*, 678. [CrossRef]
29. Gibson, T.B.; Nguyen, M.D.; Burrell, T.; Yoon, F.; Wong, J.; Dharmarajan, S.; Ouellet-Hellstrom, R.; Hua, W.; Ma, Y.; Baro, E.; et al. Electronic Phenotyping of Health Outcomes of Interest Using a Linked Claims-Electronic Health Record Database: Findings from a Machine Learning Pilot Project. *J. Am. Med. Inform. Assoc.* **2021**, *28*, 1507–1517. [CrossRef]
30. Gentry, S.V.; Gauthier, A.; Ehrstrom, B.L.E.; Wortley, D.; Lilienthal, A.; Car, L.T.; Dauwels-Okutsu, S.; Nikolaou, C.K.; Zary, N.; Campbell, J.; et al. Serious Gaming and Gamification Education in Health Professions: Systematic Review. *J. Med. Internet Res.* **2019**, *21*, e12994. [CrossRef]
31. Patel, M.S.; Small, D.S.; Harrison, J.D.; Hilbert, V.; Fortunato, M.P.; Oon, A.L.; Rareshide, C.A.L.; Volpp, K.G. Effect of Behaviorally Designed Gamification with Social Incentives on Lifestyle Modification among Adults with Uncontrolled Diabetes: A Randomized Clinical Trial. *JAMA Netw. Open* **2021**, *4*, e2110255. [CrossRef] [PubMed]
32. Maurin, K.D.; Girod, C.; Consolini, J.L.; Belzeaux, R.; Etain, B.; Cochet, B.; Leboyer, M.; Genty, C.; Gamon, L.; Picot, M.C.; et al. Use of a Serious Game to Strengthen Medication Adherence in Euthymic Patients with Bipolar Disorder Following a Psychoeducational Programme: A Randomized Controlled Trial. *J. Affect. Disord.* **2020**, *262*, 182–188. [CrossRef] [PubMed]
33. Crisafulli, S.; Santoro, E.; Recchia, G.; Trifirò, G. Digital Therapeutics in Perspective: From Regulatory Challenges to Post-Marketing Surveillance. *Front. Drug Saf. Regul.* **2022**, *2*, 5. [CrossRef]

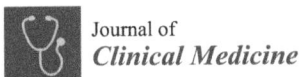
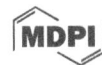

Article

Drug-Related Hypersensitivity Reactions Leading to Emergency Department: Original Data and Systematic Review

Silvia Pagani [1,†], Niccolò Lombardi [2,3,*,†], Giada Crescioli [2,3,†], Violetta Giuditta Vighi [4], Giulia Spada [4], Paola Andreetta [1], Annalisa Capuano [5,6], Alfredo Vannacci [2,3], Mauro Venegoni [1,7], Giuseppe Danilo Vighi [1] and on behalf of the MEREAFaPS Study Group [‡]

1. Department of Medicine, ASST Vimercate, 20871 Vimercate, Italy; silvia.pagani@asst-brianza.it (S.P.); paola.andreetta4@gmail.com (P.A.); mauro.venegoni@gmail.com (M.V.); giuseppedanilo.vighi@asst-brianza.it (G.D.V.)
2. Section of Pharmacology and Toxicology, Department of Neurosciences, Psychology, Drug Research and Child Health, University of Florence, 50139 Florence, Italy; giada.crescioli@unifi.it (G.C.); alfredo.vannacci@unifi.it (A.V.)
3. Tuscan Regional Centre of Pharmacovigilance, 50122 Florence, Italy
4. Hospital Pharmacy, ASST Vimercate, 20871 Vimercate, Italy; giudittavioletta.vighi@asst-brianza.it (V.G.V.); giulia.spada@asst-brianza.it (G.S.)
5. Section of Pharmacology "L. Donatelli", Department of Experimental Medicine, University of Campania "Luigi Vanvitelli", 80138 Naples, Italy; annalisa.capuano@unicampania.it
6. Campania Regional Centre for Pharmacovigilance and Pharmacoepidemiology, 80138 Naples, Italy
7. Pharmacology Unit, Department of Diagnostics and Public Health, University of Verona, 37100 Verona, Italy
* Correspondence: niccolo.lombardi@unifi.it; Tel.: +39-055-27-58-206
† These authors contributed equally to this manuscript.
‡ Membership of the MEREAFaPS Study Group is provided in Acknowledgments.

Abstract: The aim of the present study is to describe pharmacological characteristics of drug-related allergies and anaphylaxis leading to the emergency department (ED). An 8-year post hoc analysis on the MEREAFaPS Study database was performed (2012–2019). Subjects who experienced drug-related hypersensitivity leading to an ED visit were selected. Logistic regression analyses were used to estimate the reporting odds ratios (RORs) of drug-related allergies and anaphylaxis adjusting for sex, age classes, and ethnicity. In addition, a systematic review of observational studies evaluating drug-related hypersensitivity reactions leading to ED visits in outpatients was performed. Out of 94,073 ED visits, 14.4% cases were drug-related allergies and 0.6% were anaphylaxis. Females accounted for 56%. Multivariate logistic regression showed a higher risk of drug-related allergy among males and all age classes < 65 years, while a higher risk of anaphylaxis was observed for females (ROR 1.20 [1.01–1.42]) and adults (ROR 2.63 [2.21–3.14]). The systematic review included 37 studies. ED visits related to allergy and anaphylaxis ranged from 0.004% to 88%, and drug-related allergies and anaphylaxis ranged from 0.007% to 88%. Both in our analysis and in primary studies, antibacterials, analgesics, and radiocontrast agents were identified as the most common triggers of hypersensitivity.

Keywords: hypersensitivity; drug allergy; anaphylaxis; emergency department; hospitalization; pharmacovigilance

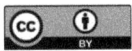

1. Introduction

Drug-related hypersensitivity reactions are a group of adverse drug events (ADEs) that are generally unexpected (Type B reactions—Bizarre) [1] and characterized by symptoms or signs initiated by exposure to a drug at dosages that are usually tolerated [2]. Following the definition proposed by the "International Consensus on Drug Allergy", hypersensitivity ADEs, which occur in the first few hours after drug administration, are usually characterized by urticaria, angioedema, rhino-conjunctivitis, bronchospasm, and, in the most serious cases, also anaphylaxis [3]. Anaphylaxis is defined as a clinically relevant, generalized, or systemic hypersensitivity ADE that can be life-threatening or fatal [3].

Although the diagnosis of the causative agent can be very difficult, pharmacological treatments are among the leading causes of allergy and anaphylaxis-related deaths in adult individuals and hypersensitivity ADEs remain a serious public health concern both in outpatient and inpatient settings worldwide, due to their high morbidity, mortality, and socioeconomic burden [4].

From an epidemiological point of view, drug-related allergies and anaphylaxis are most frequently triggered by analgesics, antibiotics, biologics, chemotherapeutics, contrast media, nonsteroidal anti-inflammatory drugs (NSAIDs), and proton pump inhibitors, again with age and geographical variations worldwide [4]. Among drug-related anaphylaxis, new triggers have been identified. These include biologics containing α-gal (i.e., cetuximab), small molecules, or novel chemotherapeutics like olaparib [5]. Disinfectants such as chlorhexidine [6], or drug ingredients such as polyethyleneglycol [7], or recently methylcellulose [8], have also been identified as novel substances inducing anaphylaxis. The global incidence of anaphylaxis was estimated to be between 50 and 112 events per 100,000 person per year, with an estimated lifetime prevalence of 0.3–5.1%, depending on the definitions used, study methodology applied, and geographical areas investigated [4,9]. Despite an increasing trend for emergency department (ED) visit and/or hospitalization due to anaphylaxis, its mortality was estimated at 0.05–0.51 per million people/year [4,10].

Taking into consideration the last update of the World Allergy Organization Anaphylaxis Guidance [4], major limitations of epidemiological studies regarding drug-related allergies and anaphylaxis reside in the lack of risk factors/triggers characterization and lack of information on large prospective population-based studies. Moreover, most studies do not differentiate between drug-related hypersensitivity ADEs and other kinds of ADEs, and the diagnosis of hypersensitivity ADEs is mostly based on a suspected clinical history or self-reporting [11].

In this context, pharmacovigilance studies, performed with an "active" approach by trained healthcare professionals, can provide detailed information about hypersensitivity ADEs and their diagnosis, especially when these studies are performed in a hospital setting (i.e., ED) [12–16]. This way, "active" pharmacovigilance studies may represent one of the best epidemiological strategies to fill the above-mentioned major limitations.

The aim of the present study was to describe pharmacological characteristics of drug-related allergies and anaphylaxis leading to ED in Italy, estimating their risk considering subjects' demographic and clinical characteristics and the most frequently reported suspected drug classes. Furthermore, to complete the evidence obtained with our post hoc analysis, a systematic review of observational studies on drug-related hypersensitivity ADEs leading to ED visit and/or hospitalization was performed.

2. Materials and Methods

2.1. Post Hoc Analysis

This is an 8-year post hoc analysis performed on the MEREAFaPS Study database [15]. A retrospective observational study was conducted by reviewing all drug-related allergies and anaphylaxis observed in the database between 1 January 2012 and 30 November 2019. Following the Italian Pharmacovigilance legislation, the MEREAFaPS Study, which was conducted in Italy since 2006 and ended in November 2020, collected all ADEs through an ad hoc ADE report form in more than 90 EDs belonging to general hospitals distributed in the national territory in five Italian Regions: Lombardy and Piedmont (north), Tuscany and Emilia-Romagna (centre), and Campania (south). As already stated, the EDs involved in the MEREAFaPS Study allowed good and widespread coverage of the ED Italian population.

For the present analysis, all ADE report forms of drug-related allergy and anaphylaxis were identified with a definite list of MedDRA terms (Supplementary Table S1). Subjects who experienced one or more hypersensitivity reactions (allergies and/or anaphylaxis) leading to ED visit were selected, retrieving the following data: demographic information (age, gender, ethnic group); suspected drugs; description of the ADE according to diagnosis and symptoms, codified as detailed by MedDRA dictionary and organized by System Organ Class (SOC) [17]. If present in the MEREAFaPS Study database, the ADE's outcome "hospitalization", ADE's management (i.e., adrenaline use), and the triage colour codes were also recorded. In Italy, the triage codes are divided into four categories and are identified with colours, as follows [18]: (1) "red code" (very critical, life threat, top priority, immediate treatment access); (2) "yellow code" (on average critical, presence of evolutionary risk, possibly life-threatening); (3) "green code" (not very critical, absence of evolutionary risks, deferred services); (4) "white code" (non-critical, non-urgent patients). Anatomical Therapeutic Chemical (ATC) classification system was used to classify suspected drugs [12]. For the pharmacologic subgroup of antibiotics, the 3rd level of ATC class was considered, whereas the 5th level of ATC class was considered for NSAIDs, radiology contrast agents, analgesics, and antineoplastic agents.

Data were summarized using descriptive statistics. Categorical data were reported as frequencies and percentages, while continuous data were reported as median values with the related interquartile ranges (IQRs). Age classes were defined as follows: newborns (from 0 to 1 years); children (from 2 to 11 years); adolescents (from 12 to 17 years); adults (from 18 to 65 years); and elderly (older than 65 years). For each drug class, univariate logistic regression was used to calculate the reporting odds ratios (RORs) of drug-related allergy and anaphylaxis with 95% confidence intervals (CIs) compared to subjects who experienced non-allergy ADEs. Multivariate logistic regression was performed and adjusted for sex, age classes, and ethnicity. All results were statistically significant at $p < 0.05$. Data management and statistical analysis were carried out using STATA 16.1.

The coordinating centre of Lombardy Region (Vimercate, Italy) approved the MEREAFaPS Study in 2006, and the local institutional ethics committee (ASST Monza Ethic Committee) approved the MEREAFaPS Study (Notification number 3724—6 May 2021) according to the legal requirements concerning observational studies [12–16]. Due to the retrospective nature of the present analysis and data anonymization, patient's consent to participate was not required.

2.2. Systematic Review

This is a systematic review conducted following the Preferred Reporting Items for Systematic Reviews and Meta-Analyses [19]. A literature search was performed in PubMed and Embase (last search performed on 25 March 2022). The PubMed search strategy was adapted to the syntax and subject headings of Embase. Records were retrieved on the same day from all sources and the search strategy was updated toward the end of the review, after being validated to ensure it retrieved a high proportion of eligible studies.

We considered for inclusion observational studies, either prospective or retrospective performed in EDs and specifically concerning outpatients, published in English. Randomized clinical trials, reviews and meta-analyses, letters to the editor, case reports, case series, and expert opinions were excluded. We included only articles focusing on drug-related hypersensitivity, anaphylactic reactions, and allergies in outpatients. Moreover, we excluded articles focusing on specific syndromes, such as Steven Johnson and toxic epidermal necrolysis. Two review authors (NL and SP) have independently screened the extracted records and identified the studies for inclusion by screening titles and abstracts yielded by search, eliminating those deemed irrelevant. Full-text articles were retrieved for all references that at least one of two review authors identified for potential inclusion. We selected studies for inclusion based on review of full-text articles. Any discrepancy between the findings of two review authors was resolved through discussion with a third expert (GC).

Data were independently extracted from each article by two authors (SP and GC) using a data collection form. Extracted data included the name of the study authors, year of publication, the country in which participants were recruited, the period of observation, and study design. For each included study, researchers retrieved information regarding: (a) the type of health facility (i.e., community hospitals, tertiary centres, university hospitals); (b) patients' selection criteria, age, and sex (percentage of females); (c) number of patients analysed in the study, the percentage of ED visits for allergy or anaphylaxis and the number of those related to drugs; (d) number of hospitalization events for drug-related allergy or anaphylaxis; (e) percentage of each causative drug class (if available). Authors of primary studies were contacted to retrieve missing data and/or for additional information. Studies with missing data for two or more of the abovementioned criteria were excluded.

Two review authors (NL and SP) independently assessed the included studies for bias, following the Joanna Briggs Institute Critical Appraisal Checklist for analytical cross-sectional study (last amended in 2017) [20]. For each domain in the tool, a judgment as to the possible risk of bias was made from the information reported in the body of papers. The judgements were made independently by two review authors (NL and SP); disagreements were resolved first by discussion and then by consulting a third author (GC). A graphic representation of potential bias was created using the software RevMan 5.4.1 (https://training.cochrane.org/, accessed on 25 March 2022).

3. Results

3.1. Post Hoc Analysis

During the study period (2012–2019), out of 94,073 ED visits, 13,532 (14.4%) cases were drug-related allergies, while 548 (0.6%) were anaphylactic events. Females accounted for 56.16%. The mean age was 46 and 55 years for patients who experienced allergies and anaphylaxis, respectively. Overall, 2105 (15.6% out of 13,532) subjects who experienced a drug-related allergy and 371 (67.7% out of 548) subjects who experienced anaphylaxis were hospitalized (Table 1).

As for drug-related allergies, the majority of subjects were female (59.2%), with a mean age of 46.3 ± 22.9 years, and Caucasian (81.72%). The most frequently reported triage colour codes were "green" (46.1%) and "yellow" (17.6%). Multivariate logistic regression showed that females (ROR 0.88 [0.84–0.91]) and subjects aged > 65 years (ROR 0.28 [0.27–0.29]) were at lower risk of drug-related allergies compared to males and other age classes, respectively. On the contrary, a higher risk of drug-related allergy was observed among all age classes < 65 years, in particular in children (age 2–11 years: ROR 2.97 [2.74–3.22]) and in adults (age 18–65 years: ROR 2.48 [2.39–2.58]). "Green" (ROR 1.29 [1.24–1.34]) and "white" (ROR 1.25 [1.15–1.37]) triage colour codes were significantly assigned to subjects experiencing an allergy compared to other triage codes.

Considering anaphylaxis, the majority of subjects were female (52.4%), with a mean age of 55.7 ± 17.7 years, and Caucasian (82.3%). The most frequently reported triage colour codes were "yellow" (33.4%) and "red" (23.5%). Considering anaphylaxis, children (ROR 0.21 [0.07–0.67]) and elderly (ROR 0.45 [0.37–0.53]) were at lower risk of this acute event, while a higher risk was observed for females (ROR 1.20 [1.01–1.42]) and adults (ROR 2.63 [2.21–3.14]). "Red" (ROR 10.68 [8.69–13.13]) and "yellow" (ROR 2.00 [1.68–2.39]) triage colour codes were significantly assigned to subjects experiencing anaphylaxis compared to other triage codes. Subjects who experienced anaphylaxis were statistically associated with a higher risk of hospitalization (ROR 5.62 [4.66–6.79]).

The majority of cases of anaphylaxis were treated with hydration, parenteral steroids, and antihistamines (data not shown). Overall, 58.94% of anaphylaxis (323 out of 548 cases) also reported adrenaline use during ED management (Table 2).

Suspected drug classes and active principles associated with anaphylaxis are reported in Table 3. In our sample, antibacterials for systemic use (ROR 8.75 [7.47–10.25]), NSAIDs (ROR 2.18 [1.71–2.78]), and radiology contrast agents (ROR 11.52 [8.33–15.92]) were significantly associated with a higher risk of anaphylaxis. Among antibacterials, the risk of anaphylaxis was significantly higher for pen, mainly represented by amoxicillin/clavulanate, and cephalosporins, particularly ceftriaxone. Among NSAIDs, the risk of anaphylaxis was significantly higher for dexibuprofen, followed by flurbiprofen, diclofenac, and ketorolac, while among radiology contrast agents, the risk of anaphylaxis was significantly higher for ioprimide, followed by ibitridol, iopamidol, and iomeprol. All other most frequently reported active principles involved in cases of anaphylaxis are depicted in Supplementary Table S2.

Table 1. Risk of drug-related allergy and anaphylaxis by patients' characteristics.

		Overall N = 94,073 (%)	Non-Allergy N = 79,993 (%)	Allergy N = 13,532 (%)	Anaphylaxis N = 548 (%)	Adjusted ROR of Allergy (95% CI)	Adjusted ROR of Anaphylaxis (95% CI)
Sex	Male	41,075 (43.66)	35,307 (44.14)	5507 (40.70)	261 (47.60)	1	1
	Female	52,832 (56.16)	44,531 (55.67)	8014 (59.22)	287 (52.40)	0.88 (0.84–0.91)	1.20 (1.01–1.42)
	Missing	166 (0.18)	155 (0.19)	11 (0.08)	-	-	-
Age, years	0–1	2174 (2.31)	1816 (2.27)	358 (2.70)	-	1.19 (1.06–1.34)	-
	2–11	2954 (3.14)	2003 (2.50)	948 (7.00)	3 (0.55)	2.97 (2.74–3.22)	0.21 (0.07–0.66)
	12–17	1616 (1.72)	1222 (1.53)	386 (2.90)	8 (1.46)	1.88 (1.68–2.12)	0.97 (0.48–1.95)
	18–65	42,303 (44.97)	33,289 (41.61)	8657 (64.00)	357 (65.14)	2.48 (2.39–2.58)	2.63 (2.21–3.14)
	>65	44,866 (47.69)	41,518 (51.90)	3170 (23.40)	178 (32.48)	0.28 (0.27–0.29)	0.44 (0.37–0.53)
	Missing	160 (0.17)	145 (0.19)	13 (0.09)	2 (0.37)	-	-
	Mean (±SD)	58.50 ± 23.90	60.59 ± 23.46	46.28 ± 22.98	55.70 ± 17.67	-	-
Ethnicity	Caucasian	75,668 (80.44)	64,158 (80.20)	11,059 (81.72)	451 (82.30)	1.12 (1.07–1.78)	1.16 (0.93–1.45)
	Other	2953 (3.14)	2330 (2.92)	603 (4.46)	20 (3.65)	-	-
	Missing	15,452 (16.42)	13,505 (16.88)	1870 (13.82)	77 (14.05)	-	-
Triage codes	Red	2672 (2.84)	2251 (2.81)	292 (2.16)	129 (23.54)	0.86 (0.76–0.97)	10.68 (8.69–13.13)
	Yellow	18,596 (19.77)	16,037 (20.05)	2376 (17.56)	183 (33.39)	0.92 (0.88–0.97)	2.00 (1.68–2.39)
	Green	36,045 (38.32)	29,748 (37.19)	6235 (46.07)	62 (11.31)	1.29 (1.24–1.34)	0.22 (0.17–0.28)
	White	3436 (3.65)	2719 (3.40)	717 (5.30)	-	1.25 (1.15–1.37)	-
	Missing	33,324 (35.42)	29,238 (36.55)	3912 (28.91)	174 (31.76)	-	-
Hospitalization	Yes	26,644 (28.32)	24,168 (30.20)	2105 (15.60)	371 (67.70)	0.53 (0.50–0.55)	5.62 (4.66–6.79)
	No	67,429 (71.68)	55,825 (69.80)	11,427 (84.40)	177 (32.30)	-	-

CI: confidence interval; IQR: interquartile range; ROR: reporting odds ratio; SD: standard deviation. Logistic regression analyses were used to estimate the reporting odds ratios (RORs) with 95% confidence intervals (CIs) of drug-related allergies and anaphylaxis adjusting for sex, age classes, and ethnicity.

Table 2. Variation of adrenaline use in the management of drug-related anaphylaxis events over the study period.

Year	Allergy Events N = 13,532	Anaphylaxis Events N = 548	Adrenaline Use N = 323 (% Row)
2012	1610	59	37 (62.71)
2013	2552	108	61 (56.48)
2014	2737	101	50 (49.50)
2015	1609	52	36 (69.23)
2016	804	36	19 (52.78)
2017	1206	65	41 (63.08)
2018	1838	64	45 (70.31)
2019	1176	63	34 (53.97)

The percentage of adrenaline use refers only to anaphylaxis cases. Overall, 58.94% of anaphylaxis (323 out of 548 cases) reported adrenaline use during ED management.

Table 3. Suspected drug classes associated with anaphylaxis.

	Anaphylaxis N = 608 (%)	Non-Allergy N = 104,366 (%)	Unadjusted ROR (95% CI)	Adjusted ROR (95% CI)
Antibacterials	327 (53.78)	10,744 (10.29)	9.99 (8.51–11.75)	8.75 (7.47–10.25)
Penicillins	218 (66.67)	5503 (51.22)	9.91 (8.37–11.73)	8.98 (7.57–10.65)
Cephalosporins	69 (21.10)	1291 (12.02)	10.09 (7.80–13.05)	10.75 (8.32–13.88)
Fluoroquinolones	28 (8.56)	1881 (17.51)	2.60 (1.77–3.80)	2.30 (1.57–3.38)
Macrolides	6 (1.83)	1155 (10.75)	0.88 (0.39–1.97)	0.75 (0.34–1.68)
Glycopeptides	5 (1.53)	347 (3.23)	2.45 (1.01–5.96)	2.28 (0.94–5.53)
Sulfamet./Trimetop.	1 (0.31)	337 (3.14)	0.50 (0.07–3.58)	0.42 (0.06–2.99)
NSAIDs	78 (12.83)	4980 (4.77)	2.88 (2.27–3.66)	2.18 (1.71–2.78)
Diclofenac	32 (41.03)	1058 (21.24)	5.33 (3.71–7.65)	4.45 (3.11–6.39)
Ketoprofen	24 (30.77)	1727 (34.68)	2.40 (1.59–3.62)	1.65 (1.08–2.52)
Ketorolac	5 (6.41)	291 (5.84)	2.91 (1.20–7.08)	2.26 (0.93–5.49)
Flurbiprofen	4 (5.13)	101 (2.03)	6.72 (2.47–18.31)	5.21 (1.91–14.25)
Indometacin	3 (3.85)	191 (3.84)	2.66 (0.85–8.34)	2.09 (0.66–6.60)
Nimesulide	2 (2.56)	581 (11.67)	0.58 (0.14–2.33)	0.43 (0.11–1.74)
Etoricoxib	2 (2.56)	234 (4.70)	1.44 (0.36–5.82)	1.30 (0.32–5.26)
Dexibuprofen	2 (2.56)	39 (0.78)	8.68 (2.09–36.02)	7.88 (1.90–32.68)
Radiology contrast agents	42 (6.92)	554 (0.53)	13.73 (9.92–19.00)	11.52 (8.33–15.92)
Iomeprol	16 (38.10)	201 (36.28)	13.83 (8.26–23.17)	11.52 (6.89–19.25)
Iopromide	12 (28.57)	88 (15.88)	25.56 (12.81–43.33)	20.26 (11.04–37.19)
Iobitridol	4 (9.52)	40 (7.22)	17.06 (6.08–47.84)	14.96 (5.41–41.41)
Iodixanol	3 (7.14)	52 (9.39)	9.82 (3.06–31.54)	8.62 (2.70–27.53)
Iopamidol	3 (7.14)	36 (6.50)	14.91 (4.36–46.22)	13.40 (4.05–44.40)
Other contrast agents	4 (9.52)	68 (12.27)	10.03 (3.65–27.59)	7.44 (2.71–20.47)
Analgesic drugs	32 (5.26)	11,131 (10.67)	0.46 (0.33–0.66)	0.47 (0.33–0.67)
Paracetamol *	15 (46.88)	2152 (19.33)	1.19 (0.71–1.98)	1.02 (0.61–1.71)
Acetylsalicylic acid	11 (34.38)	5589 (50.21)	0.32 (0.18–0.58)	0.38 (0.21–0.68)
Tramadol	2 (6.25)	859 (7.72)	0.39 (0.10–1.58)	0.34 (0.09–1.39)
Pethidine	2 (6.25)	12 (0.11)	28.34 (6.33–126.95)	22.99 (4.92–107.37)
Other analgesics	2 (6.25)	254 (2.28)	1.34 (0.33–5.38)	1.44 (0.36–5.86)
Antineoplastic drugs	23 (3.78)	7887 (7.56)	0.47 (0.31–0.72)	0.41 (0.27–0.63)
Paclitaxel	7 (30.43)	645 (8.18)	1.85 (0.87–3.91)	1.56 (0.73–3.30)
Oxaliplatin	5 (21.74)	486 (6.16)	1.75 (0.72–4.24)	1.53 (0.63–3.72)
Cetuximab	2 (8.70)	101 (1.28)	3.36 (0.83–13.67)	3.35 (0.83–13.54)
Trastuzumab	2 (8.70)	166 (2.10)	2.05 (0.51–8.27)	1.78 (0.44–7.15)
Rituximab	2 (8.70)	546 (6.92)	0.62 (0.15–2.49)	0.59 (0.14–2.37)
Other antineoplas. drugs	5 (21.74)	1226 (15.54)	0.69 (0.28–1.66)	0.59 (0.25–1.43)

CI: confidence interval; NSAID: non-steroidal anti-inflammatory drug; ROR: reporting odds ratio. * Alone or in combinations. The total number of suspected drugs involved in anaphylaxis and non-allergy events is bigger than the number of cases because more than one suspected drug can be reported in a pharmacovigilance report form. Logistic regression analyses were used to estimate the reporting odds ratios (RORs) with 95% confidence intervals (CIs) of drug-related allergies and anaphylaxis adjusting for sex, age classes, and ethnicity.

For all suspected drug classes, the most frequently reported drug-related hypersensitivity reactions affected the skin and subcutaneous tissue (data not shown). In particular, we observed several cases of urticaria, localized or general pruritus, erythema, and rash. These dermatological manifestations showed a different degree of seriousness among patients. Considering the most severe cases, these were represented by systemic reactions, including respiratory distress and anaphylactic shock.

3.2. Systematic Review

A total of 832 citations were identified through PubMed and Embase searching. After removing duplicates, 745 citations were screened, of which 657 were excluded as they were deemed irrelevant after title and abstract screening. Eighty-eight citations met inclusion criteria for full-text review (Figure 1).

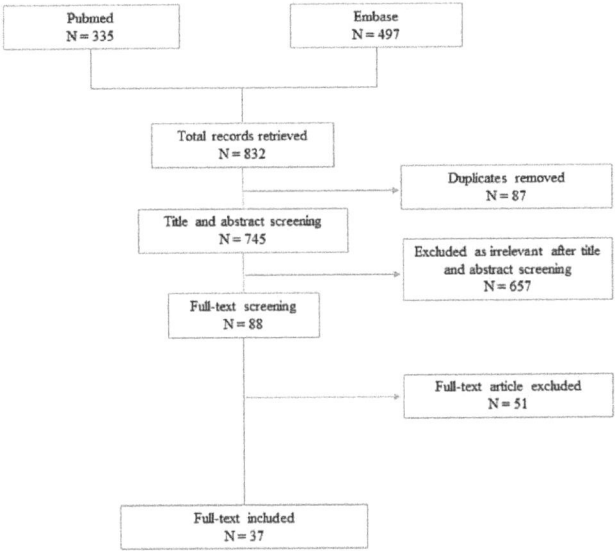

Figure 1. Flowchart depicting article selection.

After full-text review, 37 manuscripts were included in the systematic review (Table 4). Most of the primary studies (57%) were performed in USA and/or Canada [21–41], followed by 10 (27%) studies performed in Asia [42–51], 5 (13%) studies in Europe [52–56], and 1 (3%) study in Australia [57]. Overall, 17 (46%) were multicentre studies, either retrospective or retrospective/prospective [23–26,28–31,33–35,40–42,44,48,57].

Four (10%) studies did not specify whether they were multicentre or single centre studies, while 16 studies were performed in a single ED [21,27,32,39,43,46,47,49–56]. Eight (22%) studies were performed on electronic databases, selecting patients mainly using the International Classification of Diseases (ICD-9 or ICD-10) codes [22–24,26,30,36,37,45]. Seven studies (19%) [30,33–35,40,56,57] focused on specific drug classes, in particular antibiotics, psychiatric medications, antivirals, and NSAIDs. Twelve studies (32%) included paediatric patients [23,24,26,28,34–36,40,41,43,45,55], and females accounted for 34.7% to 73% of selected participants. Overall, female was the most represented sex in the majority of the included studies (24 studies out of 37). The number of included patients varied among the studies, ranging from 21 to 10,848,695. ED visits related to allergy and anaphylaxis accounted for a minimum of 0.004% to a maximum of 88%. According to the study design and selection criteria, drug-related allergies and anaphylaxis ranged from 0.007% to 88%. Eight studies (22%) [21,42,47,48,51,54–56] did not report the number of hospitalizations, which varied from 1 to 22,646 patients. The most frequently reported causative drug classes were antibiotics, analgesics and NSAIDs, radiology contrast agents, and anticancer agents.

Table 4. Characteristics of studies included in the systematic review.

Author, Year	Country	Period of Observation and Study Design	Participating Centres	Patients' Selection	Age and Sex	Total of Patients	ED Visits for Allergy or Anaphylaxis	Drug-Related Allergy or Anaphylaxis	Hospitalization for Drug-Related Allergy or Anaphylaxis	Causative Drug Classes
Asai, 2014 [21]	Canada	2011–2012 Retrospective single centre study	Adult tertiary care ED	Diagnosis of anaphylaxis or allergic reactions (ICD-10 codes)	Median (IQR): 31.5 (26.4–44.0) years Females 66.3%	37,730	98	18	NR	Amoxicillin 16.7%
Banerji, 2014 [22]	USA	2006–2008 Retrospective database analysis	Truven Health MarketScan Commercial and Medicare Supplemental Databases (Truven, Ann Arbor, Mich)	Diagnosis of anaphylaxis (ICD9-CM codes)	Mean ± SD 48 ± 19 years Females 71%	716	716	716	205	NR
Bellou, 2003 [52]	France	1 year (1998) Retrospective single centre study	General hospital ED	Cases of suspected allergic reaction	Mean ± SD 55 ± 18.5 years Females 51%	324	324	25	Overall, 90	Beta-lactams 28% Macrolides 20% NSAIDs 52%
Bielen, 2019 [53]	Croatia	2012–2015 Retrospective single centre study	Tertiary care university hospital ED	Cases of hypersensitivity (SMQ)	<29 years: 8005 30–39 years: 7875 40–49 years: 8095 50–64 years: 17611 65–74 years: 13414 >75 years: 16982 Females 54.6%	71,982	3039	627	38	Antibiotics 44.7% Analgesics and NSAIDs 18.7%
Budnitz, 2005 [23]	USA	3 months Retrospective multicentre study; database analysis	NEISS-CADES database	Cases of ADE	<2 years: 56; 2–9 years: 62; 10–19 years: 44; 20–29: 66; 30–39 years: 59; 40–49 years: 84; 50–59 years: 65; 60–69 years: 57; 70–79: 58; ≥80 years: 47 Females 63.9%	598	155	155	4	Antibiotics 42.9% Non-opioid analgesics 29.3% Cardiovascular agents 24%
Budnitz, 2006 [24]	USA	2004–2005 Retrospective multicentre study; database analysis	NEISS-CADES database	Cases of ADE	0–4 years: 104,185; 5–17 years: 225,082; 18–44 years: 362,044; 45–64: 147,178; ≥65 years: 83,549 Females 44.7%	701,547 estimated annual ED visits	235,202 estimated annual ED visits	235,202 estimated annual ED visits	13,232 estimated annual ED visits	NR
Budnitz, 2011 [25]	USA	2007–2009 Retrospective multicentre study; database analysis	NEISS-CADES database	Cases of ADE	65–69 years: 2470; 70–74 years: 1840; 75–79 years: 2629; 80–84 years: 2476; ≥85 years: 2621 Females 59%	265,802 estimated annual ED visits	39,455 estimated annual ED visits	39,455 estimated annual ED visits	5617 estimated annual hospitalization	Cardiovascular agents Antibiotics
Cho, 2019 [42]	Korea	2012–2016 Cross-sectional multicentre study	7 community hospitals EDs	Cases of anaphylaxis (ICD-10 codes)	Mean ± SD 51.5 ± 16.0 Females 34.7%	325,857	1021	135	NR	NSAIDs 28.1% Antibiotics 15.6% Antibiotics and NSAIDs 3.7% Radiocontrast media 2.2%

Table 4. Cont.

Author, Year	Country	Period of Observation and Study Design	Participating Centres	Patients' Selection	Age and Sex	Total of Patients	ED Visits for Allergy or Anaphylaxis	Drug-Related Allergy or Anaphylaxis	Hospitalization for Drug-Related Allergy or Anaphylaxis	Causative Drug Classes
Cianferoni, 2001 [54]	Italy	1985–1996 Retrospective chart review	University hospital ED	Diagnosis of acute anaphylaxis	Mean ± SD 42 ± 18 Females 45%	113	113	52	NR	Antibiotics 48% NSAIDs 35%
Cohen, 2008 [26]	USA	2004–2005 Retrospective multicentre study; database analysis	NEISS-CADES database	Cases of ADE	<1 year: 386; 1–4 years: 703; 5–8 years: 302; 9–12 years: 216; 13–18 years: 475 Females NR	6681	2802	2802	Overall, 5.1	Antibiotics 60.8% Analgesics 9.2% Multiple agents 6.7% Respiratory medications 5.9% Psychotropic medications 2.2%
Cohen, 2018 [43]	Israel	2013–2016 Retrospective single centre study	Paediatric hospital ED	Cases of allergic reactions or anaphylaxis (Anaphylaxis Criteria, Sampson et al.)	Mean 6.8 years (range 0–16 years) Females 34.7%	113,067	428	10	8 (1 of which in ICU)	NR
Dennehy, 1996 [27]	USA	30 days (1994) Single centre study	General hospital ED	Cases of drug-related illness	Mean ± SD 41.7 ± 22.5 years Females 50%	50	7	7	Overall, 8	NR
Gabrielli, 2018 [28]	Canada	2012–2016 Retrospective/prospective multicentre study	3 paediatric hospital and 1 general hospital EDs	Cases of anaphylaxis (diagnosis at ED presentation or ICD codes)	Median 49.4 (IQR 40.1–62.9) adults; median 8.00 (IQR 3.79–15.36) children Females: 71.9% adults; 47.1% children	884,000	1913	115 (64 adults; 51 children)	Admitted (5/51 = 9.8% children, 3/64 = 4.7% adults) Admitted ICU (1/51 = 2.0% children, 1/64 = 1.6% adults) Admitted hospital ward (4/51 = 7.8% children, 2/64 = 3.1% adults)	Beta-lactams (28.1% adults, 31.4% children) Quinolones (20.3% adults, 2% children) Other antibiotics (6.3% adults, 0% children) NSAIDs (20.3% adults, 21.6% children) Radiocontrast media (3.1% adults, 3.9% children)
Goh, 2018 [44]	Singapore	2014–2015 Prospective multicentre study	3 general hospital EDs	Cases of anaphylaxis (ICD-9 codes)	Median 23 years (range 3 months to 88 years and 9 months) Females 49.1%	7373	426	85 (66 adults; 19 children)	3	NSAIDs (24.2% adults, 52.6% children) Antibiotics (21.2% adults, 5.3% children) Paracetamol (3.0% adults, 10.5% children)
Grunau, 2015 [29]	USA and Canada	2007–2012 Retrospective multicentre cohort study	2 teaching hospital EDs	Diagnosis of allergic reaction	Median (IQR): 34 (27–47) years patients treated with steroids; 35 (26–49) years patients treated without steroids Females 60.9%	2701	2701	702	11	Anti-infective agents 48.9% Nervous system agents 10.3% (analgesics 2%) Radiocontrast media 3.7% NSAIDs 2.4%

Table 4. Cont.

Author, Year	Country	Period of Observation and Study Design	Participating Centres	Patients' Selection	Age and Sex	Total of Patients	ED Visits for Allergy or Anaphylaxis	Drug-Related Allergy or Anaphylaxis	Hospitalization for Drug-Related Allergy or Anaphylaxis	Causative Drug Classes
Hall, 2020 [57]	Australia	2010–2015 Retrospective multicentre cohort study	5 university tertiary hospital EDs	Cases of antimicrobial anaphylaxis (ICD-10 codes)	Median 51 years (IQR 36–67) Females 61%	293	185	185	7 ICU admission	Overall (out of 185) Penicillins 39.9% Cephalosporins 35.1% Amino-penicillins 18.5% Amino-cephalosporins 17.0%
Hampton, 2014 [30]	USA	2009–2011 Retrospective multicentre study; database analysis	Administrative database 63 centres	Cases of psychiatric medication-related ADE	19–44 years: 49.4 (46.5–52.4) 45–64 years: 33.3 (30.7–35.9) ≥65 years: 17.3 (14.7–19.8) Females 61.9%	89,094 estimated annual ED visits	11,493 estimated annual ED visits	11,493 estimated annual ED visits	Overall, 17,188 estimated annual hospitalization	Zolpidem Quetiapine Alprazolam Lorazepam Haloperidol Clonazepam Trazodone Citalopram Lithium Risperidone
Han, 2018 [45]	Korea	2009–2014 Retrospective cohort study; database analysis	National insurance claim database of the Health Insurance Review and Assessment (HIRA)	Cases of drug hypersensitivity reactions (ICD-10 codes)	88,003 ≤19 years 169,103 20–44 years 180,535 45–64 years 97,408 ≥65 years Females 57.5%	535,049	3984 (T88.6 code)	3984 (T88.6 code)	184 (T88.6 code)	NR
Harduar-Morano, 2011 [31]	USA	2005–2006 Retrospective multicentre study	General hospital EDs	Diagnosis of anaphylaxis (ICD9-CM codes)	Mean ± SD 38.7 ± 21.46 Females 57%	2751	2751	228	54	NR
Hitti, 2015 [46]	Lebanon	July–December 2009 Retrospective single centre study	Tertiary care centre ED	Cases of acute allergic reaction (ICD-9 codes)	Mean ± SD 31.8 ± 19.2 years Females 42%	293	245	58	Overall, 1 patient was hospitalized	Antibiotics 8.2% NSAIDs 4.9%
Hsin, 2011 [47]	India	2000–2010 Retrospective single centre cohort study	General hospital ED	Diagnosis of anaphylaxis (ICD9 codes)	Mean age overall 43.3 years Female 47%	201	86	Overall, 161	NR	NSAIDs Antibiotics Chemotherapy Anti-epileptics Contrast media Immunotherapy Biologics H1N1 Vaccine Anaesthesia
Huang, 2012 [32]	USA	2004–2008 Retrospective single centre study	Paediatric hospital ED	Cases of anaphylaxis	Median (IQR) 8 (4 months–18 years) years Females 49%	192 (20 had multiple reactions)	192	19	Overall, 28	NR

Table 4. Cont.

Author, Year	Country	Period of Observation and Study Design	Participating Centres	Patients' Selection	Age and Sex	Total of Patients	ED Visits for Allergy or Anaphylaxis	Drug-Related Allergy or Anaphylaxis	Hospitalization for Drug-Related Allergy or Anaphylaxis	Causative Drug Classes
Jones, 2013 [33]	USA	2004–2013 Retrospective multicentre study; database analysis	NEISS-CADES database	Cases of fluoroquinolone-associated hypersensitivity ADEs	Mean age overall 48.22 years Females 73.7%	102,536	1659	1422	96	Ciprofloxacin Levofloxacin Moxifloxacin Gemifloxacin Ofloxacin
Kim MY, 2018 (a) [48]	Korea	2011–2013 Retrospective multicentre study	2 tertiary hospitals and 1 secondary hospital EDs	Cases of anaphylaxis (ICD codes)	Mean ± SD 46 ± 17.1 Females 55.2%	194	194	151	NR	Antibiotics Acetylsalicylic acid Radiocontrast media NSAIDs
Kim MY, 2018 (b) [49]	South Korea	2003–2016 Retrospective single centre study	Tertiary university hospital ED	Cases of anaphylaxis (Korean Standard Classification of Disease)	Mean ± SD 41.1 ± 23.4 Females 48.2%	199	199	72	13	Overall (out of 199) Antibiotics 40.2% NSAIDs 33.3% Radiocontrast media 11.1%
Ko, 2015 [50]	Korea	2007–2014 Single centre study	Tertiary teaching hospital ED	Cases of anaphylaxis (Skin or mucosal tissue involvement; Respiratory compromise; Systolic blood pressure <90 mmHg or syncope; Gastrointestinal symptoms)	Mean ± SD 48.4 ± 15.7 years Females 54.9%	655	415	187	Overall, 3 patients were hospitalized	Radiocontrast media 70 NSAIDs 39 Cephalosporins 34 Anticancer agents 16
Losappio, 2014 [55]	Italy	2011 Retrospective single centre study	General hospital ED	Cases of allergic urticaria (ICD-9 codes)	Mean 35.4 years (range 0–90 years) Females 49.2%	44,112	459	92 (79 adults; 13 children)	NR	NSAIDs Beta-lactams
Lovegrove, 2011 [34]	USA	2006–2009 Retrospective multicentre study	Drug Abuse Warning Network (DAWN), 250 non-federal, short-stay general hospitals	Cases of antivirals-related ADE	<6 years: 139; 6–11 years: 103; 12–17 years: 58; 18–44 years: 332; 45–64 years: 161; ≥65 years: 89 Female 59.3%	879	274	274	Overall, 125	Amantadine Rimantadine Oseltamivir Zanamivir
Lovegrove, 2019 [35]	USA	2011–2015 Retrospective multicentre study; database analysis	NEISS-CADES database	Cases of antibiotics-related ADE in children (MedDRA)	2870 <1–2 years 743 3–4 years 1187 5–9 years 1742 10–19 years Females 52.1%	6542	5763	5763	Overall, 265	Overall (out of 6542) Penicillins 59.7% Cephalosporins 11.2% Sulfonamides 9.5%
Motosue, 2018 (a) [36]	USA	2005–2014 Prospective observational study; database analysis	OLDW administrative database	Cases of anaphylaxis (ICD-9 codes)	Median 36 years (interquartile range 17–52) Females 57.5%	56,212	56,212	6720	Inpatient 717 and ICU 409	NR

Table 4. Cont.

Author, Year	Country	Period of Observation and Study Design	Participating Centres	Patients' Selection	Age and Sex	Total of Patients	ED Visits for Allergy or Anaphylaxis	Drug-Related Allergy or Anaphylaxis	Hospitalization for Drug-Related Allergy or Anaphylaxis	Causative Drug Classes
Motosue, 2018 (b) [37]	USA	2008–2012 Retrospective study; database analysis	Administrative claims database (OptumLabs Data Warehouse)	Cases of anaphylaxis and anaphylactic shock (ICD-9 codes)	Median 42 years (range 1–87 years) Females 58.3%	7367	7367	1076	Overall, 532 ICU admission	NR
Quiralte, 1997 [56]	Spain	1992–1995 Prospective single centre study	University hospital ED	Cases of NSAIDs-related anaphylaxis	Mean ± SD 35.7 ± 13.9 Females 71%	21	21	21	NR	Dipyrone 57.1% Propyphenazone 14.2% Acetic derivatives (diclofenac and indomethacin) 14.2%
Rangkakulnuwat, 2020 [51]	Thailand	2007–2016 Retrospective single centre study	University hospital ED	Cases of anaphylaxis (ICD-10 codes)	Median 24.0 years (IQR 19.0–43.0) Females 57.2%	10,848,695	441	79	NR	NSAIDs 7.4% Antimicrobial Agents 4.0% Radiocontrast media 0.9%
Russell, 2010 [38]	USA	2002–2006 Retrospective single centre cross-sectional study	Tertiary care paediatric hospital ED	Diagnosis of anaphylaxis (ICD-9 codes)	Mean ± SD 9.49 ± 5.56 Females 36%	103	103	15	4	Antibiotics Intravenous contrast
Schneitman Mcintire, 1996 [39]	USA	1992–1993 Retrospective single centre study	General hospital ED	Patients who experienced medication misadventures	15–44 years 38% 65 years or older 33% Females 62%	62,216	221	204	7	Trimetoprim sulfametoxazol 34% Amoxicillin 21% Ibuprofen 5.4%
Shehab, 2008 [40]	USA	2004–2005 Retrospective multicentre study; database analysis	NEISS-CADES database	Cases of antibiotics-related ADE	<1 years: 545; 1–4 years: 976; 5–14 years: 656; 15–44 years: 2577; 45–64 years: 1143; 65–79 years: 507; ≥80 years: 210 Females 64.4%	142,505 estimated annual ED visits	112,116 estimated annual ED visits	112,116 estimated annual ED visits	8738 estimated annual hospitalization	Penicillins 36.9% Cephalosporins 12.2% Fluoroquinolones 13.5% Sulfonamide trimethoprim 11.8% Macrolides and Ketolides 6.9% Tetracyclines 3.1% Vancomycin Linezolid 0.8%
Willy, 2009 [41]	USA	2004–2005 Retrospective multicentre study; database analysis	NEISS-CADES database	Cases of analgesics-related ADE	0–9 years: 32,222; 10–19 years: 17,012; 20–29 years: 28,298; 30–39 years: 23,165; 40–49 years: 22,706; 50–59 years: 18,767; 60–69 years: 14,590; 70–79 years: 15,030; 80–89 years: 14,933; ≥90 years: 1998 Females 57%	188,721	58,101	58,101	Overall, 22,646	Acetaminophen Non-narcotic-acetaminophen combination Narcotic-acetaminophen combination Acetylsalicylic acid Ibuprofen Naproxen

ADE: adverse drug event; ED: emergency department; ICD-CM: International Classification of Diseases-Clinical Modification; ICU: intensive care unit; IQR: interquartile range; MedDRA: Medical Dictionary for Regulatory Activities Terminology; NR: not reported; NSAIDs: non-anti-inflammatory drugs; SD: standard deviation; SMQ: standardized MedDRA query; T88.6 code: Anaphylactic shock due to adverse effect of correct drug or medication properly administered.

Quality assessment is depicted in Figure 2. Only 11 studies [23,28,29,31,37,42,45,46,51,55,57] were at low risk of bias for all considered domains. Identification of confounding factors and strategies to deal with them were unclear or at high risk of bias for most of the included studies. In particular, several papers did not report any clear identification of variables for analysis adjustment. Only one study [39] was judged at unclear risk of bias for incomplete description of inclusion criteria, two studies [22,39] for the domain "Exposure measurement", and only one [40] for "outcome measurement". Statistical analysis was properly performed in the majority of studies.

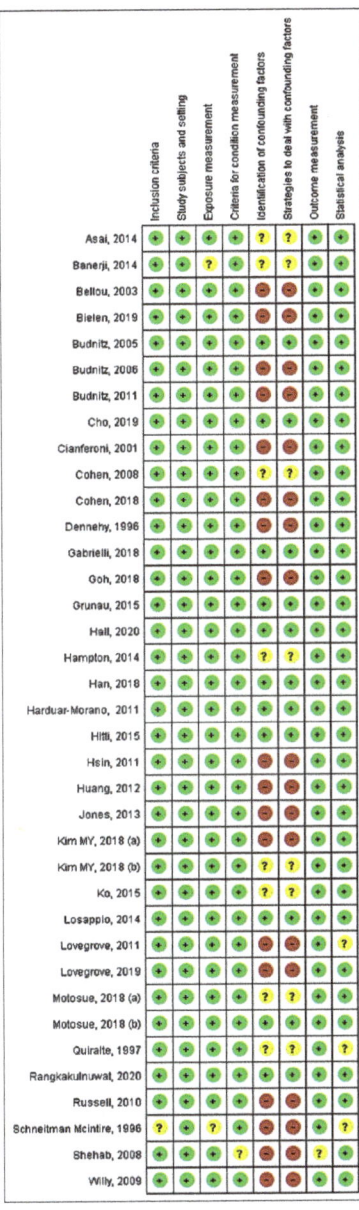

Figure 2. Risk of bias graph assessment, performed according to Cochrane Collaboration's risk of bias tool [21–57].

4. Discussion

The current study summarizes the up-to-date evidence on drug-related allergies and anaphylaxis causing ED visit and hospitalization. Antibacterials for systemic use, NSAIDs, and radiology contrast agents were the most reported drug classes associated with drug-related hypersensitivity reactions.

Although our post hoc analysis showed that female was the sex most represented in allergy events, women seem to be associated with a lower risk of drug-related allergy but a higher risk of anaphylaxis, even if at the limit of statistical significance. Considering drug-related allergy, this evidence is comparable with real-world data coming from observational studies, in which a higher risk of ADEs was usually observed in women [58,59]. Nevertheless, there are no conclusive data that drug-related allergies are more common in females than in males [60]. In general, discrepancy exists regarding the sex difference in allergy caused by different triggers, including pharmacological treatments, with females reporting significantly more allergic reactions in questionnaire studies [61]. Moreover, we also observed that women experienced anaphylaxis more frequently than men. This evidence is comparable with hospital-based studies that suggested a female predominance regarding drug-induced anaphylaxis or a history of immediate penicillin allergy [62,63]. Furthermore, some studies reported that females are twice as likely to have drug-induced anaphylaxis than males [64]. However, the reasons for this sex discrepancy are still incompletely understood [65].

Considering patients' age, we observed that most drug-related allergies occurred in adults (age 18–65 years). This result can be compared with the evidence published in the literature where it is reported that drug-related allergies typically occur in young and middle-aged adults [66]. In fact, with regards to children, it is well known that they are less likely to be exposed repeatedly to medications, especially due to the absence or lower incidence of comorbidities [59,66]. In our sample, drug-related anaphylaxis was also reported more frequently by adults (age 18–65 years), an age group known to be associated with these serious events, which occur mainly in subjects with a mean age of around 58–60 years [67,68]. Of note, the mean age of patients experiencing an allergy or anaphylaxis in our sample was even lower. Although age is consistently associated with severity of anaphylaxis in many studies [64,69], we did not observe a higher risk of drug-related allergy and anaphylaxis in elderly (>65 years). This may be due to the presence of a relatively low number of elderly subjects who experienced an allergy or anaphylaxis as the cause of ED visits and hospitalization in our sample. Moreover, we hypothesize that the elderly included in our analysis may be represented by subjects mainly exposed to long-term pharmacological treatments (i.e., chronic treatment), which can be considered to be less associated with hypersensitivity reactions.

In Italy, triage assessment is made on a colour code basis, with highest priority given to a red code, followed by yellow, green, and white [70]. Although triage is a very useful tool for prioritizing patients upon their arrival to the ED, limited data relating to the triage assessment colour code for drug-related hypersensitivity reactions are available [71]. Nevertheless, our analysis found that more serious events, in particular anaphylaxis, were correctly coded and were mainly associated with "red" and "yellow" triage codes.

With respect to drug classes most frequently associated with anaphylaxis, striking geographical differences exist and are likely caused by local prescription patterns and are influenced by other less characterized factors, such as genetic differences [64]. Despite this, as highlighted by the results of our systematic review, the findings of the active pharmacovigilance study MEREAFaPS were in line with those of studies already published in literature on this topic. Both in our post hoc analysis and in the studies included in the systematic review, most cases of anaphylaxis were caused by the administration of antibacterials for systemic use, NSAIDs, and radiology contrast agents. In general, the best strategy for drug-related hypersensitivity management is avoidance or discontinuation of the suspected medication. Alternative medications with unrelated chemical structures should be substituted, always considering the presence of drugs cross-reactivity [72]. Antibacterials for systemic use, in particular penicillins, are the most common triggers observed in drug-related allergy, affecting approximately 10% of patients [73]. Another group of antibiotics frequently associated with hypersensitivity are cephalosporins, which are generally causative of maculopapular rashes and drug fever, while urticaria and anaphylaxis are uncommon [74]. Analgesics, in particular NSAIDs, can cause hypersensitivity reactions, including exacerbations of underlying respiratory diseases, urticaria, angioedema, and anaphylaxis [72]. Finally, radiology contrast agents are associated with both allergic and pseudoallergic reactions. The incidence of these reactions, including anaphylaxis, appears to be lower with non-ionic versus ionic agents. Drug-related hypersensitivity reactions to radiology contrast agents can be prevented through pre-treatment regimens with corticosteroids and H1-antihistamines [72]. Intramuscular epinephrine (adrenaline) represents the first-line treatment for anaphylaxis. However, even if its use remains suboptimal [4], in our population epinephrine was used in a relatively high percentage of cases of anaphylaxis. After anaphylaxis occurrence, patients should be referred to a specialist to assess the potential cause and to be educated on prevention of recurrences and self-management. The limited availability of epinephrine auto-injectors remains a major problem worldwide, especially in low- and middle-income countries [75].

Strengths and Limitations

Our study has some limitations. First, the retrospective nature of the study may have led to an underestimation of allergic and anaphylactic ADEs, because ED physicians could not report the reaction or could not recognize the allergic nature of the reaction. This possibility has been evidenced by several studies, such those published by Sundquist et al. [76] and Martelli et al. [77], who evidenced a reduced capacity to recognize anaphylaxis in ED. Another cause of underestimation of anaphylaxis could be the death of serious cases before their arrival in ED. However, considering that the ADEs were collected through a national active pharmacovigilance initiative, the issue of underreporting, especially for anaphylaxis, can be considered of relatively low relevance. Moreover, we did not evaluate the effect of concomitant medications and comorbidities on hypersensitivity reactions and the seriousness of each drug-related allergy. It should be of great importance to have information on concomitant medications since they may potentiate anaphylaxis symptoms or reduce the efficacy of its treatment [78,79]. Even some comorbidities, such as respiratory and cardiovascular diseases, have been associated with poorer prognosis as they may lead to insufficient compensatory mechanisms to endure anaphylaxis complications [80]. Furthermore, we cannot exclude a partial lack of additional data mainly due to the specific condition of each ED (i.e., lack of time, general conditions of patients, and other emergencies). Our analysis is based on ADE reports that are affected by limits that include inaccurate and incomplete information on patients (i.e., sex, age, ethnicity, triage colour code), also mainly related to lack of clinical data in the ED electronic sources. Finally, we cannot have data on the recurrence of anaphylaxis, which involves 3% of patients within one year [37].

Despite these shortcomings, our study overcomes the limitations listed by the World Allergy Organization Anaphylaxis Guidance [4]. As for lack of large prospective population-based studies, this is the first nationwide multicentre study investigating allergic ADEs as the cause of ED visits in Italy. Our analysis included five Italian Regions located in northern, central, and southern Italy, allowing us to reach an estimated coverage of over 45% of the Italian population (more than 28 million inhabitants) [15]. Few multicentre studies examined such a large population with an active pharmacovigilance approach in ED. Most studies were carried out in single hospitals, involving few EDs, and larger studies have usually been performed on administrative databases (i.e., insurance claims), using ICD-9 and ICD-10 codes [22–24,26,30,36,37,45]. The use of ICD codes in observational studies may have been associated with a misclassification of patients, with the possible introduction of a selection bias. Moreover, these codes cover anaphylaxis definition as reported by Regateiro et al. [64] only partially. On the contrary, the use of MedDRA standardized medical terminology in our study allowed us to reach a proper differentiation between drug-related hypersensitivity ADEs and other kinds of ADEs, with a certainty of the diagnosis. In fact, each ADE and diagnosis in pharmacovigilance report forms were identified and then coded by trained monitors, and additional information was requested to ensure the greatest correspondence between what occurred and what was entered in the database, thus minimizing the misclassification and the selection bias in this post hoc analysis. Moreover, while several studies concerning allergies and anaphylaxis did not always report risk factors and triggers [22,24,27,31,32,36,37,43,45], the use of the ATC classification system allowed us to record all active principles causative of the hypersensitivity event with certainty.

5. Conclusions

In conclusion, drug-related hypersensitivity reactions represent a relevant clinical issue worldwide. Despite the large number of available marketed medications, pharmacological triggers associated with hypersensitivity are mostly well-known drug classes. Both our post hoc analysis and the systematic review confirmed the association between allergy and anaphylaxis and antibiotics for systemic use, NSAIDs, and radiology contrast agents, especially in women and adults. This information should always be taken into consideration by general practitioners, patients and their caregivers, and ED healthcare professionals, to both minimize the occurrence of drug-related hypersensitivity reactions and improve their management.

Supplementary Materials: The following supporting information can be downloaded at: https://www.mdpi.com/article/10.3390/jcm11102811/s1, Table S1: MedDRA preferred terms attributable to allergic reactions or anaphylaxis. Table S2: Most frequently reported active principles involved in cases of anaphylaxis.

Author Contributions: Conceptualization, S.P., N.L. and G.C.; methodology, S.P. and G.C.; formal analysis, S.P. and G.C.; data curation, V.G.V., G.S. and P.A.; writing—original draft preparation, S.P., N.L. and G.C.; writing—review and editing, A.C. and A.V.; supervision, A.C., A.V., M.V. and G.D.V. All authors have read and agreed to the published version of the manuscript.

Funding: This study was funded by a research grant from the AIFA (the Italian Medicines Agency), Rome, Italy, Tuscan County resolution DGRT 790/2016 All. C. The funder of the study had no role in the collection, analysis, and interpretation of data, in the writing of the report, or in the decision to submit the article for publication.

Institutional Review Board Statement: The coordinating centre of Lombardy Region (Vimercate, Italy) approved the MEREAFaPS Study in 2006, and the local institutional ethics committee (ASST Monza Ethic Committee) approved the MEREAFaPS Study (Notification number 3724—6 May 2021) according to the legal requirements concerning observational studies.

Informed Consent Statement: Due to the retrospective nature of the present study and data anonymization, patients' consent to participate was not required.

Data Availability Statement: Data that support the findings of this study are available upon reasonable request from the corresponding author, N.L.

Acknowledgments: We thank members of the MEREAFaPS Study group who provided patient data for this study: Maria Luisa Aiezza (Naples), Alessandra Bettiol (Florence), Daria Bettoni (Brescia), Corrado Blandizzi (Pisa), Roberto Bonaiuti (Florence), Valentina Borsi (Florence), Annalisa Capuano (Naples), Errica Cecchi (Prato), Irma Convertino (Pisa), Giada Crescioli (Florence), Martina Del Lungo (Florence), Cristina Di Mauro (Naples), Gabriella Farina (Milan), Sara Ferraro (Pisa), Annamaria Fucile (Naples), Elena Galfrascoli (Milan), Elisabetta Geninatti (Turin), Linda Giovannetti (Florence), Luca Leonardi (Pisa), Rosa Liccardo (Naples), Niccolò Lombardi (Florence), Anna Marra (Ferrara), Eleonora Marrazzo (Turin), Giovanna Monina (Gallarate), Alessandro Mugelli (Florence), Silvia Pagani (Vimercate), Maria Parrilli (Florence), Concetta Rafaniello (Naples), Francesco Rossi (Naples), Marco Rossi (Siena), Stefania Rostan (Naples), Marco Ruocco (Vimercate), Marita Sironi (Vimercate), Giulia Spada (Vimercate), Liberata Sportiello (Naples), Marco Tuccori (Pisa), Alfredo Vannacci (Florence), Mauro Venegoni (Vimercate), Giuditta Violetta Vighi (Vimercate), Giuseppe Danilo Vighi (Vimercate).

Conflicts of Interest: The authors declare no conflict of interest.

References

1. Edwards, I.R.; Aronson, J.K. Adverse drug reactions: Definitions, diagnosis, and management. *Lancet* **2000**, *356*, 1255–1259. [CrossRef]
2. Aun, M.V.; Kalil, J.; Giavina-Bianchi, P. Drug-Induced Anaphylaxis. *Immunol. Allergy Clin. N. Am.* **2017**, *37*, 629–641. [CrossRef]
3. Demoly, P.; Adkinson, N.F.; Brockow, K.; Castells, M.; Chiriac, A.M.; Greenberger, P.A.; Khan, D.A.; Lang, D.M.; Park, H.-S.; Pichler, W.; et al. International Consensus on drug allergy. *Allergy* **2014**, *69*, 420–437. [CrossRef] [PubMed]
4. Cardona, V.; Ansotegui, I.J.; Ebisawa, M.; El-Gamal, Y.; Fernandez Rivas, M.; Fineman, S.; Geller, M.; Gonzalez-Estrada, A.; Greenberger, P.A.; Borges, M.S.; et al. World allergy organization anaphylaxis guidance 2020. *World Allergy Organ. J.* **2020**, *13*, 100472. [CrossRef] [PubMed]
5. Grabowski, J.P.; Sehouli, J.; Glajzer, J.; Worm, M.; Zuberbier, T.; Maurer, M.; Fluhr, J.W. Olaparib Desensitization in a Patient with Recurrent Peritoneal Cancer. *N. Engl. J. Med.* **2018**, *379*, 2176–2177. [CrossRef] [PubMed]
6. Toletone, A.; Dini, G.; Massa, E.; Bragazzi, N.L.; Pignatti, P.; Voltolini, S.; Durando, P. Chlorhexidine-induced anaphylaxis occurring in the workplace in a health-care worker: Case report and review of the literature. *Med. Del Lav.* **2018**, *109*, 68–76. [CrossRef]
7. Wylon, K.; Dölle, S.; Worm, M. Polyethylene glycol as a cause of anaphylaxis. *Allergy Asthma Clin. Immunol.* **2016**, *12*, 67. [CrossRef]
8. Ohnishi, A.; Hashimoto, K.; Ozono, E.; Sasaki, M.; Sakamoto, A.; Tashiro, K.; Moriuchi, H. Anaphylaxis to carboxymethylcellulose: Add food additives to the list of elicitors. *Pediatrics* **2019**, *143*, e20181180. [CrossRef]
9. Tejedor Alonso, M.A.; Moro Moro, M.; Múgica García, M.V. Epidemiology of anaphylaxis. *Clin. Exp. Allergy* **2015**, *45*, 1027–1039. [CrossRef]
10. Turner, P.J.; Campbell, D.E.; Motosue, M.S.; Campbell, R.L. Global Trends in Anaphylaxis Epidemiology and Clinical Implications. *J. Allergy Clin. Immunol. Pract.* **2020**, *8*, 1169–1176. [CrossRef]
11. Gomes, E.R.; Kuyucu, S. Epidemiology and Risk Factors in Drug Hypersensitivity Reactions. *Curr. Treat Options Allergy* **2017**, *4*, 239–257. [CrossRef]
12. Crescioli, G.; Bettiol, A.; Bonaiuti, R.; Tuccori, M.; Rossi, M.; Capuano, A.; Pagani, S.; Spada, G.; Venegoni, M.; Vighi, G.D.; et al. Risk of Hospitalization Associated with Cardiovascular Medications in the Elderly Italian Population: A Nationwide Multicenter Study in Emergency Departments. *Front. Pharmacol.* **2021**, *11*, 611102. [CrossRef] [PubMed]
13. Pagani, S.; Lombardi, N.; Crescioli, G.; Vighi, G.V.; Spada, G.; Romoli, I.; Andreetta, P.; Capuano, A.; Marrazzo, E.; Marra, A.; et al. Analysis of fatal adverse drug events recorded in several Italian emergency departments (the MEREAFaPS study). *Intern. Emerg. Med.* **2021**, *16*, 741–748. [CrossRef] [PubMed]
14. Lombardi, N.; Bettiol, A.; Crescioli, G.; Ravaldi, C.; Bonaiuti, R.; Venegoni, M.; Vighi, G.D.; Mugelli, A.; Mannaioni, G.; Vannacci, A.; et al. Risk of hospitalisation associated with benzodiazepines and z-drugs in Italy: A nationwide multicentre study in emergency departments. *Intern. Emerg. Med.* **2020**, *15*, 1291–1302. [CrossRef]
15. Lombardi, N.; Crescioli, G.; Bettiol, A.; Tuccori, M.; Capuano, A.; Bonaiuti, R.; Mugelli, A.; Venegoni, M.; Vighi, G.D.; Vannacci, A.; et al. Italian Emergency Department Visits and Hospitalizations for Outpatients' Adverse Drug Events: 12-Year Active Pharmacovigilance Surveillance (The MEREAFaPS Study). *Front. Pharmacol.* **2020**, *11*, 412. [CrossRef] [PubMed]
16. Lombardi, N.; Crescioli, G.; Bettiol, A.; Marconi, E.; Vitiello, A.; Bonaiuti, R.; Calvani, A.M.; Masi, S.; Lucenteforte, E.; Mugelli, A.; et al. Characterization of serious adverse drug reactions as cause of emergency department visit in children: A 5-years active pharmacovigilance study. *BMC Pharmacol. Toxicol.* **2018**, *19*, 16. [CrossRef]
17. MedDRA Hierarchy—Medical Dictionary for Regulatory Activities n.d. Available online: https://www.meddra.org/how-to-use/basics/hierarchy (accessed on 25 March 2022).
18. Cremonesi, P.; di Bella, E.; Montefiori, M.; Persico, L. The Robustness and Effectiveness of the Triage System at Times of Overcrowding and the Extra Costs due to Inappropriate Use of Emergency Departments. *Appl. Health Econ. Health Policy* **2015**, *13*, 507–514. [CrossRef]
19. Moher, D.; Liberati, A.; Tetzlaff, J.; Altman, D.G.; PRISMA Group. Preferred reporting items for systematic reviews and meta-analyses: The PRISMA statement. *PLoS Med.* **2009**, *6*, e1000097. [CrossRef]
20. Ma, L.L.; Wang, Y.Y.; Yang, Z.H.; Huang, D.; Weng, H.; Zeng, X.T. Methodological quality (risk of bias) assessment tools for primary and secondary medical studies: What are they and which is better? *Mil. Med. Res.* **2020**, *7*, 7. [CrossRef]
21. Asai, Y.; Yanishevsky, Y.; Clarke, A.; La Vieille, S.; Scott Delaney, J.; Alizadehfar, R.; Joseph, L.; Mill, C.; Morris, J.; Ben-Shoshan, M. Rate, triggers, severity and management of anaphylaxis in adults treated in a Canadian emergency department. *Int. Arch. Allergy Immunol.* **2014**, *164*, 246–252. [CrossRef]
22. Banerji, A.; Rudders, S.; Clark, S.; Wei, W.; Long, A.A.; Camargo, C.A. Retrospective study of drug-induced anaphylaxis treated in the emergency department or hospital: Patient characteristics, management, and 1-year follow-up. *J. Allergy Clin. Immunol. Pract.* **2014**, *2*, 46–51. [CrossRef] [PubMed]
23. Budnitz, D.S.; Pollock, D.A.; Mendelsohn, A.B.; Weidenbach, K.N.; McDonald, A.K.; Annest, J.L. Emergency department visits for outpatient adverse drug events: Demonstration for a national surveillance system. *Ann. Emerg. Med.* **2005**, *45*, 197–206. [CrossRef] [PubMed]

24. Budnitz, D.S.; Pollock, D.A.; Weidenbach, K.N.; Mendelsohn, A.B.; Schroeder, T.J.; Annest, J.L. National surveillance of emergency department visits for outpatient adverse drug events. *J. Am. Med. Assoc.* **2006**, *296*, 1858–1866. [CrossRef]
25. Budnitz, D.S.; Lovegrove, M.C.; Shehab, N.; Richards, C.L. Emergency Hospitalizations for Adverse Drug Events in Older Americans. *N. Engl. J. Med.* **2011**, *365*, 2002–2012. [CrossRef] [PubMed]
26. Cohen, A.L.; Budnitz, D.S.; Weidenbach, K.N.; Jernigan, D.B.; Schroeder, T.J.; Shehab, N.; Pollock, D.A. National Surveillance of Emergency Department Visits for Outpatient Adverse Drug Events in Children and Adolescents. *J. Pediatr.* **2008**, *152*, 416–421. [CrossRef] [PubMed]
27. Dennehy, C.E.; Kishi, D.T.; Louie, C. Drug-related illness in emergency department patients. *Am. J. Heal. Pharm.* **1996**, *53*, 1422–1426. [CrossRef]
28. Gabrielli, S.; Clarke, A.E.; Eisman, H.; Morris, J.; Joseph, L.; La Vieille, S.; Small, P.; Lim, R.; Enarson, P.; Zelcer, M.; et al. Disparities in rate, triggers, and management in pediatric and adult cases of suspected drug-induced anaphylaxis in Canada. *Immun. Inflamm. Dis.* **2018**, *6*, 3–12. [CrossRef]
29. Grunau, B.E.; Wiens, M.O.; Rowe, B.H.; McKay, R.; Li, J.; Yi, T.W.; Stenstrom, R.; Schellenberg, R.R.; Grafstein, E.; Scheuermeyer, F.X. Emergency Department Corticosteroid Use for Allergy or Anaphylaxis Is Not Associated with Decreased Relapses. *Ann. Emerg. Med.* **2015**, *66*, 381–389. [CrossRef]
30. Olfson, M. Surveillance of adverse psychiatric medication events. *JAMA J. Am. Med. Assoc.* **2014**, *313*, 1256–1257. [CrossRef]
31. Harduar-Morano, L.; Simon, M.R.; Watkins, S.; Blackmore, C. A population-based epidemiologic study of emergency department visits for anaphylaxis in Florida. *J. Allergy Clin. Immunol.* **2011**, *128*, 594–600. [CrossRef]
32. Huang, F.; Chawla, K.; Järvinen, K.M.; Nowak-Węgrzyn, A. Anaphylaxis in a New York City pediatric emergency department: Triggers, treatments, and outcomes. *J. Allergy Clin. Immunol.* **2012**, *129*, 162–168.e3. [CrossRef]
33. Jones, S.C.; Budnitz, D.S.; Sorbello, A.; Mehta, H. US-based emergency department visits for fluoroquinolone-associated hypersensitivity reactions. *Pharmacoepidemiol. Drug Saf.* **2013**, *22*, 1099–1106. [CrossRef] [PubMed]
34. Lovegrove, M.C.; Shehab, N.; Hales, C.M.; Poneleit, K.; Crane, E.; Budnitz, D.S. Emergency department visits for antiviral adverse events during the 2009 H1N1 influenza pandemic. *Public Health Rep.* **2011**, *126*, 312–317. [CrossRef] [PubMed]
35. Lovegrove, M.C.; Geller, A.I.; Fleming-Dutra, K.E.; Shehab, N.; Sapiano, M.R.P.; Budnitz, D.S. US Emergency Department visits for adverse drug events from antibiotics in children, 2011–2015. *J. Pediatric. Infect. Dis. Soc.* **2019**, *8*, 384–391. [CrossRef] [PubMed]
36. Motosue, M.S.; Bellolio, M.F.; Van Houten, H.K.; Shah, N.D.; Li, J.T.; Campbell, R.L. Outcomes of Emergency Department Anaphylaxis Visits from 2005 to 2014. *J. Allergy Clin. Immunol. Pract* **2018**, *6*, 1002–1009.e2. [CrossRef] [PubMed]
37. Motosue, M.S.; Bellolio, M.F.; Van Houten, H.K.; Shah, N.D.; Campbell, R.L. Risk factors for recurrent anaphylaxis-related emergency department visits in the United States. *Ann. Allergy Asthma Immunol.* **2018**, *121*, 717–721.e1. [CrossRef] [PubMed]
38. Russell, S.; Monroe, K.; Losek, J.D. Anaphylaxis management in the pediatric emergency department: Opportunities for improvement. *Pediatr. Emerg. Care* **2010**, *26*, 71–76. [CrossRef]
39. Schneitman-McIntire, O.; Farnen, T.A.; Gordon, N.; Chaaan, J.; Toy, W.A. Medication misadventures resulting in emergency department visits at an HMO medical center. *Am. J. Heal. Pharm.* **1996**, *53*, 1416–1422. [CrossRef]
40. Shehab, N.; Patel, P.R.; Srinivasan, A.; Budnitz, D.S. Emergency department visits for antibiotic-associated adverse events. *Clin. Infect. Dis.* **2008**, *47*, 735–743. [CrossRef]
41. Willy, M.E.; Kelly, J.P.; Nourjah, P.; Kaufman, D.W.; Budnitz, D.S.; Staffa, J. Emergency department visits attributed to selected analgesics, United States, 2004–2005. *Pharmacoepidemiol. Drug Saf.* **2009**, *18*, 188–195. [CrossRef]
42. Cho, H.; Kim, D.; Choo, Y.; Park, J.; Choi, J.; Jang, D.; Kim, T.; Jeong, J.W.; Kwon, J.-W. Common causes of emergency department visits for anaphylaxis in Korean community hospitals: A cross-sectional study. *Medicine* **2019**, *98*, e14114. [CrossRef] [PubMed]
43. Cohen, N.; Capua, T.; Pivko, D.; Ben-Shoshan, M.; Benor, S.; Rimon, A. Trends in the diagnosis and management of anaphylaxis in a tertiary care pediatric emergency department. *Ann. Allergy Asthma Immunol.* **2018**, *121*, 348–352. [CrossRef] [PubMed]
44. Goh, S.H.; Soh, J.Y.; Loh, W.; Lee, K.P.; Tan, S.C.; Heng, W.J.K.; Ibrahim, I.; Lee, B.W.; Chiang, W.C. Cause and clinical presentation of anaphylaxis in Singapore: From infancy to old age. *Int. Arch. Allergy Immunol.* **2018**, *175*, 91–98. [CrossRef]
45. Han, J.E.; Ye, Y.M.; Lee, S. Epidemiology of drug hypersensitivity reactions using 6-year national health insurance claim data from Korea. *Int. J. Clin. Pharm.* **2018**, *40*, 1359–1371. [CrossRef] [PubMed]
46. Hitti, E.A.; Zaitoun, F.; Harmouche, E.; Saliba, M.; Mufarrij, A. Acute allergic reactions in the emergency department: Characteristics and management practices. *Eur. J. Emerg. Med.* **2015**, *22*, 253–259. [CrossRef]
47. Hsin, Y.C.; Hsin, Y.C.; Huang, J.L.; Yeh, K.W. Clinical features of adult and pediatric anaphylaxis in Taiwan. *Asian Pacific J. Allergy Immunol.* **2011**, *29*, 307–312.
48. Kim, M.Y.; Park, C.S.; Jeong, J.W. Management and educational status of adult anaphylaxis patients at emergency department. *Korean J. Intern. Med.* **2018**, *33*, 1008–1015. [CrossRef]
49. Kim, S.Y.; Kim, M.H.; Cho, Y.J. Different clinical features of anaphylaxis according to cause and risk factors for severe reactions. *Allergol. Int.* **2018**, *67*, 96–102. [CrossRef]
50. Ko, B.S.; Kim, W.Y.; Ryoo, S.M.; Ahn, S.; Sohn, C.H.; Seo, D.W.; Lee, Y.-S.; Lim, K.S.; Kim, T.-B. Biphasic reactions in patients with anaphylaxis treated with corticosteroids. *Ann. Allergy Asthma Immunol.* **2015**, *115*, 312–316. [CrossRef]
51. Rangkakulnuwat, P.; Sutham, K.; Lao-Araya, M. Anaphylaxis: Ten-year retrospective study from a tertiary-care hospital in Asia. *Asian Pacific J. Allergy Immunol.* **2020**, *38*, 31–39. [CrossRef]

52. Bellou, A.; Manel, J.; Samman-Kaakaji, H.; De Korwin, J.D.; Moneret-Vautrin, D.A.; Bollaert, P.E.; Lambert, H. Spectrum of acute allergic diseases in an emergency department: An evaluation of one years' experience. *Emerg. Med.* **2003**, *15*, 341–347. [CrossRef] [PubMed]
53. Bielen, C.; Bielen, L.; Likić, R. Incidence, etiology, pred.dictors and outcomes of suspected drug hypersensitivity reactions in a tertiary care university hospital's emergency department: A retrospective study. *Wien. Klin. Wochenschr.* **2019**, *131*, 329–336. [CrossRef]
54. Cianferoni, A.; Novembre, E.; Mugnaini, L.; Lombardi, E.; Bernardini, R.; Pucci, N.; Vierucci, A. Clinical features of acute anaphylaxis in patients admitted to a university hospital: An 11-year retrospective review (1985–1996). *Ann. Allergy Asthma Immunol.* **2001**, *87*, 27–32. [CrossRef]
55. Losappio, L.; Heffler, E.; Bussolino, C.; Cannito, C.D.; Carpentiere, R.; Raie, A.; Di Biase, M.; Bugiani, M.; Rolla, G. Acute urticaria presenting in the emergency room of a general hospital. *Eur. J. Intern. Med.* **2014**, *25*, 147–150. [CrossRef]
56. Quiralte, J.; Blanco, C.; Castillo, R.; Ortega, N.; Carrillo, T. Anaphylactoid reactions due to nonsteroidal antiinflammatory drugs: Clinical and cross-reactivity studies. *Ann. Allergy Asthma Immunol.* **1997**, *78*, 293–296. [CrossRef]
57. Hall, V.; Wong, M.; Munsif, M.; Stevenson, B.R.; Elliott, K.; Lucas, M.; Baird, A.J.; Athan, E.; Young, M.; Pickles, R. Antimicrobial anaphylaxis: The changing face of severe antimicrobial allergy. *J. Antimicrob. Chemother.* **2020**, *75*, 229–235. [CrossRef] [PubMed]
58. Crescioli, G.; Boscia, E.; Bettiol, A.; Pagani, S.; Spada, G.; Vighi, G.V.; Bonaiuti, R.; Venegoni, M.; Vighi, G.D.; Vannacci, A.; et al. Risk of Hospitalization for Adverse Drug Events in Women and Men: A Post Hoc Analysis of an Active Pharmacovigilance Study in Italian Emergency Departments. *Pharmaceuticals* **2021**, *14*, 678. [CrossRef]
59. Thong, B.Y.H.; Tan, T.C. Epidemiology and risk factors for drug allergy. *Br. J. Clin. Pharmacol.* **2011**, *71*, 684–700. [CrossRef]
60. Bernard, T.; Daniel, V.; Maria, J.T.J. *Drug Allergies*; WAO: Milwaukee, WI, USA, 2021.
61. Chen, W.; Mempel, M.; Schober, W.; Behrendt, H.; Ring, J. Gender difference, sex hormones, and immediate type hypersensitivity reactions. *Allergy Eur. J. Allergy Clin. Immunol.* **2008**, *63*, 1418–1427. [CrossRef]
62. Romano, A.; Blanca, M.; Mayorga, C.; Venuti, A.; Gasbarrini, G. Immediate hypersensitivity to penicillins. *Stud. Ital. Subj. Allergy Eur. J. Allergy Clin. Immunol.* **1997**, *52*, 89–93. [CrossRef]
63. International Collaborative Study of Severe Anaphylaxis. Risk of anaphylaxis in a hospital population in relation to the use of various drugs: An international study. *Pharmacoepidemiol. Drug Saf.* **2003**, *12*, 195–202. [CrossRef] [PubMed]
64. Regateiro, F.S.; Marques, M.L.; Gomes, E.R. Drug-Induced Anaphylaxis: An Update on Epidemiology and Risk Factors. *Int. Arch. Allergy Immunol.* **2020**, *181*, 481–487. [CrossRef] [PubMed]
65. Castells, M.C. Capturing Drug-Induced Anaphylaxis Through Electronic Health Records: A Step Forward. *J. Allergy Clin. Immunol. Pract.* **2019**, *7*, 112–113. [CrossRef] [PubMed]
66. Warrington, R.; Silviu-Dan, F.; Wong, T. Drug allergy. *Allergy Asthma Clin. Immunol.* **2018**, *14*, 60. [CrossRef] [PubMed]
67. Turner, P.J.; Gowland, M.H.; Sharma, V.; Ierodiakonou, D.; Harper, N.; Garcez, T.; Pumphrey, R.; Boyle, R.J. Increase in anaphylaxis-related hospitalizations but no increase in fatalities: An analysis of United Kingdom national anaphylaxis data, 1992–2012. *J. Allergy Clin. Immunol.* **2015**, *135*, 956–963.e1. [CrossRef] [PubMed]
68. Oussalah, A.; Mayorga, C.; Blanca, M.; Barbaud, A.; Nakonechna, A.; Cernadas, J.; Gotua, M.; Brockow, K.; Caubet, J.-C.; Bircher, A. Genetic variants associated with drugs-induced immediate hypersensitivity reactions: A PRISMA-compliant systematic review. *Allergy Eur. J. Allergy Clin. Immunol.* **2016**, *71*, 443–462. [CrossRef]
69. Jerschow, E.; Lin, R.Y.; Scaperotti, M.M.; McGinn, A.P. Fatal anaphylaxis in the United States, 1999–2010, Temporal patterns and demographic associations. *J. Allergy Clin. Immunol.* **2014**, *134*, 1318–1328.e7. [CrossRef]
70. Fabbian, F.; Melandri, R.; Borsetti, G.; Micaglio, E.; Pala, M.; De Giorgi, A.; Menegatti, A.M.; Boccafogli, A.; Manfredini, R. Color-coding triage and allergic reactions in an Italian ED. *Am. J. Emerg. Med.* **2012**, *30*, 826–829. [CrossRef]
71. D'Antonio, C.D.; Galimberti, M.; Barbone, B.; Calamari, M.; Airoldi, G.; Campanini, M.; Di Pietrantonj, C.; Avanzi, G.C. Suspected acute allergic reactions: Analysis of admissions to the Emergency Department of the AOU Maggiore della Carità Hospital in Novara from 2003 to 2007. *Eur. Ann. Allergy Clin. Immunol.* **2008**, *40*, 122–129.
72. Khan, D.A.; Solensky, R. Drug allergy. *J. Allergy Clin. Immunol.* **2010**, *125*, S126–S137. [CrossRef]
73. Tanno, L.K.; Chalmers, R.; Bierrenbach, A.L.; Simons, F.E.R.; Martin, B.; Molinari, N.; Annesi-Maesano, I.; Worm, M.; Cardona, V.; Papadopoulos, N.G. Changing the history of anaphylaxis mortality statistics through the World Health Organization's International Classification of Diseases–11. *J. Allergy Clin. Immunol.* **2019**, *144*, 627–633. [CrossRef] [PubMed]
74. Kelkar, P.S.; Li, J.T.-C. Cephalosporin Allergy. *N. Engl. J. Med.* **2001**, *345*, 804–809. [CrossRef] [PubMed]
75. Tanno, L.K.; Simons, F.E.R.; Sanchez-Borges, M.; Cardona, V.; Moon, H.B.; Calderon, M.A.; Sisul, J.C.; Muraro, A.; Casale, T.; Demoly, P.; et al. Applying prevention concepts to anaphylaxis: A call for worldwide availability of adrenaline auto-injectors. *Clin. Exp. Allergy* **2017**, *47*, 1108–1114. [CrossRef] [PubMed]
76. Sundquist, B.K.; Jose, J.; Pauze, D.; Pauze, D.; Wang, H.; Järvinen, K.M. Anaphylaxis risk factors for hospitalization and intensive care: A comparison between adults and children in an upstate New York emergency department. *Allergy Asthma Proc.* **2019**, *40*, 41–47. [CrossRef]
77. Martelli, A.; Ghiglioni, D.; Sarratud, T.; Calcinai, E.; Veehof, S.; Terracciano, L.; Fiocchi, A. Anaphylaxis in the emergency department: A paediatric perspective. *Curr. Opin. Allergy Clin. Immunol.* **2008**, *8*, 321–329. [CrossRef]
78. Clark, S.; Wei, W.; Rudders, S.A.; Camargo, C.A. Risk factors for severe anaphylaxis in patients receiving anaphylaxis treatment in US emergency departments and hospitals. *J. Allergy Clin. Immunol.* **2014**, *134*, 1125–1130. [CrossRef]

79. Worm, M.; Francuzik, W.; Renaudin, J.M.; Bilo, M.B.; Cardona, V.; Scherer Hofmeier, K.; Köhli, A.; Bauer, A.; Christoff, G.; Cichocka-Jarosz, E.; et al. Factors increasing the risk for a severe reaction in anaphylaxis: An analysis of data from The European Anaphylaxis Registry. *Allergy Eur. J. Allergy Clin. Immunol.* **2018**, *73*, 1322–1330. [CrossRef]
80. Triggiani, M.; Patella, V.; Staiano, R.I.; Granata, F.; Marone, G. Allergy and the cardiovascular system. *Clin. Exp. Immunol.* **2008**, *153*, 7–11. [CrossRef]

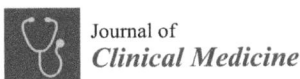 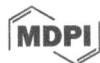

Article

Evaluating the Medication Regimen Complexity Score as a Predictor of Clinical Outcomes in the Critically Ill

Mohammad A. Al-Mamun [1,*], Jacob Strock [2], Yushuf Sharker [3], Khaled Shawwa [4], Rebecca Schmidt [4], Douglas Slain [1], Ankit Sakhuja [4] and Todd N. Brothers [5]

1. School of Pharmacy, University of West Virginia, 706 Health Sciences Ctr S, Morgantown, WV 26506, USA
2. Graduate School of Oceanography, University of Rhode Island, 215 S Ferry Rd, Narragansett, RI 02882, USA
3. Children's National Hospital, 111 Michigan Ave. NW, Washington, DC 20010, USA
4. School of Medicine, University of West Virginia, 1 Medical Center Dr, Morgantown, WV 26506, USA
5. College of Pharmacy, University of Rhode Island, 7 Greenhouse Road Kingston, Narragansett, RI 02881, USA
* Correspondence: mohammad.almamun@hsc.wvu.edu

Abstract: Background: Medication Regimen Complexity (MRC) refers to the combination of medication classes, dosages, and frequencies. The objective of this study was to examine the relationship between the scores of different MRC tools and the clinical outcomes. Methods: We conducted a retrospective cohort study at Roger William Medical Center, Providence, Rhode Island, which included 317 adult patients admitted to the intensive care unit (ICU) between 1 February 2020 and 30 August 2020. MRC was assessed using the MRC Index (MRCI) and MRC for the Intensive Care Unit (MRC-ICU). A multivariable logistic regression model was used to identify associations among MRC scores, clinical outcomes, and a logistic classifier to predict clinical outcomes. Results: Higher MRC scores were associated with increased mortality, a longer ICU length of stay (LOS), and the need for mechanical ventilation (MV). MRC-ICU scores at 24 h were significantly ($p < 0.001$) associated with increased ICU mortality, LOS, and MV, with ORs of 1.12 (95% CI: 1.06–1.19), 1.17 (1.1–1.24), and 1.21 (1.14–1.29), respectively. Mortality prediction was similar using both scoring tools (AUC: 0.88 [0.75–0.97] vs. 0.88 [0.76–0.97]. The model with 15 medication classes outperformed others in predicting the ICU LOS and the need for MV with AUCs of 0.82 (0.71–0.93) and 0.87 (0.77–0.96), respectively. Conclusion: Our results demonstrated that both MRC scores were associated with poorer clinical outcomes. The incorporation of MRC scores in real-time therapeutic decision making can aid clinicians to prescribe safer alternatives.

Keywords: critical care; outcomes; patient safety; medication therapy management; electronic health records

1. Introduction

Medication Regimen Complexity (MRC) refers to multiple features of a patient's medication drug regimen rather than an absolute number of medications consumed per day [1]. MRC incorporates features such as the number of agents, dosages, administration time intervals, and additional instructions (i.e., take on an empty stomach) [2–4]. An increase in MRC burden has been associated with poorer medication noncompliance and caregiver quality of life measures, as well as an increase in healthcare resource utilization [5–9]. Critical illness has been referred to as a subset of hospitalized individuals who are commonly afflicted with severe respiratory, cardiovascular, or neurological impairment, reflected in abnormal physiological observations. These patients are at a significant risk of higher MRC due to the severity of illness, the management of multiple chronic conditions, and the complex pharmacotherapies prescribed. It has been estimated that a critically ill adult may receive up to 13 medications per day and the chances of experiencing an adverse drug event are greater than 25% [10–12]. Therefore, examining only the quantity of medications

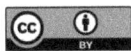

administered may not accurately describe the complex and intricate nature of critical care medication therapy [13].

Numerous methods have been used to quantify the complexity of medication use. Yet, the most commonly utilized and validated objective scoring tool is the 65-item, weighted MRC Index (MRCI), which has been developed for outpatient use only [14–18]. The MRCI has been used to evaluate conditions such as neurological impairment in children and hypertension, diabetes, chronic obstructive pulmonary disease, and chronic kidney disease in adults [19–24]. The MRC for the intensive care unit (ICU) scoring tool has been developed and intended for use in critically ill patients [25,26]. MRC-ICU is the first validated quantitative weighted scoring tool intended to predict clinical events such as mortality [27,28]. A recent study demonstrates that the prediction of patient outcomes can be improved by incorporating the MRC-ICU score into the previously established severity-of-disease classification system Acute Physiology and Chronic Health Evaluation (APACHE II) scoring tool [29].

MRC scoring tools have the potential to aid in the identification of which patients may benefit from subsequent interventions (i.e., comprehensive medication review) [23,24]. In the critical care setting, the tool can further support the need for clinical pharmaceutical expertise and workload assignment to address the complex pharmacotherapeutic needs of the patient. However, the utilization of these tools has been limited due to the narrowly defined scope of the MRCI tool and the lack of substantial validation. To date, no studies have assessed the association between these two MRC scoring tools and clinical outcomes within the critical care setting.

In this study, we created two custom MRC scoring algorithms and several statistical and prediction models using the MRCI and MRC-ICU tools to investigate whether MRC scores are important predictors of clinical outcomes (i.e., ICU mortality, length of stay (LOS), and need for mechanical ventilation (MV)). We aimed to (1) examine how MRC scores correlate with clinical characteristics, (2) test the hypothesis that higher MRC scores are associated with poorer clinical outcomes, and (3) determine the utility of MRC scores as predictors of clinical outcomes.

2. Methods

2.1. Study Design and Setting

This was a single-center, STROBE-compliant retrospective cohort study of 322 patients enrolled into the ICU in a 220-bed community hospital in Providence, Rhode Island, USA, between 1 February 2020 and 30 August 2020. Due to the retrospective nature of the data, informed consent was not deemed necessary as all patient data were de-identified prior to use. The study was granted exemption by the Human Research Review Committee Roger Williams Medical Center (RWMC) Institutional Review Board (IRB: 00000058) and University of Rhode Island Institutional Review Board (IRB: 00000559). The data were curated and reviewed for accuracy by the RWMC data-extraction team.

2.2. Participants

All adults admitted to the ICU with general admission criteria were included in this study.

2.3. Inclusion and Exclusion Criteria

The patients were included if the following conditions were met: $\geq$18 years of age and admission to the ICU > 24 h. A total of 317 patients were included in the final analysis, five of whom were excluded due to extensive LOS (>40 days) and missing laboratory values.

2.4. Variables

Demographics, vital signs, laboratories, medication classes, and MV data were collected for each patient from the electronic health records (EHR) (Tables S1 and S2).

2.5. Data Sources

MRC Scoring Tools

MRC can be defined by the number of drugs and their dosing frequency. Two medication scoring indexes, the MRCI and MRC-ICU, have been developed for outpatient and critical care use, respectively. The total MRCI score is the weighted sum of 3 sections (dosage form, dosing frequency, and additional administration information), in which a higher score reflects a higher MRC burden. In computing the MRCI, both scheduled and 'as needed' medications and supplements are considered (see supplementary material). Despite the established use of the MRCI tool in the outpatient setting, we aimed to explore its utility in the ICU setting in this study [8].

Conversely, MRC-ICU is a 39-item, weighted, critically ill medication scoring tool comprising specific agents and classes (i.e., vancomycin—3 point; continuous intravenous saline—1 point) [26,30]. The MRC-ICU scoring calculation and individually assigned medication weights are provided in the supplementary material. The score has undergone validation testing for both internal and external validity [26,30]. Although an MRC-ICU score can be determined at any time during ICU admission, daily historical evaluation at 24 h intervals is most commonly utilized and was applied to our study. These two scores were calculated using custom codes for each patient at 24 and 48 h intervals.

2.6. Definitions

We defined cutoff values for both MRC scores based upon their distribution 24 h after ICU admission. We chose the median values as cutoff values, as there are no standardized cutoff values available for critically ill patients. The 'high' MRCI scoring cohort and the 'high' MRC-ICU cohort were defined as having cutoff scores of >63 and >6, respectively. Three clinical outcomes were measured: mortality, LOS, and need for MV for the ICU setting. We created a binary variable for LOS = 0 when LOS was < 48 h and LOS = 1 when LOS > 48 h. The need for MV was defined using a binary variable after 48 h of ICU admission (MV = 0, not mechanically ventilated; MV = 1, mechanically ventilated). Hemodynamic instability was defined as a hypotension (i.e., systolic blood pressure < 100 mmHg), mean arterial pressure < 65 mmHg, or an abnormal heart rate (i.e., arrhythmia or heart rate < 60 bpm or > 100 bpm).

2.7. Statistical Analysis

Descriptive statistics were used to describe the study population where continuous values were represented using means and interquartile ranges (IQRs). Categorical variables were described using frequencies and proportions. We conducted a descriptive analysis comparing survivor and non-survivor and low- and high-MRC-scoring groups using Student's t, chi-squared (χ^2), or Fisher's exact tests to examine the relationships between clinical characteristics and the respective cohorts. Physiological and clinical characteristics were compared among the survivor and non-survivor cohorts. To account for the severity of illness, we included the following scoring tools: Simplified Acute Physiology Score (SAPS II), APACHE II, and Charlson comorbidity index (CCI). The MRCI and MRC-ICU were analyzed for mortality, need for MV, and SARS-CoV-2 (COVID-19) infection using the Wilcoxon signed-rank test. Four multivariable logistic regression models were utilized to identify the predictors of clinical outcomes (i.e., mortality, LOS, and need for MV) using severity scores, MRCI, MRC-ICU, and all the variables. The four models were: Model I—demographics, APACHE II, SAPS II, CCI, and 15 drug classes; Model II—demographics, MRCI_24 h, MRCI_48 h, CCI, and drug classes; Model III—demographics, MRC-ICU_24 h, MRC-ICU_48 h, CCI, and drug classes; and Model IV—all variables (see Table S3). In the LOS models, we excluded MRCI and MRC-ICU values at 48 h, as our threshold for binary values was 48 h after ICU admission. Significant predictors ($p < 0.05$) were selected for each model using a stepwise forward selection method. To further assess variable selection, we used an L1 penalization technique (LASSO). LASSO allows a more restrictive parameter selection to be performed that is minimally influenced by multicollinearity. The demographic variables included were age, sex, height, weight, body mass index (BMI), and race. Odds Ratios (OR) were calculated for each outcome of interest. All analyses were conducted using R, Version 4.0.0 (R Project for Statistical Computing), and the *glm, glmnet, and ggplot2 R* packages were used [31–33].

2.8. Prediction Model Development

To test the prediction ability of MRC scores for mortality, LOS, and need for MV, seven logistic classifier models were constructed without any variable selection (see Table S3). A 'no imputation' approach was used when preparing the data for the prediction model. We assessed correlated variables using the Pearson correlation coefficient. The SAPS II severity score was used in the prediction models due to a high correlation within the APACHE II classification system (Figure S1). The best fit models were selected using the best Akaike information criterion (AIC) measurement through an interactive process during cross-validation. We included all the predictor variables in each prediction model setup for exploring their individual role explicitly. Model performance was assessed via the area under the receiver operating characteristic (ROC) curve (AUC). An AUC of at least 0.7 was regarded as acceptable. We applied a 'leave-one-out' cross-validation method with 10,000 repetitions, and the AUC was selected as an overall performance measure. Additionally, sensitivity and specificity analyses were included for the three outcomes. Lastly, all prediction models recorded variable importance rankings for each clinical outcome.

3. Results

3.1. Demographic and Clinical Characteristics

Of the 317 patients included in the analysis, most were male (175 patients (55.2%)); and White (205 patients (65%)), with a median (interquartile range (IQR)) age of 62 (51–75) years. A total of 77% patients survived; 51% had an LOS > 48 h; and 31% required MV. Vital signs, serum electrolytes, and blood-cell values were similar among the survivor and non-survivor cohorts. Conversely, serum blood urea nitrogen (BUN) and creatinine values were significantly worse in the non-survivor cohort (25.7 mg/dL and 1.5 mg/dL vs. 38.7 mg/dL and 1.8 mg/dL), respectively. Non-survivors had a significantly longer duration on MV (147.2 h vs. 34.6 h) and a prolonged LOS (191.4 h vs. 87.4 h) than the survivor cohort. There was a high prevalence among both cohorts of acute respiratory failure with hypoxia (125 (39.4%)), COVID infection (52 (16.4%)), lactic acidosis (101 (31.9%)), kidney failure (96 (30.3%)), and acute myocardial infarction (78 (24.6%)) (Table 1).

Table 1. Demographic and clinical characteristics between survivor and non-survivor cohorts.

Characteristics	Survivors (n = 243)	Non-Survivors (n = 74)	p-Value
Demographics			
Age, median (IQR), y	60.8 (48–73.5)	65.8 (58–76)	0.81
Sex, No. (%)			
Male	134 (55)	41 (55)	>0.99
Race, No. (%)			
White	163 (67)	42 (57)	0.14
Black	19 (8)	7 (9)	0.83
Hispanic	25 (10)	12 (16)	0.24
Asian	4 (2)	0 (0)	0.61
BMI, median (IQR)	29 (23–32)	28.5 (23–31.8)	0.44

Table 1. Cont.

Characteristics	Survivors (n = 243)	Non-Survivors (n = 74)	p-Value
Vital Signs			
Systolic blood pressure (mm Hg)	122.8 (108–133.7)	107.1 (96.1–118.4)	0.22
Diastolic blood pressure (mm Hg)	71.6 (62.3–80.4)	64.2 (55.4–71.6)	0.38
Mean arterial pressure (mm Hg)	88.7 (77.7–97.5)	78.5 (69.4–86.4)	0.22
Heart rate (beats/min)	88.7 (78–99.1)	99.4 (86.2–113.5)	0.82
Respiratory rate (breaths/min)	19.2 (16–21)	25.2 (21.4–28)	0.09
Temperature (°C)	98.2 (97.7–98.7)	97.8 (96.8–99.2)	0.74
SaO$_2$ (mm Hg)	96.7 (95.1–98.7)	93.9 (92.5–97)	0.77
Serum Laboratory Values			
Sodium (mEq/L)	136.3 (134–139)	138.1 (134.6–143)	0.58
Potassium (mEq/L)	4 (3.6–4.4)	4.4 (3.9–4.9)	0.16
Chloride (mg/dL)	103.9 (101–108)	102.7 (98–108.5)	0.35
Carbon dioxide (mEq/L)	23.6 (21–26)	20.7 (14.2–25.9)	0.96
BUN (mg/dL)	25.7 (12–30)	38.7 (21.2–50)	0.03
SCr (mg/dL)	1.5 (0.7–1.4)	1.8 (0.9–2.5)	0.05
Glucose (mg/dL)	168.5 (110.5–198)	219.5 (124–251.2)	0.30
Calcium (mg/dL)	8.2 (7.7–8.7)	8.1 (7.2–8.5)	0.21
Magnesium (mg/dL)	1.9 (1.6–2.1)	2.3 (1.9–2.5)	0.12
Phosphate (mg/dL)	3.5 (2.8–4)	6.1 (3.8–7.6)	0.26
White blood cell ($\times 10^3$/mL)	11 (7.2–13.8)	15.6 (8.4–19.4)	0.51
Hemoglobin (g/dL)	10.2 (8.6–11.8)	9.7 (8.1–11.6)	0.31
Hematocrit (%)	31.8 (27.6–36.2)	31.4 (24.9–36)	0.35
Platelets ($\times 10^3$/mL)	211.3 (143–268)	215.5 (128.5–271.8)	0.57
Lactate (U/L)	3 (1.4–3.3)	8.2 (3.1–13.5)	0.41
PT (s)	17.6 (11.5–16.1)	19.9 (13.3–27.8)	0.56
INR	1.7 (1.1–1.6)	2 (1.3–2.8)	0.56
Albumin (g/L)	3.1 (2.8–3.5)	2.8 (2.3–3.2)	0.71
Total bilirubin (mg/dL)	1.3 (0.5–1.2)	2.5 (0.5–1.2)	0.87
Urine Output every 6 h (mL/h)	60.4 (7–96.5)	56.5 (10.3–58.4)	0.49
eGFR (mL/min/1.73 m^2)	71.2 (42–99.2)	50.3 (26.8–70.5)	0.11
Durations			
Time on mechanical ventilation (h)	34.6 (0–0)	147.2 (4–197.5)	0.08
ICU length of stay (h)	87.4 (21–86)	191.4 (22–282.5)	0.08
Scoring Assessment on ICU admission			
APACHE II	17 (13–20)	27.1 (21–32)	0.01
SAPS II	12.5 (5–18)	27.5 (18.2–35)	0.039
MRCI	62.9 (34–84)	81.1 (43–104.5)	0.339
MRC-ICU	6 (3–8)	8.6 (4–12)	0.107
GCS at admission	13.1 (12–15)	7.2 (3–11)	0.351
Lactic acidosis (E87.2)	62 (26)	39 (53)	<0.001
Hypokalemia (E87.6)	83 (34)	19 (26)	0.22
Kidney failure (N17.9)	63 (26)	33 (45)	0.004
Hypo-osmolality hyponatremia (E87.1)	63 (26)	26 (35)	0.16
Was not resuscitated (Z66)	35 (14)	51 (69)	<0.001
Acute myocardial infarction (I21.A)	52 (21)	26 (35)	0.025
Unspecified sepsis (A41.9)	53 (22)	23 (31)	0.14

BUN, blood urea nitrogen; Scr, serum creatinine; eGFR, estimated glomerular filtration rate; PT, prothrombin time; APACHE II, Acute Physiology and Chronic Health Evaluation II; SAPS II, Simplified Acute Physiology Score II; MRCI, Medication Regimen Complexity Index; MRC-ICU, Medication Regimen Complexity in the Intensive Care Unit.

3.2. Clinical Characteristics between MRC Cohorts

3.2.1. Low- and High-MRC Cohorts

Among the higher-MRCI-scoring group, lower vital-sign values (systolic blood pressure, diastolic blood pressure, mean arterial pressure) were found to be significant ($p < 0.01$). Serum laboratory indices including phosphate, lactate, and albumin varied significantly among the MRCI cohorts. Higher MRCI scores were correlated with increased patient acuity when compared with lower-MRCI-scoring groups. Comorbidities such as hypoosmolality, acute myocardial infarction, and unspecified sepsis were significant among both MRCI and MRC-ICU cohorts (Tables S4 and S5).

3.2.2. Survivor and Non-Survivor Cohorts

When compared with the non-survivor cohort, the survivor cohort had significantly lower APACHE II and SAPS II scores and a trend towards lower MRCI and MRC-ICU scores. In the COVID-19-infected cohort, APACHE II and SAPS II had significantly lower median values than in the non-COVID-infected group. Further, MRCI and MRC-ICU scores were significantly higher in the mechanically ventilated cohort (Figure 1). When analyzing age distribution by decade of life among different comorbidity severity indexes (i.e., Charlson, APACHE II, SAPS II) patients older than sixty years of age were associated with the highest severity index scores (Figure S2).

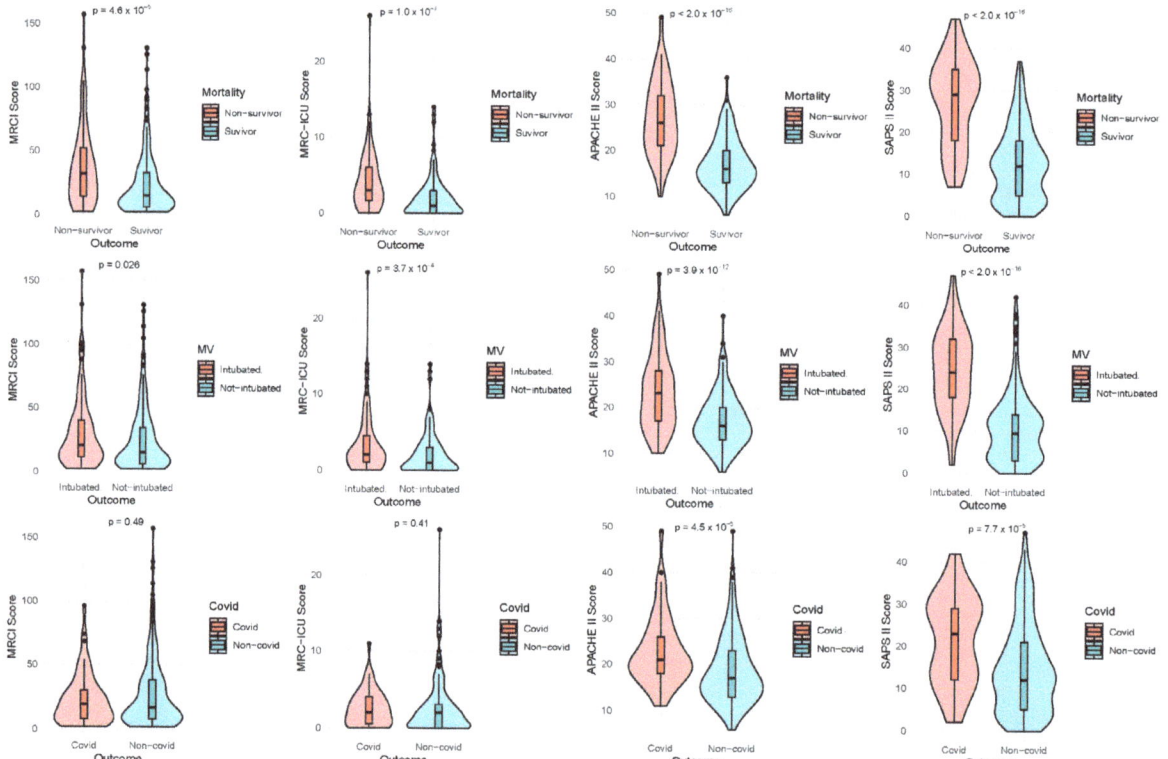

Figure 1. Comparisons among the severity score and MRC scores. Comparison of the severity-of-illness scores Acute Physiology and Chronic Health Evaluation (APACHE II), Simplified Acute Physiology Score (SAPS) II, Medication Regimen Complexity Index (MRCI), and Medication Regimen Complexity for the Intensive Care Unit (MRC-ICU) between survivors and non-survivors.

3.3. Medication Use

The top five medication classes prescribed among the high-scoring MRC cohorts (MRCI and MRC-ICU) were intravenous fluids (normal saline, 36% and 35%), gastrointestinal agents (pantoprazole, 29% and 32%), analgesics (acetaminophen, 26% and 26%), electrolytes (potassium chloride, 24% and 26%), and anti-infectives (piperacillin/tazobactam, 23%, and vancomycin, 27%). When incorporating the severity-of-illness scoring tools (APACHE II and SAPS II) with MRCI and MRC-ICU scores, patients with higher MRC scores (i.e., >63 MRCI and >6 MRC-ICU) were associated with increased mortality (14%

and 15%), a longer LOS (i.e., >48 h; 30% and 34%), and an increased need for MV (24% and 28%), respectively (Figure S3).

3.4. Associations between MRC Scores and Clinical Outcomes

At admission, SAPS II was significant for all three outcomes: mortality (OR: 1.12 (1.07–1.18)), LOS (OR: 1.04 (1.0–1.11)), and need for MV (OR: 1.17 (1.13–1.21)) (Table 2), respectively. When only incorporating MRCI scores into the model (Model II), the MRCI score at 24 h was a significant predictor but showed slight associations with all outcomes with ORs of 1.01 (95% CI: 1.0–1.02), 1.01 (1.0–1.02), and 1.01 (1.01–1.02) for mortality, LOS, and need of MV, respectively. Further, MRCI scores at 48 h were found to be significant risk factors but weakly associated with mortality and need for MV (Table 2). MRC-ICU scores at 24 h (Model III) were significant risk factors in all outcomes in Model III with ORs of 1.12 (95% CI: 1.06–1.19), 1.17 (1.1–1.24), and 1.21 (1.14–1.29) for mortality, LOS, and need of MV, respectively. Notably, in Model III, Hispanic ethnicity was significantly (*p*-value < 0.001) associated with mortality 6.44 (3.45–12.41) and need for MV (2.21 (1.29–3.85) with ORs 6.44 (3.45–12.41) and 2.21 (1.29–3.85), respectively. Complimentary results from the LASSO model confirmed the risk-factor selection trends (Table S6). The use of vasopressors was found to be a significant risk factor for all clinical outcomes in Model IV. When evaluating morality, the use of paralytic agents was significant (OR: 3.38 (1.09–11.11)). The use of anti-infectives, anticoagulants, and cardiovascular agents was significantly associated with a prolonged LOS. Lastly, the use of analgesics, sedatives, psychiatric, cardiovascular, and pulmonary agents was a significant risk factor for the need of MV.

Table 2. Four logistic regression models for three clinical outcomes: mortality, length of ICU stay (LOS), and need for mechanical ventilation (MV). List of selected variables using stepwise selection method for the four logistic regression models and their associations with mortality, LOS, and need for MV.

Selected Features	Mortality OR (95% CI)	*p*-Value	Length of ICU Stay OR (95% CI)	*p*-Value	Mechanical Ventilation OR (95% CI)	*p*-Value
Model I						
Age	1.02 (1.0–1.05)	0.12	1.02 (1.0–1.03)	0.05	-	-
Body mass index (BMI)	-	-	1.02 (1.0–1.05)	0.11	-	-
White	-	-	0.59 (0.35–0.98)	-	-	-
Hispanic	6.11 (2.84–13.85)	<0.001	-	-	-	-
SAPS II at admission	1.12 (1.07–1.18)	0.001	1.04 (1–1.11)	<0.001	1.17 (1.13–1.21)	<0.001
APACHE II at admission	1.13 (1.05–1.21)	0.002	0.92 (0.88–0.98)	0.15	-	-
CCI	-	-	1.13 (1.0–1.32)	0.14	-	-
Model II						
Age	1.03 (1.02–1.05)	<0.001	1.01 (1.0–1.03)	0.09	-	-
Height	-	-	1.14 (1.01–1.35)	0.11	1.02 (1.04–1.46)	0.03
Weight	-	-	0.95 (0.89–1.01)	0.09	0.95 (0.89–1.01)	0.1
Body mass index (BMI)	-	-	1.17 (1.0–1.41)	0.06	1.18 (1.0–1.42)	0.07
White	-	-	0.56 (0.33–0.93)	0.03	-	-
Hispanic	5.74 (3.15–10.79)	<0.001	-	-	1.84 (1.11–3.07)	0.02
MRCI score at 24 h	1.01 (1–1.02)	0.003	1.01 (1.0–1.02)	<0.001	1.01 (1.01–1.02)	<0.001
MRCI score at 48 h	1.01 (1–1.02)	0.004	-	-	1.01 (1.0–1.02)	0.03
CCI	-	-	1.13 (1.0–1.32)	0.13	-	-

Table 2. Cont.

Selected Features	Mortality OR (95% CI)	p-Value	Length of ICU Stay OR (95% CI)	p-Value	Mechanical Ventilation OR (95% CI)	p-Value
Model III						
Age	1.03 (1.02–1.05)	<0.001	1.01 (1.0–1.03)	0.1	-	-
White	-	-	0.59 (0.35–0.99)	0.04	-	-
Hispanic	6.44 (3.45–12.41)	<0.001	-	-	2.21 (1.29–3.85)	0.004
MRC-ICU at 24 h	1.12 (1.06–1.19)	<0.001	1.17 (1.1–1.24)	<0.001	1.21 (1.14–1.29)	<0.001
MRC-ICU at 48 h	1.1 (1.04–1.17)	0.002	1.05 (1.0–1.11)	0.7	1.11 (1.05–1.18)	0.001
CCI	-	-	1.14 (1.0–1.34)	0.1	0.84 (0.65–1.07)	0.155
Model IV						
Age	1.04 (1.01–1.08)	0.017	-	-	-	-
Hispanic	6.23 (2.55–16.41)	0.001	-	-	-	-
SAPS II at admission	1.09 (1.04–1.15)	0.001	1.04 (1–1.08)	0.072	1.17 (1.11–1.23)	<0.001
APACHE II at admission	1.14 (1.05–1.23)	0.002	0.94 (0.89–1)	0.038	-	-
MRCI at 24 h	-	-	0.99 (0.98–1)	0.134	0.97 (0.95–0.99)	0.001
MRC-ICU at 24 h	-	-	1.1 (1–1.22)	0.05	1.3 (1.13–1.51)	<0.001
CCI	0.79 (0.6–1.03)	0.093	-	-	0.77 (0.58–1)	0.052
Anti-infectives	-	-	2.27 (1.15–4.57)	0.019	-	-
Anticoagulants	0.38 (0.1–1.42)	0.139	2.26 (1.02–5.29)	0.05	-	-
Psychiatric agents	-	-	1.8 (0.96–3.36)	0.065	2.52 (1.01–6.64)	0.05
Pulmonary agents	-	-	-	-	3.14 (1.34–7.66)	0.01
Cardiovascular agents	-	-	2.81 (1.46–5.53)	0.002	0.4 (0.15–0.98)	0.05
Diuretics	-	-	3.35 (1.74–6.62)	<0.001	-	-
Analgesics sedatives	-	-	-	-	6.96 (1.73–36.07)	0.012
Vasopressors	5.55 (2.12–15.26)	0.001	3.49 (1.63–7.75)	0.002	5.75 (2.4–14.48)	<0.001
Paralytic agents	3.38 (1.09–11.11)	0.039	-	-	-	-
Vitamins	-	-	1.63 (0.88–3.03)	0.122	0.25 (0.09–0.62)	0.004
Others	2.54 (1.08–6.15)	0.034	-	-	-	-

The final models of logistic regression are reported using Odds Ratios (ORs) and 95% confidence intervals of risk factors for logistic regression. If the variable was not selected, the cell was marked with '-'. Bold ORs for logistic regression were significant. Model I: Demographics, Acute Physiology and Chronic Health Evaluation (APACHE II), Simplified Acute Physiology Score (SAPS II), Charlson comorbidity index (CCI), and drug classes. Model II: Demographics, Medication Regimen Complexity Index (MRCI_24 h), MRCI_48 h, CCI, and drug classes. Model III: Demographics, Medication Regimen Complexity in Intensive Care Unit (MRC-ICU_24 h), MRC-ICU_48 h, CCI, and drug classes. Model IV: all variables.

3.5. Role of MRC Scores in the Prediction of Clinical Outcomes

The Admission Model was found to be the best model (AUC: 0.88 (95% CI: 0.77–0.97)) to predict mortality (Table 3). However, models MRCI and SAPS II (AUC: 0.88 [0.75–0.97]) and MRC-ICU and SAPS (AUC: 0.88 [0.76–0.97]) performed similarly (Figure 2). In the MRCI and SAPS II Model, MRCI scores at 24 and 48 h were identified as the top variables of importance when predicting mortality (Figure 3). Further, vasopressors were the most important variable to predict mortality within the Medication Model. When predicting the LOS, the Medication Model (AUC: 0.82 [0.71–0.93]) outperformed all other models. Vasopressors and psychiatric agents were among the top five important variables to predict the LOS. Further, MRC scores at 24 h and 48 h were selected in the top 10 variable importance list for models including MRC scores (i.e., MRCI and SAPS II, and MRC-ICU and SAPS II).

Table 3. Comparison of the prediction models. Prediction evaluation for ICU mortality, LOS, and need for mechanical ventilation. (The best 3 prediction results are noted in bold font, and demographic variables are included in each of the models).

	AIC	AUC	Sensitivity	Specificity
ICU Mortality				
Admission Model	222.007 (217.45–222.15)	0.88 (0.77–0.97)	0.72 (0.60–0.82)	0.89 (0.85–0.92)
MRCI Model	313 (308–313)	0.73 (0.54–0.89)	0.73 (0.60–0.84)	0.89 (0.85–0.93)
MRCI and SAPS II Model	225 (220–225)	0.88 (0.75–0.97)	0.73 (0.63–0.83)	0.89 (0.84–0.93)
MRC-ICU Model	302 (297–302)	0.75 (0.57–0.89)	0.73 (0.62–0.83)	0.89 (0.85–0.92)
MRC-ICU and SAPS II Model	225 (221–225)	0.88 (0.76–0.97)	0.73 (0.62–0.84)	0.90 (0.85–0.94)
Medication Model	236 (232–236)	0.88 (0.78–0.96)	0.61 (0.48–0.73)	0.86 (0.82–0.90)
Full Model	226 (221–226)	0.88 (0.77–0.97)	0.73 (0.62–0.84)	0.89 (0.85–0.92)
Length of ICU Stay				
Admission Model	422.74 (421–423)	0.68 (0.53–0.82)	0.63 (0.5–0.70)	0.62 (0.54–0.70)
MRCI Model	431 (429–431)	0.64 (0.48–0.78)	0.65 (0.58–0.71)	0.62 (0.55–0.71)
MRCI and SAPS II Model	421 (419–422)	0.69 (0.53–0.83)	0.64 (0.57–0.70)	0.62 (0.55–0.69)
MRC-ICU Model	404 (402–405)	0.70 (0.52–0.83)	0.64 (0.56–0.74)	0.61 (0.55–0.70)
MRC-ICU and SAPS II Model	401 (399–402)	0.71 (0.57–0.84)	0.63 (0.57–0.70)	0.62 (0.56–0.70)
Medication Model	323 (320–324)	0.82 (0.71–0.93)	0.75 (0.69–0.81)	0.74 (0.68–0.80)
Full Model	402 (399–403)	0.71 (0.56–0.84)	0.64 (0.58–0.71)	0.62 (0.54–0.70)
Need for Mechanical Ventilation				
Admission Model	304.62 (300.23–305.0)	0.85 (0.72–0.95)	0.79 (0.70–0.86)	0.8 (0.75–0.85)
MRCI Model	408 (406–409)	0.65 (0.48–0.80)	0.79 (0.69–0.86)	0.80 (0.75–0.85)
MRCI and SAPS II Model	308 (304–308)	0.84 (0.73–0.94)	0.77 (0.69–0.86)	0.80 (0.75–0.85)
MRC-ICU Model	365 (362–366)	0.75 (0.62–0.873)	0.78 (0.69–0.86)	0.80 (0.76–0.84)
MRC-ICU and SAPS II Model	290 (286–291)	0.87 (0.77–0.96)	0.78 (0.71–0.86)	0.80 (0.75–0.86)
Medication Model	273 (269–274)	0.86 (0.75–0.96)	0.8 (0.71–0.88)	0.81 (0.76–0.86)
Full Model	286 (281–286)	0.87 (0.77–0.96)	0.78 (0.70–0.86)	0.80 (0.76–0.85)

Abbreviations: Akaike information criterion (AIC), receiver operating characteristic curve (AUC). AUC is presented as a median value and 95% CI.

When predicting the need for MV, MRC-ICU and SAPS II (AUC: 0.87 [0.77–0.96]) outperformed all other models. SAPS II and MRC-ICU at 24 and 48 h were among the top important variables to predict the need for MV. Lastly, vasopressors and pulmonary agents were among the top five medication classes identified when predicting the need for MV. Hispanic ethnicity was found to be one of the top important variables in the MRCI and MRC-ICU models for predicting mortality and need for MV (Figure 3).

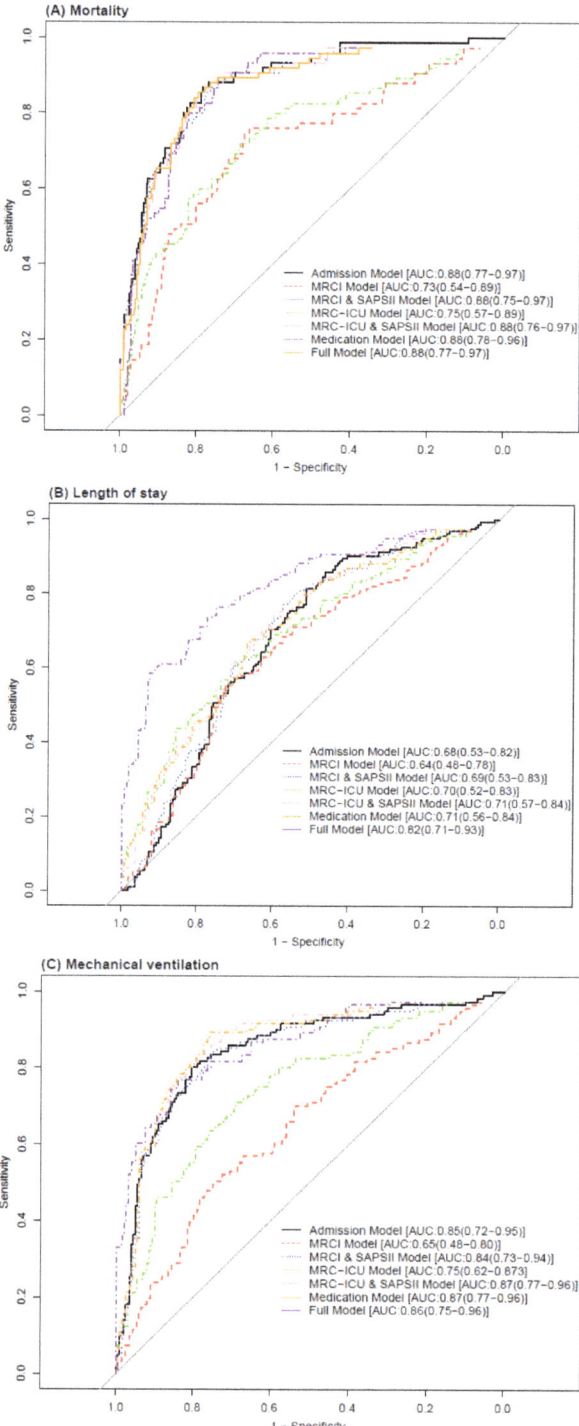

Figure 2. Performance of the prediction models for predicting the clinical outcomes. Receiver operating characteristic curves (AUCs) for (**A**) ICU mortality, (**B**) ICU length of stay, and (**C**) need for mechanical ventilation.

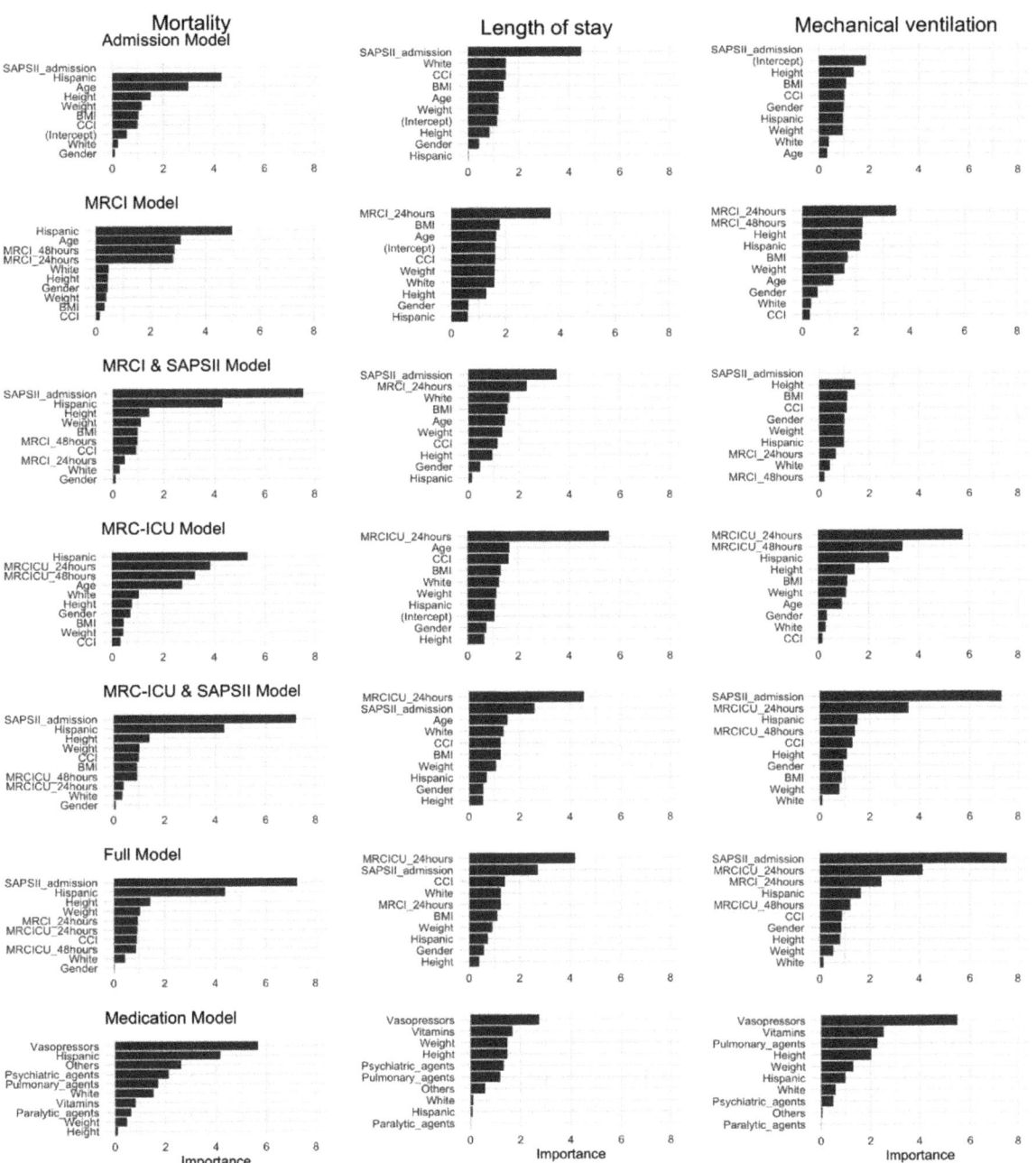

Figure 3. Variable importance of the prediction models. Top 10 variables of importance were ranked for 7 prediction models: ICU mortality (**left panel**), length of ICU stay (**middle panel**), and need for mechanical ventilation (**right panel**).

4. Discussion

4.1. Clinical Characteristics between MRC and Survivor Cohorts

We found that both MRC scores varied widely within the cohort. The regression analysis confirmed that MRCI and MRC-ICU scores at 24 h were significantly associated with all outcomes: mortality, LOS, and need for MV. Secondly, higher MRC scores were associated with hemodynamic instability and higher APACHE II scores. Survivors had significantly lower MRCI, MRC-ICU, APACHE II, and SAPS II scores. Thirdly, the MRC-ICU and SAPS II Model improved the prediction of all three outcomes. Historically, the utility of MRC scores and their relationships with clinical outcomes in the critical care setting have not been fully established. Previous studies have suggested inconsistent findings when investigating the MRCI score with medication nonadherence and hospitalization in the outpatient settings [34–36]. In the ICU, MRC-ICU scoring has been correlated with mortality, but it has not been explored for the LOS nor the need for MV. This study explored the relationship between MRC-ICU scores and all three clinical outcomes. Although it did not meet statistical significance, our study suggested that non-survivors had poorer renal function, increased time on MV, and an extended ICU LOS [37–39]. Lastly, these findings suggest that MRC scores should be further investigated to determine their association with the LOS. Importantly, our findings have several real-world implications for the identification, clinical management, and potentially prevention of poorer clinical outcomes in critically ill adults with the highest MRC scores.

4.2. Associations between MRC Scores and Clinical Outcomes

Our results clearly demonstrated that both MRC scores at 24 h were associated with mortality, suggesting they could be considered for incorporation into current practice (Table 2). It is plausible to mention that MRC-ICU scores at 24 h showed slightly higher association with all three clinical outcomes than MRCI scores at 24 h. Moreover, the previously published ML model has demonstrated that MRC-ICU scores are associated with ICU mortality [29]. Historically, MRC has been shown to be a better risk factor of mortality than polypharmacy alone [35]. Interestingly, we found that Hispanic ethnicity was one of the top 10 important variables identified for predicting mortality, LOS, and need for MV. Historically, racial inequalities in critical illnesses and outcomes have been well described [40]. For example, African American patients have the highest disease burden requiring intensive care treatments and are more likely to die from sepsis. During the COVID-19 pandemic, Hispanic patients have been found to have higher ICU utilization and mortality than non-Hispanic patients [41].

4.3. Medication Use as Predictor of Clinical Outcomes

The use of vasopressors was a significant predictor in all clinical outcome models. In practice, the use of vasopressors is indicated in patients with poorer health conditions, such as decompensated heart failure and shock [42,43]. The frequent diagnosis of ICU-related delirium has been a known contributing factor to the ICU LOS among other undesirable outcomes [44–46]. Historically, numerous medications have been used to minimize the duration of delirium, yet studies to identify a safe and effective agent are lacking. Our findings of current psychiatric medications potentially contributing to an increase in time on MV suggest the continued need to identify an agent to minimize the incidence and duration of ICU delirium leading to extended time on MV and LOS.

The association of pulmonary and paralytic agent use with mortality and the need for MV was anticipated in our findings as these therapeutic classes are commonly associated with high-acuity diseases such as acute respiratory distress syndrome (ARDS) and acute brain injury [47,48]. Therefore, our study supports the inclusion of medication-class usage to predict critically ill outcomes. Most notably, the lack of medication-use evaluation into the existing severity-of-illness scoring tools (i.e., SAPS II and APACHE II) is a major shortcoming for their prediction accuracy. MRC scores may provide valuable information to bedside clinicians, including critical care pharmacists, who have been recognized as essential members of the interdisciplinary care team by major societal organizations [49,50].

4.4. Implications of These Findings

MRC scores can be calculated and incorporated into the EHR to readily identify patients at higher risk. During the COVID-19 pandemic, it has become even more evident that the healthcare system and, in particular, the access and utilization of critical care resources have become profoundly strained [51]. The early identification of higher-risk patients based upon MRC scores can aid in triaging limited ICU resources. Currently, there is no standardized MRC method for presenting safety alerts pertaining to medication use in the ICU. The development and integration of MRC scores into clinical decision support tools can alert interdisciplinary care team members to review and modify the medication regimen to ensure safer, patient-centered care [52–55]. This study corroborates the need of standardizing MRC scores within the critically ill population. The strength of our study findings is three-fold: (1) rigorous statistical investigation to identify the MRC score as a predictor of clinical outcomes, (2) evaluating the accuracy of incorporating MRC scores to predict clinical outcomes, and (3) investigating the utility and usability of MRC scores in the critically ill population.

Despite finding an association between MRC scores and all three clinical outcomes in our regression modeling exercise, neither score is without its unique limitations [6,56]. The MRCI has been established and validated for use in the outpatient setting only, but it does not incorporate influential critical care medications for ICU patients [7,8,18,56,57]. On the contrary, MRC-ICU does include critical care medications, yet it does not incorporate the complexities of the pharmacotherapeutic regimen, such as the medication combinations, dosages, or frequencies. Further, neither previously established scores consider pre-existing comorbidities or severity of critical illness, which are crucial when assessing critical care outcomes. Our results suggest that the inclusion of MRC scores into standardized severity index scoring tools (i.e., APACHE II, SAPS II) can improve the prediction of critical care outcomes (MRCI and SAPS II, and MRC-ICU and SAPS II models). However, these MRC scoring tools need to be further validated using a larger critically ill patient cohort to compare against existing standardized mortality prediction tools. We propose adopting MRC scores, pre-existing comorbidities, and severity of illness into future modeling to improve the accuracy of prediction.

4.5. Limitations

Our study must be considered in the context of several limitations. First, the retrospective nature of the study design exposes the risk of missing data that can contribute to confounding bias. For example, our findings suggest that psychiatric medications increase time on MV. However, these results can be confounded by (a) the exclusion of the weights in MRCI score calculation for important medications (i.e., vasopressors and anti-infectives), (b) the exclusion of weights in MRC-ICU score calculation for over-the-counter medications, (c) the exclusion of patient's disease severity, and (d) the exclusion of multiple combinations of regimens. Second, we were unable to measure the previous exposure of MRC prior to ICU admission due to unconfirmed and varying pre-admission medication use. Third, these results may have been subjected to residual biases and unmeasured confounders due to the exclusion of commonly associated conditions (i.e., diabetes, hypertension, and dyslipidemia) as contributing factors to MRC scores. Fourth, selection biases could have occurred as general admission criteria applied to patient selection regardless of disease severity and prior to healthcare resource utilization. The generalizability of these findings is limited as they may not apply to patients with specific and life-threatening diseases such as ARDS, decompensated heart failure, and sepsis. Lastly, both MRC scores at 24 and 48 h can be indirectly related to the LOS, as a higher LOS may constitute higher MRC scores for the patients who remained admitted to the ICU for more than 48 h. Further research is necessary to control for the identified biases through a multi-centered randomized controlled trial among critically ill patients.

5. Conclusions

In this retrospective cohort study, our findings suggested that higher MRC scores were associated with poorer clinical outcomes (i.e., ICU mortality, LOS, and need for MV). Moreover, we found that MRC scores in conjunction with current severity-of-illness scores (i.e., APACHE II and SAPS II) improved the accuracy of the prediction of clinical outcomes. However, the future application of these findings needs to be validated using large EHR datasets from a more diverse patient population. Lastly, adopting these tools into the daily clinical practice could become the standard of care.

Supplementary Materials: The following supporting information can be downloaded at: https://www.mdpi.com/article/10.3390/jcm11164705/s1, Table S1: Variables extracted from electronic health record data. Description of the variables extracted by group: demographics, vital signs, laboratories, scoring tools, medication classes, and comorbidities, Table S2: Grouping of medication classes according to their pharmacologic classification, Table S3: Model specifications of logistic regression model and prediction models for intensive-care-unit mortality, length of stay, and mechanical ventilation, Table S4: Comparison between patient characteristics and Medication Regimen Complexity Index (MRCI) scores. Demographic and clinical characteristics between low- and high-MRC-scoring cohorts, Table S5: Comparison between patient characteristics and Medication Regimen Complexity Intensive Care Unit (MRC-ICU) score. Demographic and clinical characteristics between low-and high-MRC-ICU-score cohorts, Table S6: Alternative method for variable selection. Four L1 penalization techniques (LASSO) for ICU mortality, ICU length of stay, and need for mechanical ventilation, Figure S1: Correlation among the severity and medication regimen scores. Pearson correlation Coefficients for severity of illness scores stratified by age groups: Charlson comorbidity index (CCI), Acute Physiology and Chronic Health Evaluation (APACHE II), Simplified Acute Physiology Score (SAPS) II, Medication Regimen Complexity Index (MRCI), and Medication Regimen Complexity in Intensive Care Unit (MRC-ICU). p-values should be interpreted as *: p-value < 0.05, **: p-value < 0.01, and ***: p-value < 0.001, Figure S2: Distribution of the severity and medication regimen scores. Distribution of severity-of-illness scores stratified by age groups: Charlson comorbidity index (CCI), Acute Physiology and Chronic Health Evaluation (APACHE II), Simplified Acute Physiology Score (SAPS) II, Medication Regimen Complexity Index (MRCI), and Medication Regimen Complexity in Intensive Care Unit (MRC-ICU), Figure S3: Bivariate analysis of severity-of-illness scoring tools (APACHE II and SAPS II) with MRC scores (MRCI and MRC-ICU). Abbreviations: Acute Physiology and Chronic Health Evaluation (APACHE II), Simplified Acute Physiology Score (SAPS) II, Medication Regimen Complexity Index (MRCI), and Medication Regimen Complexity in Intensive Care Unit (MRC-ICU). References [1,29,30] are cited in the supplementary materials.

Author Contributions: Conceptualization, M.A.A.-M. and T.N.B.; Formal analysis, M.A.A.-M. and J.S.; Investigation, M.A.A.-M., T.N.B., J.S. and K.S.; Methodology, M.A.A.-M., T.N.B. and Y.S.; Visualization, M.A.A.-M. and J.S.; Writing—original draft, M.A.A.-M. and T.N.B.; Writing—review and editing, M.A.A.-M., T.N.B., R.S., K.S., D.S. and A.S. All authors have read and agreed to the published version of the manuscript.

Funding: The authors disclose receipt of the following financial support for the research study, authorship, and/or publication of this article: This study was funded by North East Big Data Innovation Hub, National Science Foundation (NSF) (OAC-1916585).

Institutional Review Board Statement: The study was granted exemption by the Human Research Review Committee Roger Williams Medical Center Institutional Review Board (IRB: 00000058) and University of Rhode Island Institutional Review Board (IRB: 00000559).

Informed Consent Statement: Due to the retrospective nature of the data, informed consent was not deemed necessary as all patient data were de-identified prior to use.

Data Availability Statement: The data supporting the findings from the study are available from the corresponding author upon a reasonable request based on the approval by the medical institution.

Conflicts of Interest: The authors declare no potential conflict of interest with respect to the research study, authorship, and/or publication of this article.

References

1. George, J.; Phun, Y.-T.; Bailey, M.J.; Kong, D.C.; Stewart, K. Development and Validation of the Medication Regimen Complexity Index. *Ann. Pharmacother.* **2004**, *38*, 1369–1376. [CrossRef]
2. Masnoon, N.; Shakib, S.; Kalisch-Ellett, L.; Caughey, G.E. What is polypharmacy? A systematic review of definitions. *BMC Geriatrics* **2017**, *17*, 230. [CrossRef] [PubMed]
3. Mortazavi, S.S.; Shati, M.; Keshtkar, A.; Malakouti, S.K.; Bazargan, M.; Assari, S. Defining polypharmacy in the elderly: A systematic review protocol. *BMJ Open* **2016**, *6*, e010989. [CrossRef]
4. Pazan, F.; Wehling, M. Polypharmacy in older adults: A narrative review of definitions, epidemiology and consequences. *Eur. Geriatr. Med.* **2021**, *12*, 443–452. [CrossRef] [PubMed]
5. Paquin, A.M.; Zimmerman, K.M.; Kostas, T.R.; Pelletier, L.; Hwang, A.; Simone, M.; Skarf, L.M.; Rudolph, J.L. Complexity perplexity: A systematic review to describe the measurement of medication regimen complexity. *Expert Opin. Drug Saf.* **2013**, *12*, 829–840. [CrossRef]
6. Alves-Conceição, V.; Rocha, K.S.S.; Silva, F.V.N.; Silva, R.O.S.; Da Silva, D.T.; De Lyra, D.P., Jr. Medication Regimen Complexity Measured by MRCI: A Systematic Review to Identify Health Outcomes. *Ann. Pharmacother.* **2018**, *52*, 1117–1134. [CrossRef] [PubMed]
7. Wimmer, B.C.; Cross, A.J.; Jokanovic, N.; Wiese, M.D.; George, J.; Johnell, K.; Diug, B.; Bell, J.S. Clinical Outcomes Associated with Medication Regimen Complexity in Older People: A Systematic Review. *J. Am. Geriatr. Soc.* **2017**, *65*, 747–753. [CrossRef] [PubMed]
8. Brysch, E.G.; Cauthon, K.A.B.; Kalich, B.A.; Sarbacker, G.B. Medication Regimen Complexity Index in the Elderly in an Outpatient Setting: A Literature Review. *Consult. Pharm.* **2018**, *33*, 484–496. [CrossRef]
9. Wurmbach, V.S.; Schmidt, S.J.; Lampert, A.; Bernard, S.; Meid, A.D.; Frick, E.; Metzner, M.; Wilm, S.; Mortsiefer, A.; Bücker, B.; et al. Prevalence and patient-rated relevance of complexity factors in medication regimens of community-dwelling patients with polypharmacy. *Eur. J. Clin. Pharmacol.* **2022**, *78*, 1127–1136. [CrossRef]
10. Pichala, P.T.; Kumar, B.M.; Zachariah, S.; Thomas, D.; Saunchez, L.; Gerardo, A.-U. An interventional study on intensive care unit drug therapy assessment in a rural district hospital in India. *J. Basic Clin. Pharm.* **2013**, *4*, 64. [CrossRef]
11. Moyen, E.; Camiré, E.; Stelfox, H.T. Clinical review: Medication errors in critical care. *Crit. Care* **2008**, *12*, 208. [CrossRef] [PubMed]
12. SCCM. Standard Medication Concentrations: An Opportunity to Reduce Medication Errors. Available online: https://www.sccm.org/Communications/Critical-Connections/Archives/2019/Standard-Medication-Concentrations-An-Opportunity (accessed on 9 December 2021).
13. Krska, J.; Corlett, S.A.; Katusiime, B. Complexity of Medicine Regimens and Patient Perception of Medicine Burden. *Pharm. J. Pharm. Educ. Pract.* **2019**, *7*, 18. [CrossRef] [PubMed]
14. Abou-Karam, N.; Bradford, C.; Lor, K.B.; Barnett, M.; Ha, M.; Rizos, A. Medication regimen complexity and readmissions after hospitalization for heart failure, acute myocardial infarction, pneumonia, and chronic obstructive pulmonary disease. *SAGE Open Med.* **2016**, *4*, 205031211663242. [CrossRef] [PubMed]
15. Colavecchia, A.C.; Putney, D.R.; Johnson, M.L.; Aparasu, R.R. Discharge medication complexity and 30-day heart failure readmissions. *Res. Soc. Adm. Pharm.* **2017**, *13*, 857–863. [CrossRef] [PubMed]
16. Willson, M.N.; Greer, C.L.; Weeks, D.L. Medication regimen complexity and hospital readmission for an adverse drug event. *Ann. Pharmacother.* **2014**, *48*, 26–32. [CrossRef]
17. Lee, S.; Jang, J.Y.; Yang, S.; Hahn, J.; Min, K.L.; Jung, E.H.; Oh, K.S.; Cho, R.; Chang, M.J. Development and validation of the Korean version of the medication regimen complexity index. *PLoS ONE* **2019**, *14*, e0216805. [CrossRef]
18. Ghimire, S.; Castelino, R.L.; Lioufas, N.M.; Peterson, G.M.; Zaidi, S.T.R. Nonadherence to Medication Therapy in Haemodialysis Patients: A Systematic Review. *PLoS ONE* **2015**, *10*, e0144119. [CrossRef]
19. Marienne, J.; Laville, S.M.; Caillard, P.; Batteux, B.; Gras-Champel, V.; Masmoudi, K.; Choukroun, G.; Liabeuf, S. Evaluation of Changes Over Time in the Drug Burden and Medication Regimen Complexity in ESRD Patients Before and After Renal Transplantation. *Kidney Int. Rep.* **2021**, *6*, 128–137. [CrossRef] [PubMed]
20. Tesfaye, W.H.; Peterson, G.M.; Castelino, R.L.; McKercher, C.; Jose, M.D.; Wimmer, B.C.; Zaidi, S.T.R. Medication Regimen Complexity and Hospital Readmission in Older Adults with Chronic Kidney Disease. *Ann. Pharmacother.* **2019**, *53*, 28–34. [CrossRef]
21. Ayele, A.A.; Tegegn, H.G.; Ayele, T.A.; Ayalew, M.B. Medication regimen complexity and its impact on medication adherence and glycemic control among patients with type 2 diabetes mellitus in an Ethiopian general hospital. *BMJ Open Diabetes Res. Care* **2019**, *7*, e000685. [CrossRef]
22. Wakai, E.; Ikemura, K.; Kato, C.; Okuda, M. Effect of number of medications and complexity of regimens on medication adherence and blood pressure management in hospitalized patients with hypertension. *PLoS ONE* **2021**, *16*, e0252944. [CrossRef] [PubMed]
23. Ab Rahman, N.; Lim, M.T.; Thevendran, S.; Ahmad Hamdi, N.; Sivasampu, S. Medication Regimen Complexity and Medication Burden Among Patients with Type 2 Diabetes Mellitus: A Retrospective Analysis. *Front. Pharmacol.* **2022**, *13*, 808190. [CrossRef] [PubMed]
24. Federman, A.D.; O'conor, R.; Wolf, M.S.; Wisnivesky, J.P. Associations of Medication Regimen Complexity with COPD Medication Adherence and Control. *Int. J. Chron. Obstruct. Pulmon. Dis.* **2021**, *16*, 2385–2392. [CrossRef]

25. Newsome, A.S.; Anderson, D.; Gwynn, M.E.; Waller, J.L. Characterization of changes in medication complexity using a modified scoring tool. *Am. J. Health-Syst. Pharm.* **2019**, *76*, S92–S95. [CrossRef]
26. Gwynn, M.E.; Poisson, M.O.; Waller, J.L.; Newsome, A.S. Development and validation of a medication regimen complexity scoring tool for critically ill patients. *Am. J. Health Syst. Pharm.* **2019**, *76*, S34–S40. [CrossRef] [PubMed]
27. Newsome, A.S.; Smith, S.E.; Jones, T.W.; Taylor, A.; van Berkel, M.A.; Rabinovich, M. A survey of critical care pharmacists to patient ratios and practice characteristics in intensive care units. *J. Am. Coll. Clin. Pharm.* **2020**, *3*, 68–74. [CrossRef]
28. Newsome, A.S.; Smith, S.E.; Olney, W.J.; Jones, T.W. Multicenter validation of a novel medication-regimen complexity scoring tool. *Am. J. Health-Syst. Pharm.* **2020**, *77*, 474–478. [CrossRef]
29. Al-Mamun, M.A.; Brothers, T.; Newsome, A.S. Development of Machine Learning Models to Validate a Medication Regimen Complexity Scoring Tool for Critically Ill Patients. *Ann. Pharmacother.* **2021**, *55*, 421–429. [CrossRef] [PubMed]
30. Newsome, A.S.; Smith, S.E.; Olney, W.J.; Jones, T.W.; Forehand, C.C.; Jun, A.H.; Coppiano, L. Medication regimen complexity is associated with pharmacist interventions and drug-drug interactions: A use of the novel MRC-ICU scoring tool. *J. Am. Coll. Clin. Pharm.* **2020**, *3*, 47–56. [CrossRef]
31. Ripley, B.D. The R Project in Statistical Computing. Available online: http://www.ltsn.gla.ac.uk/rworkshop.asp (accessed on 14 December 2021).
32. R: The R Project for Statistical Computing. Available online: https://www.r-project.org/ (accessed on 25 April 2020).
33. Villanueva, R.A.M.; Chen, Z.J.; Wickham, H. *ggplot2, Elegant Graphics for Data Analysis Using the Grammar of Graphics*; Springer: New York, NY, USA, 2016. [CrossRef]
34. Schoonover, H.; Corbett, C.F.; Weeks, D.L.; Willson, M.N.; Setter, S.M. Predicting potential postdischarge adverse drug events and 30-day unplanned hospital readmissions from medication regimen complexity. *J. Patient Saf.* **2014**, *10*, 186–191. [CrossRef] [PubMed]
35. Wimmer, B.C.; Bell, J.S.; Fastbom, J.; Wiese, M.D.; Johnell, K. Medication Regimen Complexity and Number of Medications as Factors Associated with Unplanned Hospitalizations in Older People: A Population-based Cohort Study. *J. Gerontol. Ser. A* **2016**, *71*, 831–837. [CrossRef] [PubMed]
36. Gamble, J.M.; Hall, J.J.; Marrie, T.J.; Sadowski, C.A.; Majumdar, S.R.; Eurich, D.T. Medication transitions and polypharmacy in older adults following acute care. *Ther. Clin. Risk Manag.* **2014**, *10*, 189. [CrossRef] [PubMed]
37. Moitra, V.K.; Guerra, C.; Linde-Zwirble, W.T.; Wunsch, H. Relationship Between ICU Length of Stay and Long-Term Mortality for Elderly ICU Survivors. *Crit. Care Med.* **2016**, *44*, 655–662. [CrossRef]
38. De Corte, W.; Dhondt, A.; Vanholder, R.; de Waele, J.; Decruyenaere, J.; Sergoyne, V.; Vanhalst, J.; Claus, S.; Hoste, E.A.J. Long-term outcome in ICU patients with acute kidney injury treated with renal replacement therapy: A prospective cohort study. *Crit. Care* **2016**, *20*, 256. [CrossRef]
39. Marshall, J.; Finn, C.A.; Theodore, A.C. Impact of a clinical pharmacist-enforced intensive care unit sedation protocol on duration of mechanical ventilation and hospital stay. *Crit. Care Med.* **2008**, *36*, 427–433. [CrossRef] [PubMed]
40. Chertoff, J. Racial disparities in critical care: Experience from the USA. *Lancet Respir. Med.* **2017**, *5*, e11–e12. [CrossRef]
41. Velasco, F.; Yang, D.M.; Zhang, M.; Nelson, T.; Sheffield, T.; Keller, T.; Wang, Y.; Walker, C.; Katterapalli, C.; Zimmerman, K.; et al. Association of Healthcare Access with Intensive Care Unit Utilization and Mortality in Patients of Hispanic Ethnicity Hospitalized With COVID-19. *J. Hosp. Med.* **2021**, *16*, 659–666. [CrossRef] [PubMed]
42. Evans, L.; Rhodes, A.; Alhazzani, W.; Antonelli, M.; Coopersmith, C.M.; French, C.; Machado, F.R.; Mcintyre, L.; Ostermann, M.; Prescott, H.C.; et al. Surviving sepsis campaign: International guidelines for management of sepsis and septic shock 2021. *Intensive Care Med.* **2021**, *47*, 1181–1247. [CrossRef] [PubMed]
43. Levy, B.; Buzon, J.; Kimmoun, A. Inotropes and vasopressors use in cardiogenic shock: When, which and how much? *Curr. Opin. Crit. Care* **2019**, *25*, 384–390. [CrossRef] [PubMed]
44. Li, M.; Chang, M.H.; Miranda-Valdes, Y.; Vest, K.; Kish, T.D. Impact of early home psychotropic medication reinitiation on surrogate measures of intensive care unit delirium. *Ment. Health Clin.* **2019**, *9*, 263–268. [CrossRef] [PubMed]
45. Devlin, J.W.; Skrobik, Y.; Gélinas, C.; Needham, D.M.; Slooter, A.J.C.; Pandharipande, P.P.; Watson, P.L.; Weinhouse, G.L.; Nunnally, M.E.; Rochwerg, B.; et al. Clinical Practice Guidelines for the Prevention and Management of Pain, Agitation/Sedation, Delirium, Immobility, and Sleep Disruption in Adult Patients in the ICU. *Crit. Care Med.* **2018**, *46*, e825–e873. [CrossRef]
46. Shehabi, Y.; Riker, R.R.; Bokesch, P.M.; Wisemandle, W.; Shintani, A.; Ely, E.W. Delirium duration and mortality in lightly sedated, mechanically ventilated intensive care patients. *Crit. Care Med.* **2010**, *38*, 2311–2318. [CrossRef] [PubMed]
47. Renew, J.R.; Ratzlaff, R.; Hernandez-Torres, V.; Brull, S.J.; Prielipp, R.C. Neuromuscular blockade management in the critically Ill patient. *J. Intensive Care* **2020**, *8*, 37. [CrossRef] [PubMed]
48. Murray, M.J.; Deblock, H.; Erstad, B.; Gray, A.; Jacobi, J.; Jordan, C.; McGee, W.; McManus, C.; Meade, M.; Nix, S.; et al. Clinical Practice Guidelines for Sustained Neuromuscular Blockade in the Adult Critically Ill Patient. *Crit. Care Med.* **2016**, *44*, 2079–2103. [CrossRef] [PubMed]
49. Lat, I.; Paciullo, C.; Daley, M.J.; Maclaren, R.; Bolesta, S.; McCann, J.; Stollings, J.L.; Gross, K.; Foos, S.A.; Roberts, R.J.; et al. Position Paper on Critical Care Pharmacy Services: 2020 Update. *Crit. Care Med.* **2020**, *48*, 813–834. [CrossRef] [PubMed]
50. Newsome, A.S.; Jones, T.W.; Smith, S.E. Pharmacists Are Associated with Reduced Mortality in Critically Ill Patients. *Crit. Care Med.* **2019**, *47*, e1036–e1037. [CrossRef] [PubMed]

51. Maves, R.C.; Downar, J.; Dichter, J.R.; Hick, J.L.; Devereaux, A.; Geiling, J.A.; Kissoon, N.; Hupert, N.; Niven, A.S.; King, M.A.; et al. Triage of Scarce Critical Care Resources in COVID-19 An Implementation Guide for Regional Allocation: An Expert Panel Report of the Task Force for Mass Critical Care and the American College of Chest Physicians. *Chest* **2020**, *158*, 212–225. [CrossRef] [PubMed]
52. Makam, A.N.; Nguyen, O.K.; Auerbach, A.D. Diagnostic accuracy and effectiveness of automated electronic sepsis alert systems: A systematic review. *J. Hosp. Med.* **2015**, *10*, 396–402. [CrossRef] [PubMed]
53. Page, N.; Baysari, M.T.; Westbrook, J.I. A systematic review of the effectiveness of interruptive medication prescribing alerts in hospital CPOE systems to change prescriber behavior and improve patient safety. *Int. J. Med. Inform.* **2017**, *105*, 22–30. [CrossRef] [PubMed]
54. Bright, T.J.; Wong, A.; Dhurjati, R.; Bristow, E.; Bastian, L.; Coeytaux, R.R.; Samsa, G.; Hasselblad, V.; Williams, J.W.; Musty, M.D.; et al. Effect of clinical decision-support systems: A systematic review. *Ann. Intern. Med.* **2012**, *157*, 29–43. [CrossRef] [PubMed]
55. Jaspers, M.W.M.; Smeulers, M.; Vermeulen, H.; Peute, L.W. Effects of clinical decision-support systems on practitioner performance and patient outcomes: A synthesis of high-quality systematic review findings. *J. Am. Med. Inform. Assoc.* **2011**, *18*, 327–334. [CrossRef] [PubMed]
56. Alves-Conceição, V.; Rocha, K.S.S.; Silva, F.V.N.; Silva, R.D.O.S.; Cerqueira-Santos, S.; Nunes, M.A.P.; Martins-Filho, P.R.; Da Silva, D.T.; De Lyra, D.P. Are Clinical Outcomes Associated with Medication Regimen Complexity? A Systematic Review and Meta-analysis. *Ann. Pharmacother.* **2020**, *54*, 301–313. [CrossRef] [PubMed]
57. Falch, C.; Alves, G. Pharmacists' Role in Older Adults' Medication Regimen Complexity: A Systematic Review. *Int. J. Environ. Res. Public Health.* **2021**, *18*, 8824. [CrossRef] [PubMed]

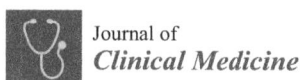 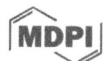

Article

Novel Method for Early Prediction of Clinically Significant Drug–Drug Interactions with a Machine Learning Algorithm Based on Risk Matrix Analysis in the NICU

Nadir Yalçın [1,*], Merve Kaşıkcı [2], Hasan Tolga Çelik [3], Karel Allegaert [4,5,6], Kutay Demirkan [1], Şule Yiğit [3] and Murat Yurdakök [3]

1. Department of Clinical Pharmacy, Faculty of Pharmacy, Hacettepe University, Ankara 06100, Turkey
2. Department of Biostatistics, Faculty of Medicine, Hacettepe University, Ankara 06100, Turkey
3. Division of Neonatology, Department of Child Health and Diseases, Faculty of Medicine, Hacettepe University, Ankara 06100, Turkey
4. Department of Pharmaceutical and Pharmacological Sciences, KU Leuven, 3000 Leuven, Belgium
5. Department of Development and Regeneration, KU Leuven, 3000 Leuven, Belgium
6. Department of Hospital Pharmacy, Erasmus Medical Center, 3000 GA Rotterdam, The Netherlands
* Correspondence: nadir.yalcin@hotmail.com; Tel.: +90-5356849300

Citation: Yalçın, N.; Kaşıkcı, M.; Çelik, H.T.; Allegaert, K.; Demirkan, K.; Yiğit, Ş.; Yurdakök, M. Novel Method for Early Prediction of Clinically Significant Drug–Drug Interactions with a Machine Learning Algorithm Based on Risk Matrix Analysis in the NICU. *J. Clin. Med.* 2022, *11*, 4715. https://doi.org/10.3390/jcm11164715

Academic Editors: Alfredo Vannacci, Niccolò Lombardi and Giada Crescioli

Received: 22 July 2022
Accepted: 10 August 2022
Published: 12 August 2022

Publisher's Note: MDPI stays neutral with regard to jurisdictional claims in published maps and institutional affiliations.

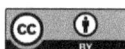

Copyright: © 2022 by the authors. Licensee MDPI, Basel, Switzerland. This article is an open access article distributed under the terms and conditions of the Creative Commons Attribution (CC BY) license (https://creativecommons.org/licenses/by/4.0/).

Abstract: *Aims:* Evidence for drug–drug interactions (DDIs) that may cause age-dependent differences in the incidence and severity of adverse drug reactions (ADRs) in newborns is sparse. We aimed to develop machine learning (ML) algorithms that predict DDI presence by integrating each DDI, which is objectively evaluated with the scales in a risk matrix (probability + severity). *Methods:* This double-center, prospective randomized cohort study included neonates admitted to the neonatal intensive care unit in a tertiary referral hospital during the 17-month study period. Drugs were classified by the Anatomical Therapeutic Chemical (ATC) classification and assessed for potential and clinically relevant DDIs to risk analyses with the Drug Interaction Probability Scale (DIPS, causal probability) and the Lexicomp® DDI (severity) database. *Results:* A total of 412 neonates (median (interquartile range) gestational age of 37 (4) weeks) were included with 32,925 patient days, 131 different medications, and 11,908 medication orders. Overall, at least one potential DDI was observed in 125 (30.4%) of the patients (2.6 potential DDI/patient). A total of 38 of these 125 patients had clinically relevant DDIs causing adverse drug reactions (2.0 clinical DDI/patient). The vast majority of these DDIs (90.66%) were assessed to be at moderate risk. The performance of the ML algorithms that predicts of the presence of relevant DDI was as follows: accuracy 0.944 (95% CI 0.888–0.972), sensitivity 0.892 (95% CI 0.769–0.962), F1 score 0.904, and AUC 0.929 (95% CI 0.874–0.983). *Conclusions:* In clinical practice, it is expected that optimization in treatment can be achieved with the implementation of this high-performance web tool, created to predict DDIs before they occur with a newborn-centered approach.

Keywords: drug–drug interactions; machine learning; neonatal intensive care unit; adverse drug reactions

1. Introduction

Undesirable effects that occur in a potential or clinically relevant way with the concurrent use of two or more drugs are drug–drug interaction (DDI) and adverse drug reactions (ADR) [1]. In the broadest sense, a DDI occurs whenever one drug affects the pharmacokinetics (PK), pharmacodynamics (PD), efficacy, or toxicity of another drug depending on various factors such as drug-related (such as the mechanism of action, route of administration, dose, dose interval, duration of treatment, dosing times) and patient-related (such as diagnosis, polypharmacy, pharmacogenetics, length of hospital stays) [2–4] factors. DDIs often lead to increased healthcare costs, morbidity, and mortality, originating from 2.5 to 4.4% of ADRs and 3 to 5% of all inpatient medication errors [5,6].

Many DDIs in neonatal intensive care unit (NICU) patients can remain unrecognized by considering these various factors as well as the workload of the health care professionals. Neonates, particularly admitted to the NICU, have increased the severity of DDIs to result in more common/severe ADR compared to other populations due to physiological/organ immaturity, congenital diseases, birth-related complications, and significant differences in PKs such as extravascular total body water, immature renal/hepatic functions, plasma protein concentrations, blood–brain barrier permeability [7,8]. As a recent illustration of this complexity of DDI in neonates, Salerno et al. explored the impact of co-administration of fluconazole on sildenafil disposition, including the PD-relevant metabolite (N-desmethyl sildenafil). Interestingly, the AUC fold change in adults (2.11-fold) was different in infants (2.82-fold), necessitating a dose reduction of about 60% to attain similar exposure [9].

With the digitalization of health and medicine and the widespread use of electronic health records (EHR), healthcare professionals have begun to adopt the latest methodologies of artificial intelligence (AI). Machine learning (ML) algorithms, a subtype of AI, can act as a kind of co-pilot and predict DDIs before they occur with a patient-centered approach. Due to the lack of comprehensive experimental data for neonates, high study cost, and long experimental duration, the use of computational prediction and DDIs assessment is an encouraging strategy to improve precision medicine: recognize the cases at higher risk to mitigate risks. [10].

Although software DDI checkers for adults are widely available, most have limited clinical utility, especially for neonates. In this context, it was aimed to develop ML algorithms and web tool that predict high-performance DDI by integrating each DDI, which is objectively evaluated with the scales in risk matrix (probability + severity) (http://www.softmed.hacettepe.edu.tr/NEO-DEER_Drug_Interaction/ (accessed on 7 August 2022)).

2. Methods

2.1. Study Design and Population

Newborns (postnatal age between 0 and 28 days), patients admitted to the NICU for at least 24 h, and patients who received at least one systemic drug during their hospital stay were included in this double-center and prospective randomized cohort study from February 2020 to June 2021. The newborns with hepatic or renal impairment excluded in the study. The Institutional Review Board of Hacettepe University ethical approved this study and written informed consent was obtained from each parent/legal guardian of the participant (decision no. 2020/11-21). This study registered with the ClinicalTrials.gov (accessed on 7 August 2022) (NCT04899960).

2.2. Data Acquisition

Patients' follow-up was performed daily to acquire the clinical status via a comprehensive assessment by the multidisciplinary team including physicians, nurses, and a clinical pharmacist. Demographical, clinical, and drug administration data were obtained from routine follow-up for each patient. International Classification of Diseases 10th Revision (ICD-10) codes for diagnoses, Anatomical Therapeutic Chemical (ATC) codes for categorization of drugs were used for all patients.

2.3. Causal Probability, Severity, a Risk Matrix Development of DDIs

Potential DDIs with all drugs prescribed simultaneously in each NICU patient until discharge was prospectively determined using the Lexicomp® DDI database, clinical and laboratory findings by the clinical pharmacist. The inhibitor/inductor and substrate (victim) drugs, mechanism of DDIs, ADRs of clinically relevant DDIs, and duration of exposure (days) were prospectively registered.

The Drug Interaction Probability Scale (DIPS) was used to determine the *causal probability* for each potential DDI. The DIPS consists of 10 questions and each question is answered as 'Yes', 'No' or 'Unknown or Not Applicable (NA)', DDIs are categorized as >8 points 'highly probable', 5–8 points 'probable', 2–4 points 'possible', and <2 points 'doubtful' [11]. By consensus, all DDIs except the 'doubtful' were considered clinically significant (any score ≥ 2). In this study, the probability categories were numbered between 1 (doubtful) to 4 (highly probable).

The Lexicomp® DDI database was used to determine the potential *severity* of each DDI. According to the Lexicomp® database, DDIs are rated as X (avoid combination), D (consider therapy modification), C (monitor therapy), B (no action needed), and A (no known interaction) [12]. In this study, the severity categories obtained were numbered between 1 (A = no known interaction) and 5 (X = avoid combination).

These categories are placed in rows (severity, 1–4) and columns (probability, 1–5) in the *risk matrix*, which consists of risk scores obtained by multiplying severity and probability values. In this risk matrix, the risk category was obtained for each DDI as low (white), moderate (light gray), and high (dark gray) risk. This risk matrix created was approved by the consensus of the clinicians involved in the study.

2.4. Establishment, Optimization, and Validation of Random Forest Model

Primarily, statistically significant correlations and differences were examined among all general and prescription information (as input variables), and the presence of DDI(s) during hospitalization (as output variables) by univariate analyses. Input variables that were found to be significant according to univariate analysis were chosen as independent variables ($p < 0.05$). Secondly, the data set containing the dependent and independent variables was randomly divided into train sets (70%) for obtain models and test set (30%) for obtaining model performance. Since the 10-fold cross-validation method separates the train data into train and validation sets, a separate validation set was not used when dividing the data set. Elastic net, random forest (RF), and support vector machine (SVM) with different kernel functions were used to compare model performances. The highest performance was provided by RF and the study was analyzed with RF. The accuracy, sensitivity (recall), specificity, positive predictive value (precision-PPV), negative predictive value (NPV), F1 score, and area under ROC curve (AUC) were used as performance measures in classification models to compare the performance of the models. A high-performance model requires these measurements of 0.70 and above.

Accuracy is the ratio of correctly classified samples to the total number of samples. Sensitivity and specificity are the ability of a model to correctly identify positive and negative samples, respectively. PPV is an indicator of how many of the samples classified as positive by the model are actually positive. NPV is an indicator of how many of the samples classified as negative by the model are actually negative. F1 score is harmonic mean of precision and recall. Lastly, AUC is an indicator of how well the classes are separated from each other according to the model obtained.

The model performances were compared after parameter optimization to avoid overfitting with the tuneLength argument in the Classification and Regression Training (caret) package [13]. Variable importance plots were used in the study to show the importance order of the variables used in the prediction models.

Finally, data were collected prospectively to examine the predictive validity of the ML-based model in a different hospital (Erasmus Medical Centre Sophia Children's Hospital) and country (The Netherlands) by the same web tool user (clinical pharmacist) to ensure quality standard.

2.5. Statistical Analysis

For predictive models based on ML, it is not possible to measure the effect size as in hypothesis testing. Instead of calculating the sample size according to the effect size of a certain power level, rules of thumb such as taking 10 or 20 times the number of independent variables as the sample size can be applied. In this study, it was planned to have a maximum of 20 independent variables in the final models, so the minimum sample size was determined as 400 patients, with 20 observations per variable [14]. Continuous variables were defined as the mean (standard deviation, SD) and median (range). The normality of continuous variables was tested using the Shapiro–Wilk test. Categorical variables were defined as percentages and were compared using the χ^2 test. Univariate analysis was carried out in *IBM SPSS Statistics Version 23* software. For all tests, $p < 0.05$ was considered statistically significant. All ML analyses were performed, using the open-source software R (version 3.6.3, http://www.rproject.org (accessed on 7 August 2022)). In terms of reproducibility, the seed number was set at 1234. Caret [13] package was used as the primary package for model training, 10-fold cross-validation, and variable importance. pROC [15], precrec [16], and ggplot2 [17] R packages were used for obtaining the ROC curve. The quantitative features were normalized before training the models.

3. Results

3.1. Clinical Characteristics

During the study period, 468 newborns were admitted to the 22-bed capacity NICU in a tertiary referral hospital. Fifty-six patients were excluded because of non-survival (n = 21, 4.5%) or not receiving any systemic drug (n = 35, 7.4%). Therefore, 412 patients were included in the study: 232 (56.3%) were males, 177 (43%) were preterm births, and 172 (41.7%) were low birth weight (<2500 g). According to the numeric variables, the median (IQR) postnatal age (PNA) was 1 (1) day and the median (IQR) length of hospital stay (LOS) was 8 (11) days. General and postnatal information about patients is given in Table 1.

Table 1. Data acquisition parameters of the study (N = 412).

Population Characteristics	
Sex, Male, n (%)	232 (56.3%)
Sex ratio (male/female)	1.29
5 min APGAR score, median (IQR)	8 (2)
Gestational age (weeks), median (IQR)	37 (4)
Extremely preterm (<28 weeks), n (%)	7 (1.7%)
Very preterm (28 to 32 weeks), n (%)	52 (12.6%)
Moderate preterm (32 to 34 weeks), n (%)	16 (3.9%)
Late preterm (34 to 37 weeks), n (%)	102 (24.8%)
Term (>37 weeks), n (%)	235 (57%)
SGA at admission, n (%)	88 (21.4%)
Birth weight (g), mean (SD)	2631.1 (877.2)
Extremely low birth weight (<1000 g), n (%)	26 (6.3%)
Very low birth weight (1000 to 1500 g), n (%)	27 (6.6%)
Low birth weight (1500 to 2500 g), n (%)	119 (28.9%)
Normal birth weight (>2500 g), n (%)	240 (58.3%)
Multiple birth, n (%)	53 (12.9%)
Caesarean section, n (%)	337 (81.8%)
Diagnosis (ICD-10), n (%)	
Complications of labor and delivery, n (%)	165 (40%)
Infectious diseases, n (%)	46 (11.2%)
Diseases of the respiratory system, n (%)	46 (11.2%)
Diseases of the circulatory system, n (%)	37 (9%)
Other disorders of fluid, electrolyte, and acid-base balance, n (%)	26 (6.3%)

Table 1. Cont.

Population Characteristics	
Diseases of the digestive system, n (%)	24 (5.8%)
Diseases of the nervous system, n (%)	20 (4.9%)
Neonatal jaundice, n (%)	19 (4.6%)
Congenital malformations, deformations and chromosomal abnormalities, n (%)	15 (3.6%)
Metabolic disorders, n (%)	9 (2.2%)
Neoplasms, n (%)	6 (1.4%)
Drugs (ATC) (N = 2280), n (%)	
J. Anti-infectives for systemic use, n (%)	905 (39.69%)
A. Alimentary tract and metabolism, n (%)	591 (25.92%)
N. Nervous system, n (%)	229 (10.05%)
B. Blood and blood-forming organs, n (%)	175 (7.67%)
C. Cardiovascular system, n (%)	170 (7.46%)
R. Respiratory system, n (%)	81 (3.55%)
H. Systemic hormonal preparations, n (%)	70 (3.07%)
S. Sensory organs, n (%)	31 (1.36%)
M. Musculo-skeletal system, n (%)	11 (0.48%)
G. Genito-urinary system and sex hormones, n (%)	10 (0.44%)
L. Antineoplastic and immunomodulating agents, n (%)	7 (0.31%)

APGAR: Appearance, Pulse, Grimace, Activity, and Respiration, SGA: Small for gestational age, ICD: International Classification of Diseases 10th Revision, ATC: Anatomical Therapeutic Chemical.

A total of 412 NICU patients (5.53 drugs/patient/day) to whom 2280 drugs were prescribed in 32,925 patient days and 11,908 medication orders (28.9 order/patient) were prescribed with the computerized physician order entry (CPOE) system were prospectively examined from prescribing to the follow-up process. The median (range) values of the total number of drugs and anti-infectives used during the hospitalization period were 3 (0–29) and 2 (0–9) respectively. According to the ATC, the most frequently prescribed drugs in these orders were anti-infective (38.82%), alimentary tract and metabolism (32.89%), and nervous system (8.07%) drugs. In the study period, a total of 131 different drugs were prescribed. The most commonly used of these agents were intravenous fluids (12.06%), gentamicin (8.03%), and ampicillin (7.81%). The rate of anti-infectives among the total number of drugs prescribed was 39.96% (Table S1).

3.2. Characteristics of Potential and Observed DDIs: Incidence and Severity

At least one potential DDI was observed in 125 (30.4%) of the patients included in the study. The total number of potential DDIs detected was 328 (2.6 potential DDI/patient, range 1–15). Of these patients, 66 (52.8%) had 1 DDI, 15 (12.0%) 2 DDIs, 19 (15.2%) 3 DDIs, 25 (20.0%) 4 or more DDIs.

Of 125 patients with potential DDIs, 38 (30.3%) had clinically relevant DDIs known to cause ADR were identified. The total number of clinically relevant DDIs observed in these 38 patients was 75 (2.0 clinically relevant DDI/patient, range: 1–5) (Figure 1). The vast majority (65/75, 99.6 %) of observed clinically relevant DDIs were found to be of moderate risk. Low- and high-risk clinically relevant DDIs were seen in 3 and 4 patients, respectively. According to the risk matrix, while the mean risk score is 10.3 in patients with potential DDIs, this score increases to 21.1 in patients with only clinically relevant DDIs.

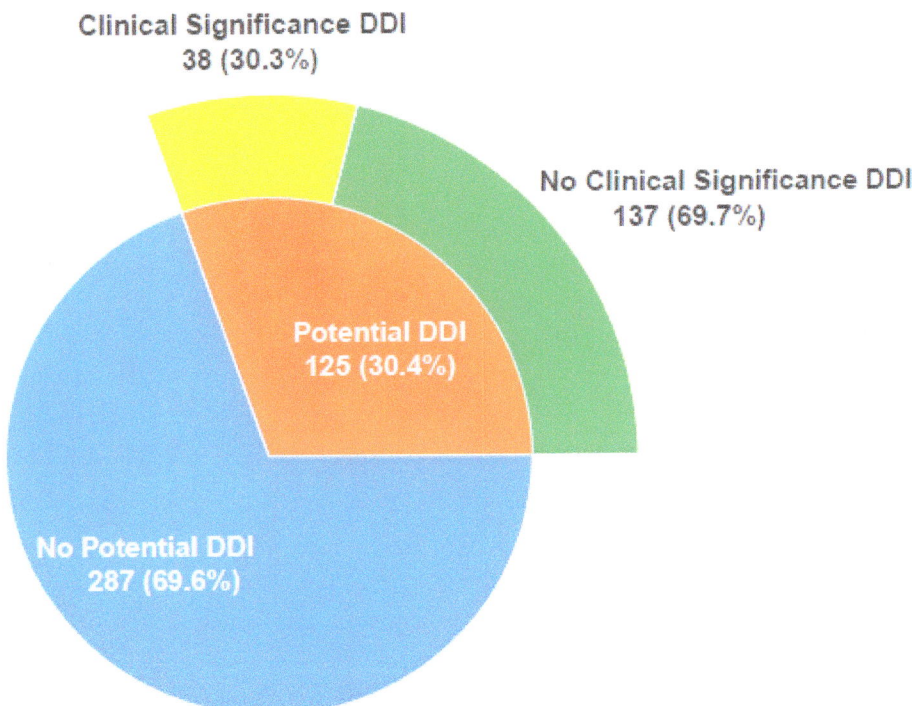

Figure 1. Distribution of potential and clinically relevant DDIs.

The most common clinically relevant DDI observed in patients was between vancomycin and amikacin (17.3%). As a result of this DDI, the mean creatinine was above the upper level to the baseline on the 17th day of this combination. It was recognized that this DDI was determined as a 'possible' probability and C (monitoring) severity level. As a result, when the probability and severity data were placed in the risk matrix, it was seen that the DDI was 'moderate' risk. DDIs with clinical findings identified as high risk were amiodarone–flecainide, caffeine–adenosine, midazolam–fentanyl, and linezolid–salbutamol (Table 2).

When the probability and severity analysis of all potential DDIs were evaluated separately, 'doubtful' probability (77.44%) and moderate (C = monitor therapy) severity (79.88%) of DDIs were most commonly observed in the risk matrix (Table 3).

3.3. Development and Optimization of a Model to Predict the Presence of Clinically Relevant DDI

The parameters that have the highest correlation with DDIs and are included in the model were: the total number of anti-infectives, total number of drugs, nervous system drugs, cardiovascular system drugs, respiratory system drugs, and anti-infectives. When considering the importance of the parameters included in the model, it was seen that the most effective variable in predicting the DDI is the total number of anti-infectives (Figure 2).

Table 2. The type, outcome, duration of exposure, probability, severity, and risk category of clinically relevant DDIs observed in the study (n = 38).

Affecting Drug (Inhibitor/Inductor)	Affected Drug (Victim)	Mechanism of DDIs	ADRs Observed as a Result of DDI *	Duration of Exposure (Mean Day)	DIPS (Probability)	Lexicomp® (Severity)	Risk Score	Risk Category
Vancomycin	Amikacin	Additive/synergistic	Increase in creatinine (13)	16.76	2	3	6	2
Dexmedetomidine	Fentanyl	Additive	Bradycardia (6) Hypotension (2)	3.25	2	3	6	2
Amikacin	Furosemide	Additive/synergistic	Increase in creatinine (4)	2	2	3	6	2
Dexmedetomidine	Furosemide	Additive	Hypotension (3)	4.33	2	3	6	2
Phenytoin	Phenobarbital	Metabolism	Decreased effect of phenytoin (2)	11	3	3	9	2
Hydrocortisone	Furosemide	Additive	Hypokalemia (2)	4.50	2	3	6	2
Phenobarbital	Furosemide	Unknown	Hypotension (2)	7.50	2	3	6	2
Salbutamol	Furosemide	Additive	Hypokalemia (2)	6.50	2	3	6	2
Amiodarone	Flecainide	Additive	QTc prolongation	2	4	4	16	3
Furosemide	Captopril	Volume depletion	Increase in creatinine Hypotension	4	2	3	5	2
Hydrocortisone	Furosemide	Additive	Hypokalemia	3	2	3	6	2
Hydrochlorothiazide	Diazoxide	Decrease in insulin secretion	Hyperglycemia	8	3	3	9	2
Nifedipine	Propranolol	Additive	Hypotension	5	2	3	6	2
Caffeine	Adenosine	Antagonism	Decreased effect of adenosine	10	3	4	12	3
Amiodarone	Fluconazole	Metabolism	QTc prolongation	3	2	4	8	2
Phenobarbital	Levetiracetam	Unknown	Decreased effect of levetiracetam	26	2	3	6	2
Ibuprofen	Amikacin	Unknown	Increase in creatinine	3	3	3	9	2
Spironolactone	Captopril	Increase in potassium retention due to aldosterone reduction	Hyperkalemia	18	3	3	9	2
Fluconazole	Midazolam	Metabolism	Prolonged sedation	1	2	3	6	2
Diazoxide	Dexmedetomidine	Additive	Hypotension	3	2	3	6	2
Dexamethasone	Hydrochlorothiazide	Additive	Hypokalemia	2	2	3	6	2
Fluconazole	Ibuprofen	Metabolism	Decrease in hemoglobin	2	2	3	6	2
Ciprofloxacin	Phenytoin	Unknown	Decreased phenytoin plasma concentration	5	4	2	8	2
Allopurinol	Phenytoin	Unknown	Increased phenytoin plasma concentration	1	3	3	9	2
Midazolam	Fentanyl	Additive	Chest rigidity	3	4	4	16	3
Adenosine	Dexmedetomidine	Additive	Bradycardia	3	2	3	6	2
Phenobarbital	Topiramate	Unknown	Decreased effect of topiramate	7	2	3	6	2

Table 2. Cont.

Affecting Drug (Inhibitor/Inductor)	Affected Drug (Victim)	Mechanism of DDIs	ADRs Observed as a Result of DDI *	Duration of Exposure (Mean Day)	DIPS (Probability)	Lexicomp® (Severity)	Risk Score	Risk Category
Phenobarbital	Dexmedetomidine	Catecholamine reduction	Hypotension	3	2	3	6	2
Fentanyl	Furosemide	Unknown	Hypotension Decreased urine output	5.50	2	3	6	2
Salbutamol	Hydrochlorothiazide	Additive	Hypokalemia	7	2	3	6	2
Phenytoin	Topiramate	Metabolism	Decreased effect of topiramate	5	2	3	6	2
Ciprofloxacin	Midazolam	Metabolism	Prolonged sedation	3	2	2	4	1
Ferrous fumarate	Levothyroxine	Absorption	Decreased effect of levothyroxine	13	2	4	8	2
Cefuroxime	Amikacin	Additive/synergistic	Increase in creatinine	1	2	3	6	2
Nitroglycerine	Furosemide	Additive	Hypotension	16	2	3	6	2
Potassium chloride	Furosemide	Unknown	Hyponatremia	1	2	2	4	1
Methylprednisolone	Furosemide	Additive	Hypokalemia	1	2	3	6	2
Linezolid	Salbutamol	Metabolism	Hypertension	10	3	4	12	3
Nitroglycerine	Dexmedetomidine	Additive	Hypotension	6	2	3	6	2
Potassium chloride	Phenobarbital	Unknown	Hyponatremia	6	2	3	6	2
Dexmedetomidine	Salbutamol	Unknown	Hypokalemia	1	2	2	4	1
Furosemide	Levothyroxine	Unknown	Increase in free T4	7	2	3	6	2
Furosemide	Levosimendan	Additive	Hypotension	1	2	3	6	2
Prednisolone	Furosemide	Additive	Hypokalemia	3	3	3	9	2
Adrenalin	Dopamine	Additive	Hypertension	3	2	3	6	2

DIPS: Drug Interaction Probability Scale, ADR: adverse drug reaction, DDI: drug–drug interaction. * The numbers in parentheses show how many times that DDI has been observed. The other ADRs were observed only once in that DDIs. Risk category column; white: low risk, light gray: moderate risk, dark gray: high risk.

Table 3. Distribution of potential drug–drug interactions detected by probability and severity.

		SEVERITY				
		A (1) n = 1 (0.30%)	B (2) n = 24 (7.32%)	C (3) n = 262 (79.88%)	D (4) n = 40 (12.20%)	X (5) n = 1 (0.30%)
P R O B A B I L I T Y	Highly Probable (4) n = 3 (0.91%)	4	8	12	16	20
	Probable (3) n = 16 (4.88%)	3	6	9	12	15
	Possible (2) n = 55 (16.77%)	2	4	6	8	10
	Doubtful (1) n = 254 (77.44%)	1	2	3	4	5

1–4 points (low risk-white), 5–10 points (moderate risk-light gray), 12–20 points (high risk-dark gray).

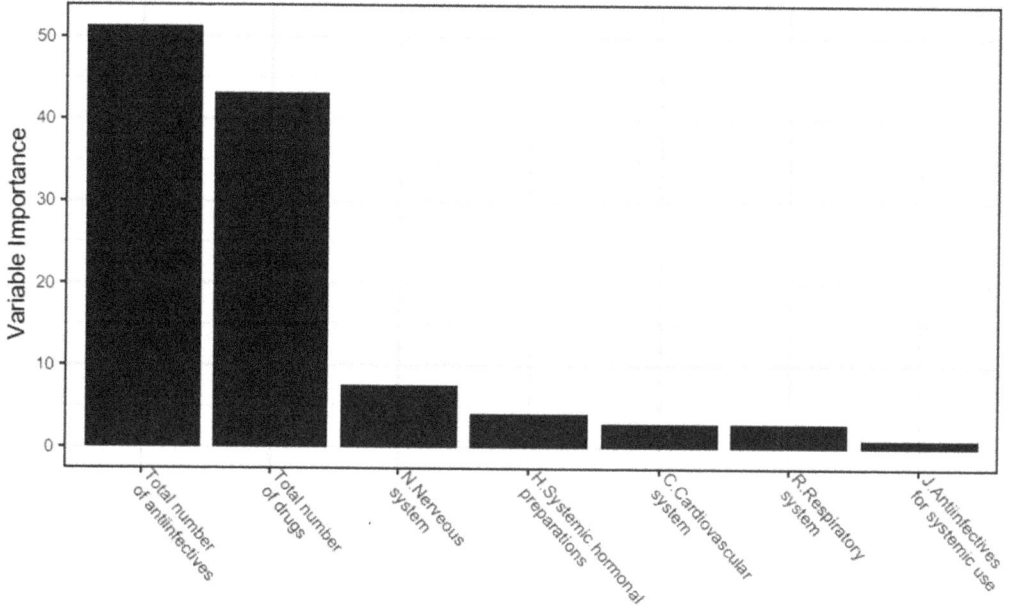

Figure 2. Variable importance plot (%) used to predict the presence of clinically relevant DDI.

The obtained model showed very high performance in predicting the presence of DDI. Performance measurements of the model were as follows: accuracy 0.944 (95% CI 0.888–0.972), sensitivity 0.892 (95% CI 0.769–0.962), selectivity 0.966 (95% CI 0.913–0.991), PPV 0.917 (95% CI 0.812–0.966), NPV 0.955 (95% CI) 0.906–0.979), F1 score 0.904, and AUC 0.929 (95% CI 0.874–0.983). The high AUC indicates that the model predicting the presence of DDI correctly classified 92.9% of the patients (Figure 3).

Data were collected prospectively to examine the predictive validity of the model. In total, a sample of 51 NICU patients was reached and 15.7% (n = 8) had observed DDI. The model correctly classified 92% of them. Sensitivity and NPV were obtained as 0.75. Sensitivity and PPV were obtained as 0.92. Similar to the results of the test data set, prospective data set results had high sensitivity and PPV.

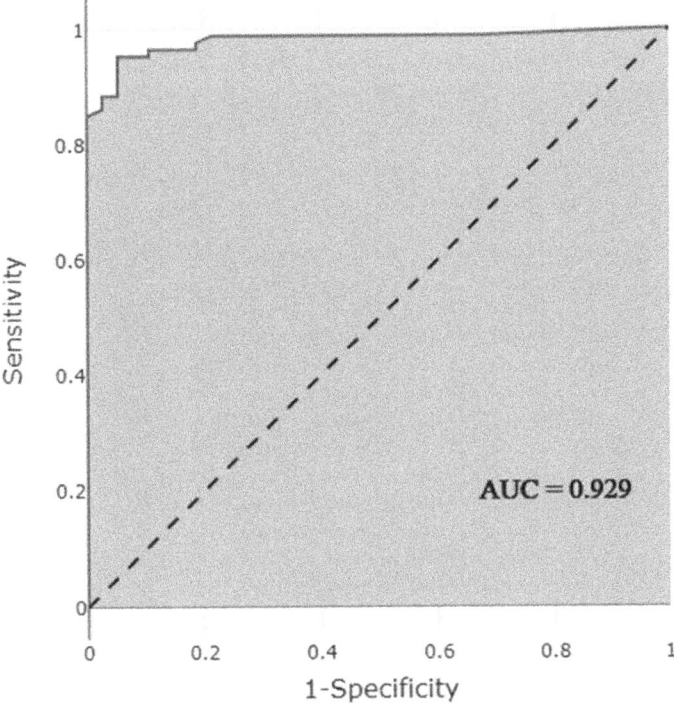

Figure 3. AUC-ROC curve showing the performance of the model predicting the presence of clinically relevant DDI.

4. Discussion

This study confirmed that the presence of ADRs (causal probability, DIPS) and risk category of each DDI (severity, Lexicomp® DDI database) varies between patients. Related to this variability, it was shown that the presence of DDIs can be predicted in neonates by using ML algorithms that show high prediction performance in such complex models.

It is estimated that >70% of neonates in the NICU are exposed to DDIs [18]. In our study, a total of 328 potential DDIs were detected in 30.4% of the patients included. More than half of the patients had only one potential DDI during hospitalization. In 30.3% of these patients with potential DDIs, clinically relevant DDIs were determined by an objective DIPS. Looking at the broader picture, a potential DDI was detected in approximately a third of the patients included in the study, and a clinically relevant DDI was detected in a third of these patients (9.2% of the study population). Similarly, Choi et al. identified clinically relevant DDIs in 16 (10.1%) PICU patients [19]. When putting our observations on DDI incidence (potential 30%, clinically relevant 9%) into perspective, other cohorts reported potential DDI incidences of 70, 13.2, or 66.2% [7,20,21].

The DIPS and Lexicomp® database are mostly used in adults in clinical practices and studies. Although there is limited research on the implementation of the DIPS [22,23] and Lexicomp® DDI database [24] in children, there is no study for its implementation in neonates in the current literature. To the best of our knowledge, this is the first study to use these measurements in neonates. Related to the causal probability and severity of each potential DDI detected with the risk analysis matrix (Table 3), 77.44% were 'doubtful' according to the DIPS, and 79.88% were in 'category C = monitor' according to the Lexicomp® database. In a study evaluating the prevalence of potential DDIs in the NICU, 61.4% of these were in category C [21]. In a single-center retrospective study evaluating the causal probability of DDIs, it was determined that 54.5% of clinically relevant DDIs were 'probable' [19]. In our study, clinically relevant DDIs were determined as 'probable' at a lower rate (31.57 %). Accordingly, it is understood that the vast majority of DDIs are potentially ongoing, and monitoring is sufficient for these DDIs without the need for any intervention such as drug change, dose change, or drug discontinuation.

While 29–50% of potential DDIs were classified as major in two studies conducted in the NICU, only 12.5% of DDIs were classified in the D or X category in our study [7,25]. In another study conducted in the NICU, 37.5% of potential DDIs were determined as severe or contraindicated [20].

When the DDIs were examined on causal probability (DIPS), only three potential DDIs were identified as 'highly probable'. These DDIs were observed for amiodarone–flecainide (day 3 of use), midazolam–fentanyl (day 3 of use), and ciprofloxacin–phenytoin (day 5 of use) (Table 2). For a full overview of the ADRs observed, refer to Table 2.

In the literature, the use of CPOE itself has not been associated with a significant decrease in the rate of DDIs [4]. Therefore, there is a need for further development of a clinical decision support system (CDSS) with ML algorithms within CPOE systems. Most of the alerts generated by the legacy CDSS were related to DDIs and dosages [26]. Although there are theoretical and review ML studies on DDI extraction from the biomedical literature [27], DrugBank and other databases [28,29], bioinformatics algorithms to predict DDI [30], and clinical safety DDI information retrieval [31], there are no real-life studies that reflect clinical practice in neonates.

In our study, due to the balanced distribution of the patients with and without the DDI, the high-performance model that predicts whether a DDI will occur in a patient with ML algorithms has been designed successfully. According to this model, the most important variables used in the prediction were, respectively: the total number of anti-infective drugs; the total number of drugs; and nervous system, endocrine system, cardiovascular system, respiratory system, and anti-infective drugs (AUC: 0.929). Our study hereby confirms previously reported cohorts, with polypharmacy as a risk factor for potential DDI in the NICU (OR: 1.60; $p < 0.01$) and PICU (≥ 11 prescribed medicines; $p < 0.001$) [7,25]. Similar to our study, polypharmacy (OR: 4.8) and respiratory system drugs (OR: 3.8) were the main risk factors associated with an increased incidence of DDIs in children with respiratory disorders [32].

According to a study in which the DIPS, which was also used in our study, was used in cardiovascular diseases, the predictive ability of probability scores showed good performance (AUC: 0.800, $p < 0.001$) [33]. In our study, the model predicting the presence of DDIs with ML algorithms showed a higher predictive ability (AUC: 0.929). In a study in which more than 74,000 DDIs from 572 different drugs in DrugBank (only theoretical information) were converted into a prediction model using deep learning techniques using protein binding, substrate, and enzyme, the accuracy and AUC were found to be, respectively, 0.885 and 0.921 [28]. In our real-life study, solely based on clinical data of newborns, accuracy and AUC values were higher (accuracy: 0.944, AUC: 0.929), although the number of patients and DDIs were lower. There are no ML-based studies in the literature that predict whether DDIs will occur during the period from hospitalization to discharge using clinical data.

It is reasonable to suggest that such prediction models could be instrumental in the evolution to precision medicine, with the identification of a subgroup of patients at high risk of DDI, instead of the alert fatigue related to an overload of automated alerts [26]. The limited duration of the study, number of patients, and absence of patient and health service (policy) heterogeneity due to the double-center study design are limitations. Due to the limited number of patients in a prospective study design, other parameters (risk category, ADRs, etc.) could not be included as output variables because it reduces the model performance.

5. Conclusions

To our knowledge, this is the first study in the literature to predict the presence of DDI using risk analysis and ML algorithms. Clinically significant DDIs were predicted with high performance according to risk analysis in neonates with PK and PD properties quite different from the pediatric and adult population. In this context, it is important to predict the likelihood of a DDI event as part of precision medicine and individualized treatment regimens.

Supplementary Materials: The following supporting information can be downloaded at: https://www.mdpi.com/article/10.3390/jcm11164715/s1, Table S1: Distribution of drugs used by patients included in the study (n = 2280).

Author Contributions: Conceptualization, N.Y. and M.K.; Methodology, N.Y.; Software, M.K.; Validation, N.Y., M.K. and K.D.; Formal Analysis, K.A.; Investigation, H.T.Ç.; Resources, N.Y.; Data Curation, N.Y.; Writing—Original Draft Preparation, N.Y. and M.K.; Writing—Review and Editing, N.Y. and K.A.; Visualization, K.D.; Supervision, Ş.Y. and M.Y.; Project Administration, K.D. All authors have read and agreed to the published version of the manuscript.

Funding: This research received no external funding.

Institutional Review Board Statement: The study was conducted according to the guidelines of the Declaration of Helsinki, and approved by the Ethics Committee of Hacettepe University (protocol code 2020/11-21 and date of approval 14.04.2020).

Informed Consent Statement: Informed consent was obtained from all subjects involved in the study.

Data Availability Statement: The data presented in this study are available on request from the corresponding author. The data are not publicly available due to restrictions privacy and ethical.

Acknowledgments: The authors would like to thank all of the study participants' parents, pediatricians, and neonatology specialists for their assistance with study data collection.

Conflicts of Interest: The authors declare no conflict of interest.

References

1. Piekos, S.; Pope, C.; Ferrara, A.; Zhong, X.B. Impact of Drug Treatment at Neonatal Ages on Variability of Drug Metabolism and Drug-drug Interactions in Adult Life. *Curr. Pharmacol. Rep.* **2017**, *3*, 1–9. [CrossRef] [PubMed]
2. Bhatt-Mehta, V. "Potential" Drug-Drug Interactions and the PICU: Should We Worry About ICU Polypharmacy? *Pediatr. Crit. Care Med.* **2016**, *17*, 470–472. [CrossRef] [PubMed]
3. Lima, E.D.C.; Camarinha, B.D.; Ferreira Bezerra, N.C.; Panisset, A.G.; de Souza, R.B.; Silva, M.T.; Lopes, L.C. Severe Potential Drug-Drug Interactions and the Increased Length of Stay of Children in Intensive Care Unit. *Front. Pharmacol.* **2020**, *11*, 555407. [CrossRef] [PubMed]
4. Lebowitz, M.B.; Olson, K.L.; Burns, M.; Harper, M.B.; Bourgeois, F. Drug-Drug Interactions Among Hospitalized Children Receiving Chronic Antiepileptic Drug Therapy. *Hosp. Pediatr.* **2016**, *6*, 282–289. [CrossRef]
5. Yeh, M.L.; Chang, Y.J.; Yeh, S.J.; Huang, L.J.; Yen, Y.T.; Wang, P.Y.; Li, Y.C.; Hsu, C.Y. Potential drug-drug interactions in pediatric outpatient prescriptions for newborns and infants. *Comput. Methods Programs Biomed.* **2014**, *113*, 15–22. [CrossRef]
6. Leape, L.L.; Bates, D.W.; Cullen, D.J.; Cooper, J.; Demonaco, H.J.; Gallivan, T.; Hallisey, R.; Ives, J.; Laird, N.; Laffel, G.; et al. Systems analysis of adverse drug events. ADE Prevention Study Group. *JAMA* **1995**, *274*, 35–43. [CrossRef]
7. Costa, H.T.; Leopoldino, R.W.D.; da Costa, T.X.; Oliveira, A.G.; Martins, R.R. Drug-drug interactions in neonatal intensive care: A prospective cohort study. *Pediatr. Neonatol.* **2021**, *62*, 151–157. [CrossRef]
8. Kearns, G.L.; Abdel-Rahman, S.M.; Alander, S.W.; Blowey, D.L.; Leeder, J.S.; Kauffman, R.E. Developmental pharmacology-Drug disposition, action, and therapy in infants and children. *N. Engl. J. Med.* **2003**, *349*, 1157–1167. [CrossRef]
9. Salerno, S.N.; Edginton, A.; Gerhart, J.G.; Laughon, M.M.; Ambalavanan, N.; Sokol, G.M.; Hornik, C.D.; Stewart, D.; Mills, M.; Martz, K.; et al. Physiologically-Based Pharmacokinetic Modeling Characterizes the CYP3A-Mediated Drug-Drug Interaction between Fluconazole and Sildenafil in Infants. *Clin. Pharmacol. Ther.* **2021**, *109*, 253–262. [CrossRef]
10. Percha, B.; Altman, R.B. Informatics confronts drug-drug interactions. *Trends Pharmacol. Sci.* **2013**, *34*, 178–184. [CrossRef]
11. Horn, J.R.; Hansten, P.D.; Chan, L.N. Proposal for a new tool to evaluate drug interaction cases. *Ann. Pharmacother.* **2007**, *41*, 674–680. [CrossRef] [PubMed]
12. Lexicomp Online, Drug Interactions Online. Waltham, MA: UpToDate. Available online: https://online.lexi.com (accessed on 7 March 2022).

13. Kuhn, M. Caret: Classification and Regression Training. R Package Version, 6, 0–85. Available online: https://cran.r-project.org/web/packages/caret/index.html (accessed on 14 March 2022).
14. Yamada, I.; Miyasaka, N.; Kobayashi, D.; Wakana, K.; Oshima, N.; Wakabayashi, A.; Sakamoto, J.; Saida, Y.; Tateishi, U.; Eishi, Y. Endometrial Carcinoma: Texture Analysis of Apparent Diffusion Coefficient Maps and Its Correlation with Histopathologic Findings and Prognosis. *Radiol. Imaging Cancer* **2019**, *1*, e190054. [CrossRef] [PubMed]
15. Robin, X.; Turck, N.; Hainard, A.; Tiberti, N.; Lisacek, F.; Sanchez, J.-C.; Müller, M. pROC: An open-source package for R and S+ to analyze and compare ROC curves. *BMC Bioinform.* **2011**, *12*, 77. [CrossRef] [PubMed]
16. Saito, T.; Rehmsmeier, M. Precrec: Fast and accurate precision–recall and ROC curve calculations in R. *Bioinformatics* **2017**, *33*, 145–147. [CrossRef]
17. Wickham, H.; Chang, W.; Henry, L.; Pedersen, T.; Takahashi, K.; Wilke, C.; Woo, K.; Yutani, H.; Dunnington, D. RStudio. Ggplot2: Elegant Graphics for Data Analysis; Springer: New York, NY, USA, 2016.
18. Stark, A.; Smith, P.B.; Hornik, C.P.; Zimmerman, K.O.; Hornik, C.D.; Pradeep, S.; Clark, R.H.; Benjamin, D.K., Jr.; Laughon, M.; Greenberg, R.G. Medication Use in the Neonatal Intensive Care Unit and Changes from 2010 to 2018. *J. Pediatr.* **2022**, *240*, 66–71.e4. [CrossRef]
19. Choi, Y.H.; Lee, I.H.; Yang, M.; Cho, Y.S.; Jo, Y.H.; Bae, H.J.; Kim, Y.S.; Park, J.D. Clinical significance of potential drug-drug interactions in a pediatric intensive care unit: A single-center retrospective study. *PLoS ONE* **2021**, *16*, e0246754. [CrossRef]
20. Rosen, K.; Wiesen, M.H.; Oberthur, A.; Michels, G.; Roth, B.; Fietz, C.; Muller, C. Drug-drug interactions in Neonatal Intensive Care Units: How to overcome a challenge. *Minerva Pediatr.* **2021**, *73*, 188–197. [CrossRef]
21. Nasrollahi, S.; Meera, N.K. Prevalence of Potential Drug-Drug Interactions in Neonatal Intensive Care Unit of a Tertiary Care Hospital: A Prospective Observational Study. *Int. J. Life Sci. Pharma Res.* **2020**, *10*, P40–P45. [CrossRef]
22. Abouelkheir, M.; Alsubaie, S. Pediatric acute kidney injury induced by concomitant vancomycin and piperacillin-tazobactam. *Pediatr. Int.* **2018**, *60*, 136–141. [CrossRef]
23. Spriet, I.; Goyens, J.; Meersseman, W.; Wilmer, A.; Willems, L.; Van Paesschen, W. Interaction between valproate and meropenem: A retrospective study. *Ann. Pharmacother.* **2007**, *41*, 1130–1136. [CrossRef]
24. Antoon, J.W.; Hall, M.; Herndon, A.; Carroll, A.; Ngo, M.L.; Freundlich, K.L.; Stassun, J.C.; Frost, P.; Johnson, D.P.; Chokshi, S.B.; et al. Prevalence of Clinically Significant Drug-Drug Interactions Across US Children's Hospitals. *Pediatrics* **2020**, *146*, e20200858. [CrossRef] [PubMed]
25. Ismail, M.; Aziz, S.; Noor, S.; Haider, I.; Shams, F.; Haq, I.; Khadim, F.; Khan, Q.; Khan, F.; Asif, M. Potential drug-drug interactions in pediatric patients admitted to intensive care unit of Khyber Teaching Hospital, Peshawar, Pakistan: A cross-sectional study. *J. Crit. Care* **2017**, *40*, 243–250. [CrossRef] [PubMed]
26. Segal, G.; Segev, A.; Brom, A.; Lifshitz, Y.; Wasserstrum, Y.; Zimlichman, E. Reducing drug prescription errors and adverse drug events by application of a probabilistic, machine-learning based clinical decision support system in an inpatient setting. *J. Am. Med. Inform. Assoc.* **2019**, *26*, 1560–1565. [CrossRef] [PubMed]
27. Zhang, T.; Leng, J.; Liu, Y. Deep learning for drug-drug interaction extraction from the literature: A review. *Brief Bioinform.* **2020**, *21*, 1609–1627. [CrossRef]
28. Deng, Y.; Xu, X.; Qiu, Y.; Xia, J.; Zhang, W.; Liu, S. A multimodal deep learning framework for predicting drug-drug interaction events. *Bioinformatics* **2020**, *36*, 4316–4322. [CrossRef]
29. Kastrin, A.; Ferk, P.; Leskosek, B. Predicting potential drug-drug interactions on topological and semantic similarity features using statistical learning. *PLoS ONE* **2018**, *13*, e0196865. [CrossRef]
30. Han, K.; Cao, P.; Wang, Y.; Xie, F.; Ma, J.; Yu, M.; Wang, J.; Xu, Y.; Zhang, Y.; Wan, J. A Review of Approaches for Predicting Drug-Drug Interactions Based on Machine Learning. *Front. Pharmacol.* **2021**, *12*, 814858. [CrossRef]
31. Xie, W.; Wang, L.; Cheng, Q.; Wang, X.; Wang, Y.; Bi, H.; He, B.; Feng, W. Integrated Random Negative Sampling and Uncertainty Sampling in Active Learning Improve Clinical Drug Safety Drug-Drug Interaction Information Retrieval. *Front. Pharmacol.* **2020**, *11*, 582470. [CrossRef]
32. Hassanzad, M.; Tashayoie Nejad, S.; Mahboobipour, A.A.; Salem, F.; Baniasadi, S. Potential drug-drug interactions in hospitalized pediatric patients with respiratory disorders: A retrospective review of clinically important interactions. *Drug Metab. Pers. Ther.* **2020**, *35*. [CrossRef]
33. Kovacevic, M.; Kovacevic, S.V.; Radovanovic, S.; Stevanovic, P.; Miljkovc, B. Adverse drug reactions caused by drug-drug interactions in cardiovascular disease patients: Introduction of a simple prediction tool using electronic screening database items. *Curr. Med. Res. Opin.* **2019**, *35*, 1873–1883. [CrossRef]

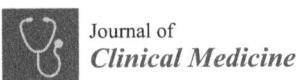

Article

Efficacy and Safety of Empagliflozin in Type 2 Diabetes Mellitus Saudi Patients as Add-On to Antidiabetic Therapy: A Prospective, Open-Label, Observational Study

Fahad M. Althobaiti [1,2,3], Safaa M. Alsanosi [1,4,*], Alaa H. Falemban [1,3], Abdullah R. Alzahrani [1,3], Salma A. Fataha [2], Sara O. Salih [2], Ali M. Alrumaih [5], Khalid N. Alotaibi [5], Hazim M. Althobaiti [6], Saeed S. Al-Ghamdi [1,3] and Nahla Ayoub [1,3,7,*]

1. Department of Pharmacology and Toxicology, Faculty of Medicine, Umm Al-Qura University (UQU), Makkah 21955, Saudi Arabia
2. Department of Endocrine and Diabetes, Armed Forces Hospital, Southern Region, Khamis Mushait 61961, Saudi Arabia
3. Saudi Toxicology Society, Umm Al-Qura University (UQU), Makkah 21955, Saudi Arabia
4. Institute of Cardiovascular and Medical Sciences, University of Glasgow, Glasgow G12 8QQ, UK
5. Ministry of Defence, Riyadh 11159, Saudi Arabia
6. King Faisal Medical City, Taif 26514, Saudi Arabia
7. Department of Pharmacognosy, Faculty of Pharmacy, Ain-Shams University, Cairo 11566, Egypt
* Correspondence: smsanosi@uqu.edu.sa (S.M.A.); naayoub@uqu.edu.sa (N.A.); Tel.: +966-504504080 (S.M.A.); +966-532190083 (N.A.)

Abstract: The Saudi Food and Drug Authority (SFDA) approved sodium-glucose cotransporter-2 (SGLT2) inhibitors in 2018. The efficacy and safety of empagliflozin (EMPA) have been confirmed in the U.S., Europe, and Japan for patients with type 2 diabetes mellitus (T2DM); however, analogous evidence is lacking for Saudi T2DM patients. Therefore, the current study aimed to assess the efficacy and safety of EMPA in Saudi patients (n = 256) with T2DM. This is a 12-week prospective, open-label, observational study. Adult Saudi patients with T2DM who had not been treated with EMPA before enrolment were eligible. The exclusion criteria included T2DM patients less than 18 years of age, adults with type one diabetes, pregnant women, paediatric population. The results related to efficacy included a significant decrease in haemoglobin A1c (HbA1c) (adjusted mean difference −0.93% [95% confidence interval (CI) −0.32, −1.54]), significant improvements in fasting plasma glucose (FPG) (−2.28 mmol/L [95% CI −2.81, −1.75]), and a reduction in body weight (−0.874 kg [95% CI −4.36, −6.10]) following the administration of 25 mg of EMPA once daily as an add-on to ongoing antidiabetic therapy after 12 weeks. The primary safety endpoints were the change in the mean blood pressure (BP) values, which indicated significantly reduced systolic and diastolic BP (−3.85 mmHg [95% CI −6.81, −0.88] and −0.06 mmHg [95% CI −0.81, −0.88], respectively) and pulse rate (−1.18 [95% CI −0.79, −3.15]). In addition, kidney function was improved, with a significant reduction in the urine albumin/creatinine ratio (UACR) (−1.76 mg/g [95% CI −1.07, −34.25]) and a significant increase in the estimated glomerular filtration rate (eGFR) (3.54 mL/min/1.73 m^2 [95% CI 2.78, 9.87]). Furthermore, EMPA reduced aminotransferases (ALT) in a pattern (reduction in ALT > AST). The adjusted mean difference in the change in ALT was −2.36 U/L [95% CI −1.031, −3.69], while it was −1.26 U/L [95% CI −0.3811, −2.357] for AST and −1.98 U/L [95% CI −0.44, −3.49] for GGT. Moreover, in the EMPA group, serum high-density lipoprotein (HDL) significantly increased (0.29 mmol/L [95% CI 0.74, 0.15]), whereas a nonsignificant increase was seen in low-density lipoprotein (LDL) (0.01 mmol/L [95% CI 0.19, 0.18]) along with a significant reduction in plasma triglyceride (TG) levels (−0.43 mmol/L [95% CI −0.31, −1.17]). Empagliflozin once daily is an efficacious and tolerable strategy for treating Saudi patients with insufficiently controlled T2DM as an add-on to ongoing antidiabetic therapy.

Keywords: empagliflozin; safety; efficacy; Saudi patients; type 2 diabetes mellitus

---

Citation: Althobaiti, F.M.; Alsanosi, S.M.; Falemban, A.H.; Alzahrani, A.R.; Fataha, S.A.; Salih, S.O.; Alrumaih, A.M.; Alotaibi, K.N.; Althobaiti, H.M.; Al-Ghamdi, S.S.; et al. Efficacy and Safety of Empagliflozin in Type 2 Diabetes Mellitus Saudi Patients as Add-On to Antidiabetic Therapy: A Prospective, Open-Label, Observational Study. *J. Clin. Med.* **2022**, *11*, 4769. https://doi.org/10.3390/jcm11164769

Academic Editors: Alfredo Vannacci, Niccolò Lombardi and Giada Crescioli

Received: 4 July 2022
Accepted: 12 August 2022
Published: 16 August 2022

Publisher's Note: MDPI stays neutral with regard to jurisdictional claims in published maps and institutional affiliations.

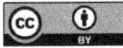

Copyright: © 2022 by the authors. Licensee MDPI, Basel, Switzerland. This article is an open access article distributed under the terms and conditions of the Creative Commons Attribution (CC BY) license (https://creativecommons.org/licenses/by/4.0/).

1. Introduction

The growing burden of type 2 diabetes mellites (T2DM) is a crucial issue in health care worldwide. T2DM continues to increase in prevalence and incidence and is a significant cause of human suffering and death. Despite sizable investments in clinical care, research, and public health interventions, there appears to be no signal of reduction in the rate of disease increase [1]. According to the World Health Organisation (WHO), Saudi Arabia has the second highest diabetes prevalence of all Middle Eastern countries (7th in the world), with an estimated population of seven million individuals living with diabetes and more than three million with prediabetes [2–4]. Moreover, by 2030, this number is expected to more than double [5].

EMPA was approved by the U.S. Food and Drug Administration (FDA) in 2014 as an adjunct to diet and exercise to improve glycaemic control in adults with T2DM [6]. EMPA is a selective sodium-glucose cotransporter 2 (SGLT2) inhibitor. It is characterised by its unique mechanism as a hypoglycaemic agent. Specifically, it depends on enhancing glycosuria away from insulin independence. This unique mechanism enables EMPA to achieve controllable hypoglycaemic action [7]. Studies conducted in the USA, Canada, UK, and Japan have recommended using EMPA alone or together with other anti-diabetic agents as a cost-effective oral treatment for T2DM once daily [8]. Many clinical trials have reported the antihyperglycemic effect of EMPA due to a reduction in haemoglobin A1c (HbA1c) and fasting plasma glucose (FPG) levels [9–12]. In addition, EMPA is reported to reduce body weight, waist circumference, and body fat index in patients with T2DM [13,14].

In 2016, the U.S. FDA approved EMPA to reduce the risk of cardiovascular death in adult patients with T2DM and cardiovascular disease. Many studies have documented the relative reductions in the risk of cardiovascular death and hospitalisation with EMPA versus placebo [7,15–18]. In addition, EMPA causes significant natriuresis [19], rapid reductions in pulmonary artery pressure, and reduced LV volumes in patients with heart failure and reduced ejection fraction (HFrEF) [20–22]. The cellular mechanism by which EMPA improves cardiovascular outcomes is its ability to stimulate erythropoiesis via an early increase in erythropoietin production in people with T2DM [23]. Early administration of EMPA may attenuate changes in extracellular water and intracellular water (ICW) in patients with acute myocardial infarction [24].

EMPA slows the progressive decline in kidney function in patients with HFrEF, with or without diabetes [25,26]. The short- and long-term benefits of EMPA on urinary albumin excretion have also been shown [27]. In addition, the haemodynamic effects of EMPA associated with lower glomerular pressure may contribute to the long-term preservation of renal function. [28]. Furthermore, EMPA improved glycaemic control in renal transplant recipients with post-transplantation diabetes mellitus (PTDM) compared with a placebo [29]. Sattar et al. proved that EMPA reduces liver enzymes ALT and AST in patients with T2DM in a pattern consistent with a reduction in liver fat, particularly when ALT levels are high [30–32].

Several studies have reported the safety and efficacy of EMPA for T2DM [11,33–35]. EMPA was the first in class to not only demonstrate safe SGLT2 inhibition but also cardio- and reno-protective effects in an adequately powered cardiovascular outcome trial [36]. However, EMPA was associated with an increased risk of hypoglycaemia and genital and urinary tract infections [37].

The Saudi Food and Drug Authority (SFDA) approved SGLT2 inhibitors in 2018 [38]. The current SFDA-approved drugs in this class include canagliflozin, dapagliflozin, and EMPA. Based on the literature, the efficacy and safety of empagliflozin have been confirmed in the U.S., Europe, and Japan for patients with T2DM; however, analogous evidence is lacking for Saudi T2DM patients. Therefore, we assessed the efficacy and safety of empagliflozin as an add-on to ongoing antidiabetic therapy in Saudi adult patients with T2DM in the Armed Forces Hospital, Southern Region between June and December 2021.

2. Materials and Methods

2.1. Study Design and Patients

This was a prospective, open-label, observational clinical study conducted at the Endocrine and Diabetes Centre of the Armed Forces Hospital, Southern Region (Saudi Arabia) between June and December 2021. The study protocol was approved by the Armed Forces Hospital, Southern Region Research Ethics Committee (Number: AFH-SRMREC/2021/PHARMACY/503). All participants provided signed and dated informed consent prior to screening.

Saudi adult participants aged ≥ 18 to <80 years were screened to determine whether they met the inclusion criteria: Adult Saudi patients with T2DM in the Endocrine and Diabetes Centre of the Armed Forces Hospital, Southern Region in Saudi Arabia. Patients who had not been treated with EMPA before enrolment were eligible. The exclusion criteria included T2DM patients less than 18 years of age, adults with type one diabetes, and pregnant women. The study population had no cardiovascular or renal disease.

This study was designed to assess the safety and efficacy of EMPA in Saudi adult patients with T2DM. Efficacy and safety analyses were based on a comparison between variables before treatment (baseline group) and in the patients treated with EMPA (25 mg/once daily) for 12 weeks (EMPA group). Efficacy measurements included changes from baseline in HbA1c levels, fasting plasma glucose (FPG) and body weight at week 12. Safety assessments included changes in BP (SBP and DBP), pulse rate, kidney markers (urine albumin/creatinine ratio (UACR) and estimated glomerular filtration rate (eGFR)), liver markers (AST, ALT, and GGT), and serum lipids (LDL-c, HDL-c, and TG) at week 12 [39].

2.2. Patient Demographics at Baseline

Sample size calculations were based on a previous study of empagliflozin with insulin, which suggested that empagliflozin would result in an HbA1c reduction of ~0.5% versus placebo after 12 weeks of treatment, and a standard deviation (SD) of 1.0% [33]. The sample size was 256 patients (113 males and 234 females) with the following characteristics: mean age 58.9 years; males 58.2 and females 59.4. Of 256 patients, 234 (91%) had been diagnosed with T2DM longer than five years, and 22 (9%) had been diagnosed for one to five years. Participating patients had insufficient glycaemic control at baseline, with HbA1c levels $\geq 7\%$ in 251 patients (97.6%). Further, 167 patients (65%) had HbA1c levels ≥ 9 despite receiving insulin (156, 64%) or OHA (93, 36%) (Table 1).

Table 1. Patient demographics.

Patient Demographics	
Sample volume, n	256
Age (years), mean (SD)	58.9 (10.75)
Sex Males, n	113
Females, n	143
Male age, mean (SD)	58.2 (11.88)
Female age, mean (SD)	59.4 (9.76)
Duration since Diagnosis of T2DM, (years)	
Mean (SD)	16.7 (8.47)
<1, n (%)	0
1 to 5	22 (9%)
>5	234 (91%)
DM Treatment before Empagliflozin	
Insulin + OHA (metformin)	156 (64%)
OHA (metformin)	93 (36%)

SD: Standard deviation, T2DM: Type 2 diabetes mellitus, DM: Diabetes mellitus, OHA: Orally administered antihyperglycemic.

2.3. Data Analysis

SPSS (Version 27.0, IBM, Armonk, NY, USA) was employed for statistical analysis using the *t*-test for two independent samples to determine the rate of change in the means of the two samples, standard deviations, and the level of confidence, which is estimated at 0.05.

Confidence domain: If the level of significance required by researchers is 5%, then the confidence level should be 95%. Thus, the confidence interval contains the possible values of the statistical parameter, which, when subjected to a statistical test using the same sample, will not be rejected. The level of statistical significance for all samples studied was less than 5%, which means that all rates of change in the mean were within the confidence range.

3. Results

3.1. Efficacy

The primary efficacy endpoints were changes in HbA1c, FPG, and body weight from baseline at week 12 (EMPA group). The mean value of HbA1c decreased from 9.77 ± 1.76 to 8.85 ± 4.83 with a change of -0.93 (-0.32, -1.54) at a rate of (-0.106) within the confidence interval estimated CI at 95%. In addition, 181 participants (72%) experienced a reduction in HbA1c $\geq 0.5\%$ from baseline. Further, the number of participants with HbA1c $\geq 9\%$ decreased from 167 (65%) to 77 (30%), corresponding to an increase in the proportion of individuals with HbA1c levels $\geq 8\%$ to $<9\%$, $\geq 7\%$ to $<8\%$, and $<7.0\%$ of (80 to 82), (4 to 76), and (5 to 21), respectively. For participants on insulin and OHA (metformin) therapies (156, 64%), there was a reduction in mean HbA1c % from 9.94 ± 1.84 to 8.66 ± 1.47, a change of -1.28 (-1.03, -1.53) at a rate -0.147, accompanied by a reduction in insulin units from 9.94 ± 1.84 to 8.67 ± 1.47 (change -1.27). Meanwhile, for those on OHA only, the reduction in HBA1c % was from 9.46 ± 1.56 to 8.31 ± 1.26 with a change of -1.11 (-0.799, -1.42).

The mean value of FPG reduced from 11.22 ± 4.79 to 8.95 ± 3.37, a change of -2.28 (-2.81, -1.75) at a rate of (-0.25) and a 95% CI. A total of 63 participants had FPG levels <7.8 at baseline increased to 115 at week 12. Individuals with FPG levels from 7.8 to <11.0 (80 to 86), while the number with FPG levels ≥ 11 decreased from 113 to 55. Mean body weight decreased from 89.99 ± 18.09 to 88.03 ± 18.47 with a change of -0.874 (-4.36, -6.10) at a rate of -0.02 (Tables 2 and 3 and Figure 1).

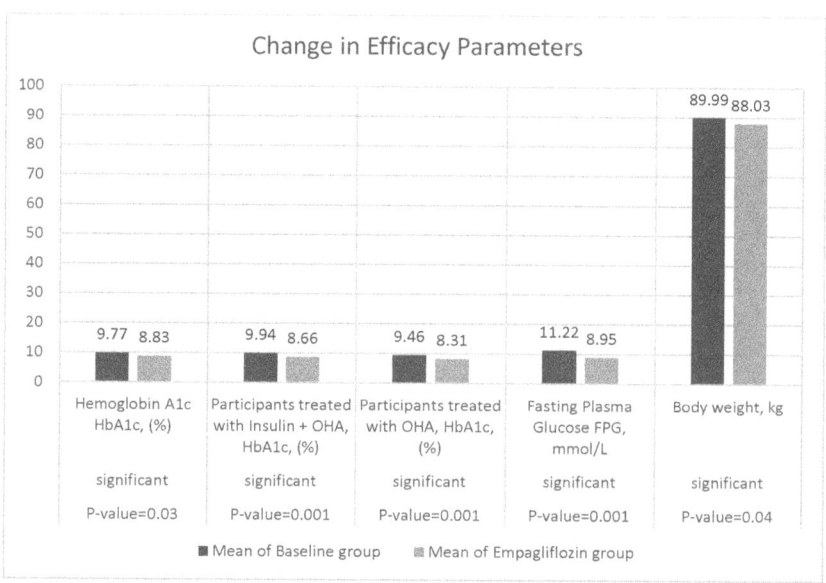

Figure 1. Change from baseline in HbA1c%, FPG mmol/L, and body weight kg at week 12 (*t*-test).

Table 2. Efficacy and Safety Parameters at baseline and week 12.

	Baseline Group Mean (SD)	Empagliflozin Group Mean (SD)	Change Amount
Efficacy:			
Haemoglobin A1c HbA1c, (%)	9.77 ± 1.76	8.85 ± 4.83	−0.92
Participants treated with Insulin + OHA, HbA1c, (%)	9.94 ± 1.84	8.66 ± 1.47	−1.27
Participants treated with OHA, HbA1c, (%)	9.46 ± 1.56	8.31 ± 1.26	−1.15
Fasting Plasma Glucose FPG, mmol/L	11.27 ± 4.79	8.95 ± 3.37	−2.32
Body weight, kg	89.99 ± 18.09	88.03 ± 18.47	−1.96
Safety:			
Systolic Blood Pressure SBP, mmHg	142.6 ± 19.45	138.8 ± 20.23	−3.8
Diastolic Blood Pressure DBP, mmHg	79.6 ± 20.32	79.4 ± 21.14	−0.2
Pulse Rate, (bpm)	85.98 ± 11.33	84.80 ± 13.52	−1.18
Kidney Function Status			
Urine Albumin/Creatinine Ratio UACR (mg/g)	20.39 ± 43.72	17.12 ± 40.05	−3.27
eGFR, mL/min/1.73 m^2	51.12 ± 120.45	72.51 ± 22.80	21.39
Liver Function Status			
Aspartate aminotransferase AST, U/L	22.92 ± 8.10	21.65 ± 6.38	−1.26
Alanine aminotransferase ALT, U/L	25.96 ± 8.09	23.91 ± 11.71	−0.70
A gamma-glutamyl transferase (GGT), U/L	30.29 ± 25.15	27.12 ± 18.32	−4.31
LDL- cholesterol, mmol/L	2.543 ± 0.93	2.544 ± 1.50	0.0009
HDL- cholesterol, mmol/L	1.69 ± 3.59	1.98 ± 0.22	0.29
Triglycerides TG, mmol/L	2.11 ± 5.90	1.66 ± 0.20	−0.45

HbA1c: haemoglobin A1c (glycosylated haemoglobin), FPG: fasting plasma glucose, SD: standard deviation, OHA: Orally administered antihyperglycemic, eGFR: Estimated glomerular filtration rate, LDL: Low-density lipoprotein, HDL: High-density lipoprotein, AST: Aspartate aminotransferase, ALT: Alanine transaminase and TG: Triglycerides. A comparison between Empagliflozin-treated group at week 12 with the same group at bassline. Data are n (%) or mean (SD).

Table 3. Change in Efficacy and Safety Parameters at week 12.

	Baseline Start Treatment Empagliflozin	Change from Baseline at Week 12	Rate of Change
Efficacy variables			
Mean change in HbA1c from baseline, % (95% CI)	−0.93 (−0.32, −1.54)		−0.106
Mean ± SD	−0.93 ± 4.93		
<7.0%	5 (0.02)	21 (0.08)	0.76
≥7% to <8%	4 (0.016)	76 (0.30)	0.95
≥8% to <9%	80 (0.31)	82 (0.32)	0.02
≥9%	167 (0.65)	77 (0.30)	−0.54
Decrease in HbA1c (%) in participants: ≥ 0.5%, n, (%)	181 (0.71)		
Treated with insulin + OHA, HbA1c, (%)	−1.28 (−1.03, −1.53)		−0.147
Treated with OHA, HbA1c (%)	−1.11 (−0.799, −1.42)		−0.139
Decrease in insulin units in participants treated with insulin + OHA	9.94 ± 1.84	8.67 ± 1.47	−1.27
Mean change in FPG from baseline (95% CI)	−2.28 (−2.81, −1.75)		−0.25
Mean ± SD	−2.27 ± 4.22		
<7.8, n, (%)	63 (0.25)	115 (0.45)	0.83
7.8 to <11.0	80 (0.32)	86 (0.34)	0.08
≥11	113 (0.44)	55 (0.21)	−0.51
Mean change in body weight from baseline (95% CI)	−0.874 (−4.36, −6.10)		−0.02
Mean ± SD	−1.96 ± 11.98		

Table 3. Cont.

	Baseline Start Treatment Empagliflozin	Change from Baseline at Week 12	Rate of Change
Safety variables			
Mean change in SBP from baseline, % (95% CI)	−3.85 (−6.81, −0.88)		−0.03
Mean ± SD	−3.82 ± 23.4		
Mean change in DBP from baseline, % (95% CI)	−0.06 (−0.81, −0.88)		−0.001
Mean ± SD	−0.05 ± 0.28		
Mean change in pulse rate from baseline (95% CI)	−1.18 (−0.79, −3.15)		−0.01
Mean ± SD	−1.18 ± 15.46		
Kidney Function Status			
Mean change in Urine Albumin/Creatinine Ratio UACR (mg/g)	−1.76 (−1.07, −34.25)		−0.067
Mean ± SD	−1.76 ± 103.5		
<30, n, (%)	126 (0.50)	177 (0.70)	0.4
30 to <300 n, (%)	51 (0.21)	67 (0.27)	0.31
≥300, n, (%)	75 (0.29)	8 (0.03)	−0.89
Mean change in body eGFR from baseline, kg (95% CI)	3.54 (2.78, 9.87)		−0.418
Mean ± SD	3.54 ± 45.98		
≥90, n, (%)	49 (0.19)	55 (0.21)	0.02
60 to < 90	120 (0.47)	116 (0.45)	−0.018
30 to < 60	87 (0.34)	84 (0.33)	−0.016
Liver Function Status			
Mean change in AST from baseline (95% CI)	−1.26 (−0.3011, −2.227)		−0.058
Mean ± SD	−1.263 ± 7.72		
Mean change in ALT from baseline (95% CI)	−2.36 (−1.031, −3.69)		−0.029
Mean ± SD	−2.36 ± 10.75		
Mean change in GGT from baseline (95% CI)	−4.31 (−2.33, −6.28)		−0.159
Mean ± SD	−4.31 ± 15.66		
Mean change in LDL from baseline (95% CI)	0.005 (0.192, 0.18)		0.0004
Mean ± SD	0.005 ± 1.46		
Mean change in HDL from baseline, kg (95% CI)	0.29 (0.74, 0.15)		0.171
Mean ± SD	0.293 ± 3.61		
Mean change in TG from baseline (95% CI)	−0.43 (−0.31, −1.17)		−0.271
Mean ± SD	−0.45 ± 5.98		

A comparison between EMPA treated group at week 12 with the same group at baseline. Data are n (%) or mean (SD).

3.2. Safety

Safety endpoints included changes in SBP, pulse rate, and kidney and liver function status at week 12. SBP decreased from 142.6 ± 19.45 to 138.8 ± 20.23, a change of −3.85 (−6.81, −0.88) at a rate of −0.03. There was a slight reduction in DBP from 79.6 ± 20.32 to 79.4 ± 21.14, a change of −0.06 (−0.81, −0.88) at a rate of −0.001. Moreover, there was a reduction in pulse rate from 85.98 ± 11.33 to 84.80 ± 13.52, a change of −1.18 (−0.79, −3.15) at a rate of −0.01 (Tables 2 and 3 and Figure 2).

It is apparent from Tables 2 and 3 that kidney function status improved, with a reduction in UACR from 20.39 ± 43.72 to 17.12 ± 40.05 at week 12, a change of −1.76 (−1.07, −34.25) at a rate of −0.067. The number of participants with UACR levels ≥300 decreased from 75 to 8, accompanied by an increase in the number of patients with UACR levels of 30 to <300 and <30 (from 51 to 67 and 126 to 177 patients, respectively). Furthermore, estimated eGFR also increased from 51.12 ± 120.45 to 72.51 ± 22.80, a change of 3.54 (2.78, 9.87) at a rate of 0.418. The number of participants with normal eGFR (≥90) increased from 49 to 55, along with a reduction in the number of participants with mild eGFR (60 to < 90;

from 120 to 116 patients) and moderate-to-severe eGFR (30 to < 60; from 86 to 84 patients). For one participant with severely decreased eGFR (<30), no change was observed (Figure 3).

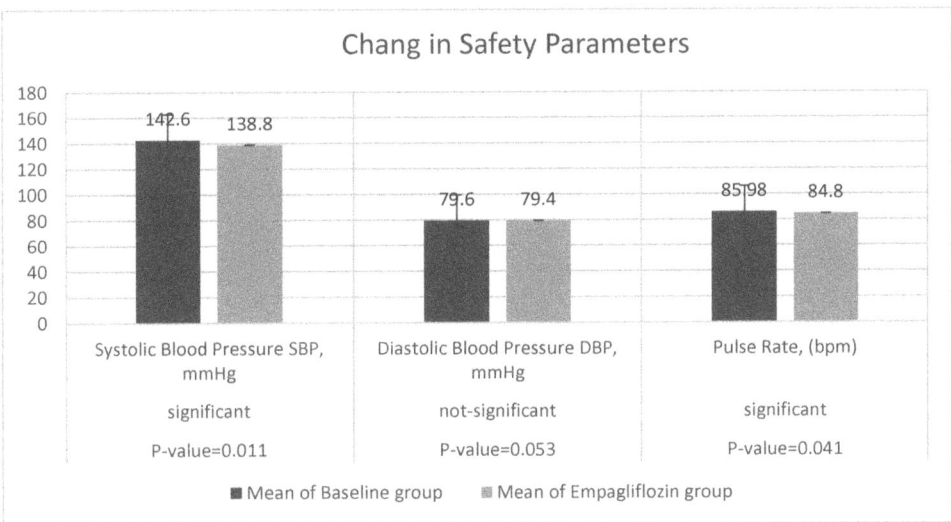

Figure 2. Change from baseline in SBP mmHg, DBP mmHg, and pulse rate bpm at week 12 (*t*-test).

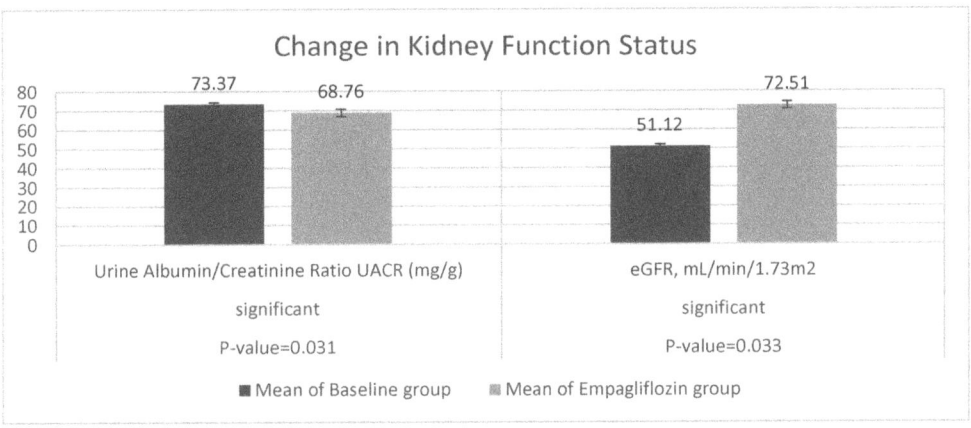

Figure 3. Change from baseline in UACR mg/g and eGFR mL/min/1.73 m^2 at week 12 (*t*-test).

The results shown in Tables 2 and 3 show the rates of change in hepatic function status between the baseline and EMPA groups. AST decreased from 22.92 ± 8.10 to 21.65 ± 6.38, a change of −1.26 (−0.3011, −2.227) at a rate of −0.06. ALT decreased from 25.96 ± 8.09 to 23.91 ± 11.71, a change of −2.36 (−1.03, −3.69) at a rate (−0.029). GGT decreased from 30.29 ± 25.15 to 27.12 ± 18.32, a change of −4.31 (−2.33, −6.28) at a rate of −0.159. Interestingly, lipid profiles improved as well (Tables 2 and 3). HDL increased significantly from 1.69 ± 3.59 to 1.98 ± 0.22, a change of 0.29 (0.74, 0.15) at a rate of 0.171, while LDL increased non-significantly from 2.543 ± 0.93 to 2.544 ±1.50, a change of 0.005 (0.192, 0.18) at a very small rate of 0.0004. Additionally, TG levels decreased from 2.11 ± 5.90 to 1.66 ± 0.20, a change of −0.43 (−0.31, −1.17) at a rate of −0.271 (Figure 4).

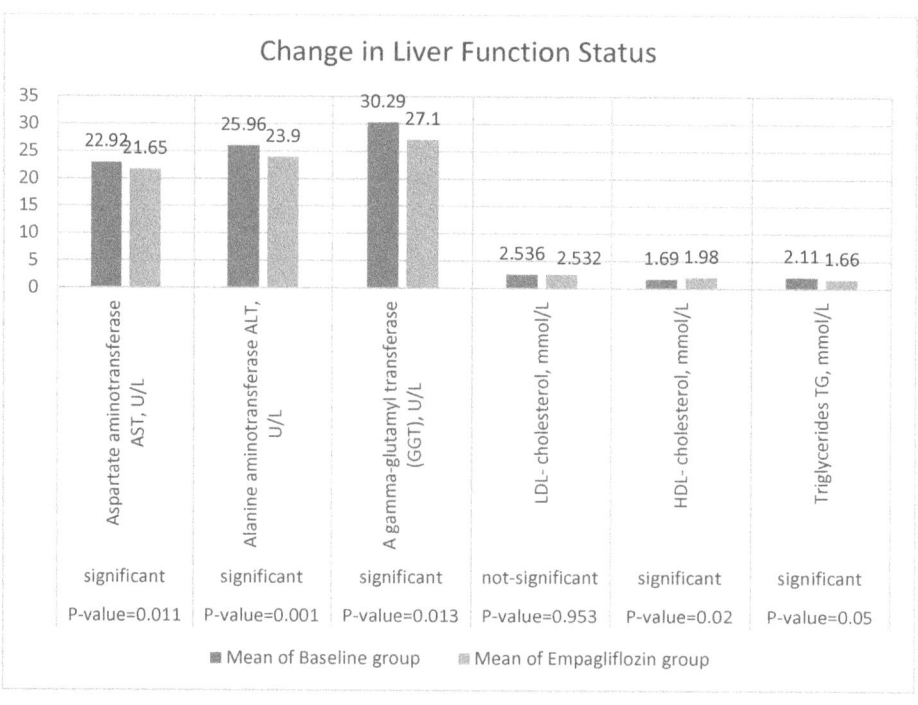

Figure 4. Change from baseline in AST U/l, ALT U/L, GGT U/L, LDL mmol/L, HDL-c mmol/L, and TG mmol/L at week 12 (*t*-test).

4. Discussion

The present study was designed to determine the efficacy and safety of EMPA for Saudi T2DM patients. In this 12-week study, once-daily add-on administration of EMPA (25 mg) resulted in significant decreases in HbA1c, FPG, and body weight for Saudi participants with insufficiently controlled T2DM on insulin or OHA. The meaningful improvement in HbA1c was seen in the participants with HbA1c $\geq$ 9.0, representing 65% of individuals at baseline group. Furthermore, after 12 weeks of treatment, a decrease in HbA1c $\geq$ 0.5% from baseline was recorded in 239 (93%) of the participants receiving 25 mg of EMPA. These findings are in line with those of another study that found that 12-week treatment with EMPA monotherapy resulted in similar reductions in HbA1c, FPG, and body weight compared to a placebo in drug-free patients with T2DM [40]. Reductions in HbA1c, FPG, and body weight were also consistent with those reported from 12-week studies on other SGLT2 inhibitors [33,41,42]. EMPA as an added therapy to insulin resulted in a significant reduction in insulin units, consistent with the results reported by [43]. Control of blood glucose levels is important in diabetic patients but often associated with weight gain [44]. The potential for a reduction in body weight is a notable feature of SGLT2 inhibitors [45,46] and may make them useful agents to combine with other antidiabetic therapies to reduce glucose levels and facilitate weight loss or mitigate any weight gain associated with improved glycaemic control [13]. Caloric loss through urinary glucose excretion may be an important contributor to this effect [22].

The reduction in BP observed in the current study is consistent with a reduction in SBP reported with a 25 mg dose of EMPA [47]. It is conceivable that EMPA stimulates osmotic diuresis through increased glycosuria rather than natriuresis, which may play a role in the potential antihypertensive effects of EMPA [48] and support its mechanism as an inhibitor of the renin–angiotensin system [49]. In addition, in Black individuals with T2DM, EMPA reduced BP although the full antihypertensive effect took $\geq$ 6 months to be fully realised [50]. Moreover, the cardioprotective mechanism of SGLT2 is reported [51]. The hypotheses on SGLT2 mechanisms of action have changed: from simple glycosuric drugs, with consequent glucose lowering, erythropoiesis enhancing, and ketogenesis stimulating, to intracellular sodium-lowering molecules. This provides their consequent cardioprotective effect, which justifies its significant reduction in CV events, especially in populations at higher risk [51]. Hyperglycaemia is a well-established cause of endothelial dysfunction (ED) in the pathophysiology of diabetic complications This abnormal vascular phenotype represents an important risk factor for the genesis of any complication of diabetes, contributing to the pathogenesis of not only macrovascular disease but also microvascular damage. Gliflozins have cardiovascular protective mechanisms of SGLT2 inhibition in patients T2DM and their impact on endothelial function [52].

The present study demonstrated an improvement in kidney function, reduced UCAR, and improved eGFR. Diabetes-associated kidney disease is the most common cause of end-stage renal disease in most countries. Diabetic kidney disease, which develops in approximately 40% of patients with T2DM, further increases the risk of cardio-vascular-related morbidity and mortality [53]. Reported kidney protection with EMPA supports our results [25,54]. It has also been shown that EMPA has a beneficial effect on key efficacy outcomes and slows the rate of kidney function decline in patients with and without chronic kidney disease CKD, regardless of the severity of kidney impairment at baseline [25]. The renal-protective effects of EMPA are likely due to a combination of several mechanisms, including EMPA-associated body weight and BP reductions, diuresis, a shift in substrate utilisation, and activation of tubuloglomerular feedback [53]. In addition, haemodynamic effects of EMPA, associated with a reduction in intraglomerular pressure, may contribute to long-term preservation of kidney function [28]. The fact that SGLT2 inhibition is also associated with small decreases in eGFR over the first 3–4 weeks' treatment suggests that reductions in intraglomerular pressure associated with EMPA may further contribute to the UCAR-lowering effects [55].

Mechanistic insights suggest that ectopic liver fat is probably part of the pathogenic process in diabetes, contributing to hepatic insulin resistance, excess gluconeogenesis, and higher fasting glucose levels [56]. Furthermore, hepatic steatosis due to non-alcoholic fatty liver disease (NAFLD) leads to and is often clinically suspected by increased levels of aminotransferases, with levels of alanine aminotransferase (ALT) exceeding those of aspartate aminotransferase (AST). Elevated ALT levels (typically >40–50 U/l) are common in individuals with type 2 diabetes and for a given serum ALT, and those with type 2 diabetes have more liver fat compared with BMI-, age-, and sex-matched individuals without diabetes [30]. The mechanisms by which empagliflozin might reduce aminotransferases or liver fat are unclear. Data from animal models support a direct effect of empagliflozin on reducing liver fat and improving hepatic glucose handling. In db/db mice, glucose uptake in the liver and kidneys has been reported to be higher in mice treated with empagliflozin than in controls [57].

In this study, EMPA was found to elicit reductions in aminotransferases ALT, AST, and GGT in Saudi patients with T2DM, and the reduction in ALT was greater than the reduction in AST. These results match those observed in an earlier study [58]. This pattern is consistent with a reduction in liver fat, especially when ALT levels are high [30].

One of the most important clinically relevant findings of the current study was the reduction in plasma TG levels and the increase in HDL-c but not LDL-c levels. These findings are in agreement with [58]. The mechanism behind this finding was also reported. Specifically, EMPA increases serum campesterol, a marker of cholesterol absorption, in patients with T2DM. This increase may be associated with SGLT2 inhibitor-induced increases in HDL cholesterol [59]. Further research is needed to investigate the adverse effects of EMPA on Saudi population with T2DM, which have not yet been documented.

5. Conclusions

This is the first study reporting the efficacy and safety of EMPA as an add-on to antidiabetic therapy (insulin or oral hypoglycaemic agent) in Saudi patients with T2DM.

Author Contributions: Conceptualization, F.M.A. and N.A.; methodology, S.A.F., A.M.A., K.N.A. and H.M.A.; software, F.M.A. and N.A.; validation, A.R.A., S.S.A.-G. and N.A.; formal analysis, S.M.A. and S.O.S.; investigation, A.H.F.; resources, F.M.A.; data curation, F.M.A. and N.A.; writing—original draft preparation, F.M.A., S.M.A. and A.H.F.; writing—review and editing, N.A. and S.M.A.; visualization, A.R.A.; supervision, S.S.A.-G.; project administration, N.A.; funding acquisition, N.A. All authors have read and agreed to the published version of the manuscript.

Funding: This research received no external funding.

Institutional Review Board Statement: The study was conducted in accordance with the Declaration of Helsinki and approved by Ethics Committee of the Armed Forces Hospital, Southern Region Research (protocol code AFHSRMREC/2021/PHARMACY/503, 30 June 2021).

Informed Consent Statement: Informed consent was obtained from all subjects involved in the study.

Data Availability Statement: The data that support the findings of this study are openly available from the corresponding author upon reasonable request.

Acknowledgments: The authors would like to thank the Deanship of Scientific Research at Umm Al-Qura University for supporting this work by Grant Code: (22UQU4331100DSR01).

Conflicts of Interest: The authors declare no conflict of interest.

References

1. Khan, M.A.B.; Hashim, M.J.; King, J.K.; Govender, R.D.; Mustafa, H.; Al Kaabi, J. Epidemiology of Type 2 Diabetes-Global Burden of Disease and Forecasted Trends. *J. Epidemiol. Glob. Health* **2020**, *10*, 107–111. [CrossRef]
2. Meo, S.A. Prevalence and future prediction of type 2 diabetes mellitus in the Kingdom of Saudi Arabia: A systematic review of published studies. *JPMA. J. Pak. Med. Assoc.* **2017**, *66*, 722–725.
3. Al Dawish, A.A.; Robert, A.; Braham, M.; Musallam, R.A.; Al Hayek, M.A.; Nasser, A.H. Type 2 Diabetes Mellitus in Saudi Arabia: Major Challenges and Possible Solutions. *Curr. Diabetes Rev.* **2017**, *133*, 59–64.
4. Alotaibi, A.; Perry, L.; Gholizadeh, L.; Al-Ganmi, A. Incidence and prevalence rates of diabetes mellitus in Saudi Arabia: An overview. *J. Epidemiol. Glob. Health* **2017**, *7*, 211–218. [CrossRef]
5. Robert, A.A.; Al Awad, A.D.; Al Dawish, M.A. Current Status of Knowledge and Awareness of Diabetes Mellitus in Saudi Arabia. *Curr. Diabetes Rev.* **2021**, *15*, e101220186818. [CrossRef]
6. FDA. US Food and Drug Adminstration: FDA Approves Jardiance (empagliflozin) to Treat Type 2 Diabetes. Available online: https://www.fda-approves-jardiance-empagliflozin-type-2-diabetes-4064.html (accessed on 1 August 2014).
7. Pan, D.; Xu, L.; Chen, P.; Jiang, H.; Shi, D.; Guo, M. Empagliflozin in Patients With Heart Failure: A Systematic Review and Meta-Analysis of Randomized Controlled Trials. *Front. Cardiovasc. Med.* **2021**, *8*, 683281. [CrossRef]
8. Frampton, J.E. Empagliflozin: A Review in Type 2 Diabetes. *Drugs* **2018**, *78*, 1037–1048. [CrossRef]
9. Ridgefield, C. *Jardiance (Empagliflozin) Tablets [Prescribing Information]*; Boehringer Ingelheim Pharmaceuticals: Ingelheim am Rhein, Germany, 2014.
10. Fala, L. Jardiance (Empagliflozin), an SGLT2 Inhibitor, Receives FDA Approval for the Treatment of Patients with Type 2 Diabetes. *Am. Health Drug Benefits* **2015**, *8*, 92–95.
11. Patorno, E.; Pawar, A.; Wexler, J.; Glynn, J.; Bessette, G.; Paik, J.M.; Najafzadeh, M.; Brodovicz, K.G.; Deruaz-Luyet, A.; Schneeweiss, S. Effectiveness and safety of empagliflozin in routine care patients: Results from the EMPagliflozin compaRative effectIveness and safEty (EMPRISE) study. *Diabetes Obes. Metab.* **2021**, *24*, 442–454. [CrossRef]
12. Liakos, A.; Karagiannis, T.; Athanasiadou, E.; Sarigianni, M.; Mainou, M.; Papatheodorou, K.; Bekiari, E.; Tsapas, A. Efficacy and safety of empagliflozin for type 2 diabetes: A systematic review and meta-analysis. *Diabetes Obes. Metab.* **2014**, *16*, 984–993. [CrossRef]
13. Neeland, I.J.; McGuire, D.K.; Chilton, R.; Crowe, S.; Lund, S.S.; Woerle, H.J.; Broedl, U.C.; Johansen, O.E. Empagliflozin reduces body weight and indices of adipose distribution in patients with type 2 diabetes mellitus. *Diab. Vasc. Dis. Res.* **2016**, *13*, 119–126. [CrossRef]
14. Cherney, D.Z.I.; Cooper, M.E.; Tikkanen, I.; Pfarr, E.; Johansen, O.E.; Woerle, H.J.; Broedl, U.C.; Lund, S.S. Pooled analysis of Phase III trials indicate contrasting influences of renal function on blood pressure, body weight, and HbA1c reductions with empagliflozin. *Kidney Int.* **2018**, *93*, 231–244. [CrossRef]

15. Fitchett, D.; Inzucchi, S.E.; Cannon, C.P.; McGuire, D.K.; Scirica, B.M.; Johansen, O.E.; Sambevski, S.; Kaspers, S.; Pfarr, E.; George, J.T.; et al. Empagliflozin Reduced Mortality and Hospitalization for Heart Failure Across the Spectrum of Cardiovascular Risk in the EMPA-REG OUTCOME Trial. *Circulation* **2019**, *139*, 1384–1395. [CrossRef]
16. Anker, S.D.; Butler, J.; Filippatos, G.; Khan, M.S.; Marx, N.; Lam, C.S.P.; Schnaidt, S.; Ofstad, A.P.; Brueckmann, M.; Jamal, W.; et al. Effect of Empagliflozin on Cardiovascular and Renal Outcomes in Patients With Heart Failure by Baseline Diabetes Status: Results From the EMPEROR-Reduced Trial. *Circulation* **2021**, *143*, 337–349. [CrossRef]
17. Packer, M.; Anker, S.D.; Butler, J.; Filippatos, G.; Pocock, S.J.; Carson, P.; Januzzi, J.; Verma, S.; Tsutsui, H.; Brueckmann, M.; et al. Cardiovascular and Renal Outcomes with Empagliflozin in Heart Failure. *N. Engl. J. Med.* **2020**, *383*, 1413–1424. [CrossRef]
18. Patorno, E.; Pawar, A.; Franklin, J.M.; Najafzadeh, M.; Deruaz-Luyet, A.; Brodovicz, K.G.; Sambevski, S.; Bessette, L.G.; Santiago Ortiz, A.J.; Kulldorff, M.; et al. Empagliflozin and the Risk of Heart Failure Hospitalization in Routine Clinical Care. *Circulation* **2019**, *139*, 2822–2830. [CrossRef]
19. Griffin, M.; Rao, V.S.; Ivey-Miranda, J.; Fleming, J.; Mahoney, D.; Maulion, C.; Suda, N.; Siwakoti, K.; Ahmad, T.; Jacoby, D.; et al. Empagliflozin in Heart Failure: Diuretic and Cardiorenal Effects. *Circulation* **2020**, *142*, 1028–1039. [CrossRef]
20. Lee, M.M.Y.; Brooksbank, K.J.M.; Wetherall, K.; Mangion, K.; Roditi, G.; Campbell, R.T.; Berry, C.; Chong, V.; Coyle, L.; Docherty, K.F.; et al. Effect of Empagliflozin on Left Ventricular Volumes in Patients With Type 2 Diabetes, or Prediabetes, and Heart Failure With Reduced Ejection Fraction (SUGAR-DM-HF). *Circulation* **2021**, *143*, 516–525. [CrossRef]
21. Abraham, W.T.; Lindenfeld, J.; Ponikowski, P.; Agostoni, P.; Butler, J.; Desai, A.S.; Filippatos, G.; Gniot, J.; Fu, M.; Gullestad, L.; et al. Effect of empagliflozin on exercise ability and symptoms in heart failure patients with reduced and preserved ejection fraction, with and without type 2 diabetes. *Eur. Heart J.* **2021**, *42*, 700–710. [CrossRef]
22. Wanner, C.; Lachin, J.M.; Inzucchi, S.E.; Fitchett, D.; Mattheus, M.; George, J.; Woerle, H.J.; Broedl, U.C.; von Eynatten, M.; Zinman, B.; et al. Empagliflozin and Clinical Outcomes in Patients With Type 2 Diabetes Mellitus, Established Cardiovascular Disease, and Chronic Kidney Disease. *Circulation* **2018**, *137*, 119–129. [CrossRef]
23. Mazer, C.D.; Hare, G.M.T.; Connelly, P.W.; Gilbert, R.E.; Shehata, N.; Quan, A.; Teoh, H.; Leiter, L.A.; Zinman, B.; Juni, P.; et al. Effect of Empagliflozin on Erythropoietin Levels, Iron Stores, and Red Blood Cell Morphology in Patients With Type 2 Diabetes Mellitus and Coronary Artery Disease. *Circulation* **2020**, *141*, 704–707. [CrossRef] [PubMed]
24. Hoshika, Y.; Kubota, Y.; Mozawa, K.; Tara, S.; Tokita, Y.; Yodogawa, K.; Iwasaki, Y.K.; Yamamoto, T.; Takano, H.; Tsukada, Y.; et al. Effect of Empagliflozin Versus Placebo on Body Fluid Balance in Patients With Acute Myocardial Infarction and Type 2 Diabetes Mellitus: Subgroup Analysis of the EMBODY Trial. *J. Card. Fail.* **2022**, *28*, 56–64. [CrossRef] [PubMed]
25. Zannad, F.; Ferreira, J.P.; Pocock, S.J.; Zeller, C.; Anker, S.D.; Butler, J.; Filippatos, G.; Hauske, S.J.; Brueckmann, M.; Pfarr, E.; et al. Cardiac and Kidney Benefits of Empagliflozin in Heart Failure Across the Spectrum of Kidney Function: Insights From EMPEROR-Reduced. *Circulation* **2021**, *143*, 310–321. [CrossRef] [PubMed]
26. Wanner, C.; Inzucchi, S.E.; Lachin, J.M.; Fitchett, D.; von Eynatten, M.; Mattheus, M.; Johansen, O.E.; Woerle, H.J.; Broedl, U.C.; Zinman, B.; et al. Empagliflozin and Progression of Kidney Disease in Type 2 Diabetes. *N. Engl. J. Med.* **2016**, *375*, 323–334. [CrossRef] [PubMed]
27. Cherney, D.Z.I.; Zinman, B.; Inzucchi, S.E.; Koitka-Weber, A.; Mattheus, M.; von Eynatten, M.; Wanner, C. Effects of empagliflozin on the urinary albumin-to-creatinine ratio in patients with type 2 diabetes and established cardiovascular disease: An exploratory analysis from the EMPA-REG OUTCOME randomised, placebo-controlled trial. *Lancet Diabetes Endocrinol.* **2017**, *5*, 610–621. [CrossRef]
28. Wanner, C.; Heerspink, H.J.L.; Zinman, B.; Inzucchi, S.E.; Koitka-Weber, A.; Mattheus, M.; Hantel, S.; Woerle, H.J.; Broedl, U.C.; von Eynatten, M.; et al. Empagliflozin and Kidney Function Decline in Patients with Type 2 Diabetes: A Slope Analysis from the EMPA-REG OUTCOME Trial. *J. Am. Soc. Nephrol.* **2018**, *29*, 2755–2769. [CrossRef] [PubMed]
29. Halden, T.A.S.; Kvitne, K.E.; Midtvedt, K.; Rajakumar, L.; Robertsen, I.; Brox, J.; Bollerslev, J.; Hartmann, A.; Asberg, A.; Jenssen, T. Efficacy and Safety of Empagliflozin in Renal Transplant Recipients With Posttransplant Diabetes Mellitus. *Diabetes Care* **2019**, *42*, 1067–1074. [CrossRef]
30. Sattar, N.; Fitchett, D.; Hantel, S.; George, J.T.; Zinman, B. Empagliflozin is associated with improvements in liver enzymes potentially consistent with reductions in liver fat: Results from randomised trials including the EMPA-REG OUTCOME(R) trial. *Diabetologia* **2018**, *61*, 2155–2163. [CrossRef]
31. Kuchay, M.S.; Krishan, S.; Mishra, S.K.; Farooqui, K.J.; Singh, M.K.; Wasir, J.S.; Bansal, B.; Kaur, P.; Jevalikar, G.; Gill, H.K.; et al. Effect of Empagliflozin on Liver Fat in Patients With Type 2 Diabetes and Nonalcoholic Fatty Liver Disease: A Randomized Controlled Trial (E-LIFT Trial). *Diabetes Care* **2018**, *41*, 1801–1808. [CrossRef]
32. Taheri, H.; Malek, M.; Ismail-Beigi, F.; Zamani, F.; Sohrabi, M.; Reza Babaei, M.; Khamseh, M.E. Effect of Empagliflozin on Liver Steatosis and Fibrosis in Patients With Non-Alcoholic Fatty Liver Disease Without Diabetes: A Randomized, Double-Blind, Placebo-Controlled Trial. *Adv. Ther.* **2020**, *37*, 4697–4708. [CrossRef]
33. Sone, H.; Kaneko, T.; Shiki, K.; Tachibana, Y.; Pfarr, E.; Lee, J.; Tajima, N. Efficacy and safety of empagliflozin as add-on to insulin in Japanese patients with type 2 diabetes: A randomized, double-blind, placebo-controlled trial. *Diabetes Obes. Metab.* **2020**, *22*, 417–426. [CrossRef]
34. Kaku, K.; Chin, R.; Naito, Y.; Iliev, H.; Ikeda, R.; Ochiai, K.; Yasui, A. Safety and effectiveness of empagliflozin in Japanese patients with type 2 diabetes: Interim analysis from a post-marketing surveillance study. *Expert Opin. Drug Saf.* **2020**, *19*, 211–221. [CrossRef]

35. Monteiro, P.; Bergenstal, R.M.; Toural, E.; Inzucchi, S.E.; Zinman, B.; Hantel, S.; Kis, S.G.; Kaspers, S.; George, J.T.; Fitchett, D. Efficacy and safety of empagliflozin in older patients in the EMPA-REG OUTCOME(R) trial. *Age Ageing* **2019**, *48*, 859–866. [CrossRef]
36. Herat, L.Y.; Matthews, V.B.; Magno, A.L.; Kiuchi, M.G.; Carnagarin, R.; Schlaich, M.P. An evaluation of empagliflozin and it's applicability to hypertension as a therapeutic option. *Expert Opin. Pharmacother.* **2020**, *21*, 1157–1166. [CrossRef]
37. Devi, R.; Mali, G.; Chakraborty, I.; Unnikrishnan, M.K.; Abdulsalim, S. Efficacy and safety of empagliflozin in type 2 diabetes mellitus: A meta-analysis of randomized controlled trials. *Postgrad. Med.* **2017**, *129*, 382–392. [CrossRef]
38. SFDA. Saudi vigilance, Saudi Food & Drug Authority (SFDA): The Risk of Rare but Serious Infection in the Genital Area with Sodium Glucose Cotransporter-2 (SGLT2) Inhibitors. 2018. Available online: https://www.sfda.gov.sa/sites/default/files/2021-02/Jardiance%C2%AE%20SAFTEY%20COMM.pdf (accessed on 1 June 2018).
39. Kadowaki, T.; Haneda, M.; Inagaki, N.; Terauchi, Y.; Taniguchi, A.; Koiwai, K.; Rattunde, H.; Woerle, H.J.; Broedl, U.C. Empagliflozin monotherapy in Japanese patients with type 2 diabetes mellitus: A randomized, 12-week, double-blind, placebo-controlled, phase II trial. *Adv. Ther.* **2014**, *31*, 621–638. [CrossRef]
40. Ferrannini, E.; Berk, A.; Hantel, S.; Pinnetti, S.; Hach, T.; Woerle, H.J.; Broedl, U.C. Long-term safety and efficacy of empagliflozin, sitagliptin, and metformin: An active-controlled, parallel-group, randomized, 78-week open-label extension study in patients with type 2 diabetes. *Diabetes Care* **2013**, *36*, 4015–4021. [CrossRef]
41. Rosenstock, J.; Aggarwal, N.; Polidori, D.; Zhao, Y.; Arbit, D.; Usiskin, K.; Capuano, G.; Canovatchel, W.; Canagliflozin, D.I.A.S.G. Dose-ranging effects of canagliflozin, a sodium-glucose cotransporter 2 inhibitor, as add-on to metformin in subjects with type 2 diabetes. *Diabetes Care* **2012**, *35*, 1232–1238. [CrossRef]
42. Rosenstock, J.; Seman, L.J.; Jelaska, A.; Hantel, S.; Pinnetti, S.; Hach, T.; Woerle, H.J. Efficacy and safety of empagliflozin, a sodium glucose cotransporter 2 (SGLT2) inhibitor, as add-on to metformin in type 2 diabetes with mild hyperglycaemia. *Diabetes Obes. Metab.* **2013**, *15*, 1154–1160. [CrossRef]
43. Kishimoto, M.; Yamaoki, K.; Adachi, M. Combination Therapy with Empagliflozin and Insulin Results in Successful Glycemic Control: A Case Report of Uncontrolled Diabetes Caused by Autoimmune Pancreatitis and Subsequent Steroid Treatment. *Case Rep. Endocrinol.* **2019**, *2019*, 9415347. [CrossRef]
44. Al-Goblan, A.S.; Al-Alfi, M.A.; Khan, M.Z. Mechanism linking diabetes mellitus and obesity. *Diabetes Metab. Syndr. Obes.* **2014**, *7*, 587–591. [CrossRef] [PubMed]
45. Rosenstock, J.; Jelaska, A.; Frappin, G.; Salsali, A.; Kim, G.; Woerle, H.J.; Broedl, U.C.; Investigators, E.-R.M.T. Improved glucose control with weight loss, lower insulin doses, and no increased hypoglycemia with empagliflozin added to titrated multiple daily injections of insulin in obese inadequately controlled type 2 diabetes. *Diabetes Care* **2014**, *37*, 1815–1823. [CrossRef] [PubMed]
46. Bolinder, J.; Ljunggren, O.; Kullberg, J.; Johansson, L.; Wilding, J.; Langkilde, A.M.; Sugg, J.; Parikh, S. Effects of dapagliflozin on body weight, total fat mass, and regional adipose tissue distribution in patients with type 2 diabetes mellitus with inadequate glycemic control on metformin. *J. Clin. Endocrinol. Metab.* **2012**, *97*, 1020–1031. [CrossRef] [PubMed]
47. Zhao, D.; Liu, H.; Dong, P. Empagliflozin reduces blood pressure and uric acid in patients with type 2 diabetes mellitus: A systematic review and meta-analysis. *J. Hum. Hypertens.* **2019**, *33*, 327–339. [CrossRef] [PubMed]
48. Boorsma, E.M.; Beusekamp, J.C.; Ter Maaten, J.M.; Figarska, S.M.; Danser, A.H.J.; van Veldhuisen, D.J.; van der Meer, P.; Heerspink, H.J.L.; Damman, K.; Voors, A.A. Effects of empagliflozin on renal sodium and glucose handling in patients with acute heart failure. *Eur. J. Heart Fail.* **2021**, *23*, 68–78. [CrossRef] [PubMed]
49. Schork, A.; Saynisch, J.; Vosseler, A.; Jaghutriz, B.A.; Heyne, N.; Peter, A.; Haring, H.U.; Stefan, N.; Fritsche, A.; Artunc, F. Effect of SGLT2 inhibitors on body composition, fluid status and renin-angiotensin-aldosterone system in type 2 diabetes: A prospective study using bioimpedance spectroscopy. *Cardiovasc. Diabetol.* **2019**, *18*, 46. [CrossRef] [PubMed]
50. Ferdinand, K.C.; Izzo, J.L.; Lee, J.; Meng, L.; George, J.; Salsali, A.; Seman, L. Antihyperglycemic and Blood Pressure Effects of Empagliflozin in Black Patients With Type 2 Diabetes Mellitus and Hypertension. *Circulation* **2019**, *139*, 2098–2109. [CrossRef]
51. Palmiero, G.; Cesaro, A.; Vetrano, E.; Pafundi, P.C.; Galiero, R.; Caturano, A.; Moscarella, E.; Gragnano, F.; Salvatore, T.; Rinaldi, L.; et al. Impact of SGLT2 Inhibitors on Heart Failure: From Pathophysiology to Clinical Effects. *Int. J. Mol. Sci.* **2021**, *22*, 5863. [CrossRef]
52. Salvatore, T.; Caturano, A.; Galiero, R.; Di Martino, A.; Albanese, G.; Vetrano, E.; Sardu, C.; Marfella, R.; Rinaldi, L.; Sasso, F.C. Cardiovascular Benefits from Gliflozins: Effects on Endothelial Function. *Biomedicines* **2021**, *9*, 1356. [CrossRef]
53. Perrone-Filardi, P.; Avogaro, A.; Bonora, E.; Colivicchi, F.; Fioretto, P.; Maggioni, A.P.; Sesti, G.; Ferrannini, E. Mechanisms linking empagliflozin to cardiovascular and renal protection. *Int. J. Cardiol.* **2017**, *241*, 450–456. [CrossRef]
54. Pabel, S.; Wagner, S.; Bollenberg, H.; Bengel, P.; Kovacs, A.; Schach, C.; Tirilomis, P.; Mustroph, J.; Renner, A.; Gummert, J.; et al. Empagliflozin directly improves diastolic function in human heart failure. *Eur. J. Heart Fail.* **2018**, *20*, 1690–1700. [CrossRef]
55. Cherney, D.; Lund, S.S.; Perkins, B.A.; Groop, P.H.; Cooper, M.E.; Kaspers, S.; Pfarr, E.; Woerle, H.J.; von Eynatten, M. The effect of sodium glucose cotransporter 2 inhibition with empagliflozin on microalbuminuria and macroalbuminuria in patients with type 2 diabetes. *Diabetologia* **2016**, *59*, 1860–1870. [CrossRef] [PubMed]
56. Perry, R.J.; Samuel, V.T.; Petersen, K.F.; Shulman, G.I. The role of hepatic lipids in hepatic insulin resistance and type 2 diabetes. *Nature* **2014**, *510*, 84–91. [CrossRef] [PubMed]
57. Kern, M.; Kloting, N.; Mark, M.; Mayoux, E.; Klein, T.; Bluher, M. The SGLT2 inhibitor empagliflozin improves insulin sensitivity in db/db mice both as monotherapy and in combination with linagliptin. *Metabolism* **2016**, *65*, 114–123. [CrossRef]

58. Hattori, S. Empagliflozin decreases remnant-like particle cholesterol in type 2 diabetes patients with insulin resistance. *J Diabetes Investig.* **2018**, *9*, 870–874. [CrossRef]
59. Jojima, T.; Sakurai, S.; Wakamatsu, S.; Iijima, T.; Saito, M.; Tomaru, T.; Kogai, T.; Usui, I.; Aso, Y. Empagliflozin increases plasma levels of campesterol, a marker of cholesterol absorption, in patients with type 2 diabetes: Association with a slight increase in high-density lipoprotein cholesterol. *Int. J. Cardiol.* **2021**, *331*, 243–248. [CrossRef]

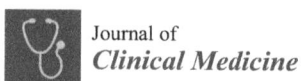

Article

Effect of Dipeptidyl Peptidase-4 Inhibitors vs. Metformin on Major Cardiovascular Events Using Spontaneous Reporting System and Real-World Database Study

Yoshihiro Noguchi [1,*], Shunsuke Yoshizawa [1], Tomoya Tachi [1] and Hitomi Teramachi [1,2,*]

1. Laboratory of Clinical Pharmacy, Gifu Pharmaceutical University, 1-25-4, Daigakunishi, Gifu-shi 501-1196, Japan
2. Laboratory of Community Healthcare Pharmacy, Gifu Pharmaceutical University, 1-25-4, Daigakunishi, Gifu-shi 501-1196, Japan
* Correspondence: noguchiy@gifu-pu.ac.jp (Y.N.); teramachih@gifu-pu.ac.jp (H.T.); Tel.: +81-230-8100 (Y.N.); +81-230-8100 (H.T.)

Abstract: Background: Metformin had been recommended as the first-line treatment for type 2 diabetes since 2006 because of its low cost, high efficacy, and potential to reduce cardiovascular events, and thus death. However, dipeptidyl peptidase-4 (DPP-4) inhibitors are the most commonly prescribed first-line agents for patients with type 2 diabetes in Japan. Therefore, it is necessary to clarify the effect of DPP-4 inhibitors on preventing cardiovascular events, taking into consideration the actual prescription of antidiabetic drugs in Japan. Methods: This study examined the effect of DPP-4 inhibitors on preventing cardiovascular events. The Japanese Adverse Drug Event Report (JADER) database, a spontaneous reporting system in Japan, and the Japanese Medical Data Center (JMDC) Claims Database, a Japanese health insurance claims and medical checkup database, were used for the analysis. Metformin was used as the DPP-4 inhibitor comparator. Major cardiovascular events were set as the primary endpoint. Results: In the analysis using the JADER database, a signal of major cardiovascular events was detected with DPP-4 inhibitors (IC: 0.22, 95% confidence interval: 0.03–0.40) but not with metformin. In the analysis using the JMDC Claims Database, the hazard ratio of major cardiovascular events for DPP-4 inhibitors versus metformin was 1.01 (95% CI: 0.84–1.20). Conclusions: A comprehensive analysis using two different databases in Japan, the JADER and the JMDC Claims Database, showed that DPP-4 inhibitors, which are widely used in Japan, have a non-inferior risk of cardiovascular events compared to metformin, which is used as the first-line drug in the United States and Europe.

Keywords: dipeptidyl peptidase-4 inhibitors; metformin; major cardiovascular events; disproportionality analysis; real-world evidence study

Citation: Noguchi, Y.; Yoshizawa, S.; Tachi, T.; Teramachi, H. Effect of Dipeptidyl Peptidase-4 Inhibitors vs. Metformin on Major Cardiovascular Events Using Spontaneous Reporting System and Real-World Database Study. *J. Clin. Med.* **2022**, *11*, 4988. https://doi.org/10.3390/jcm11174988

Academic Editor: Niccolò Lombardi

Received: 11 August 2022
Accepted: 23 August 2022
Published: 25 August 2022

Publisher's Note: MDPI stays neutral with regard to jurisdictional claims in published maps and institutional affiliations.

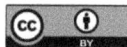

Copyright: © 2022 by the authors. Licensee MDPI, Basel, Switzerland. This article is an open access article distributed under the terms and conditions of the Creative Commons Attribution (CC BY) license (https://creativecommons.org/licenses/by/4.0/).

1. Introduction

Type 2 diabetes is associated with a variety of complications that not only worsen an individual's quality of life [1], but also place a significant burden on medical and social welfare systems [2]. Therefore, achieving and maintaining target blood glucose levels is essential in the treatment of diabetes. The American Diabetes Association and the European Association for the Study of Diabetes [3,4] have recommended metformin as the first-line treatment for type 2 diabetes since 2006 because of its low cost, high efficacy, and potential to reduce cardiovascular events, and thus death [5]. Several studies have demonstrated the effect of metformin on reducing cardiovascular complications [6–9].

However, not only do the genetic backgrounds of diabetes onset differ between Japanese and European people [10], but Japanese type 2 diabetics are also less susceptible to insulin secretion disorders, less obese, and have a lower prevalence of cardiovascular complications than type 2 diabetics in Europe and North America [11,12]. Therefore, the Japanese Diabetes Society recommends considering the differences in the pathogenesis of type 2 diabetes between Japanese and European people, and antidiabetic therapeutic agents should be selected according to the pathogenesis of the disease, rather than using specific drugs such as metformin as a first-line treatment [13].

Several studies have reported on the trends of antidiabetic drugs in Japan and compared their efficacy and cost [14,15]. An analysis of the National Database of Health Insurance Claims and Specific Health Checkups of Japan reported that, unlike in the United States and Europe, dipeptidyl peptidase-4 (DPP-4) inhibitors are the most frequently prescribed first-line drugs for patients with type 2 diabetes in Japan [15]. Furthermore, randomized placebo-controlled cardiovascular outcome trials on DPP-4 inhibitors including the SAVOR-TIMI 53 trial (where DPP-4 inhibition with saxagliptin did not increase or decrease the rate of ischemic events) [16], the TECOS trial (where adding sitagliptin to a patient's usual care did not appear to increase the risk of major adverse cardiovascular events) [17], the EXAMINE trial (where the rates of major adverse cardiovascular events were not increased with alogliptin as compared with a placebo) [18], and the CARMELINA trial [19] (where linagliptin being added to a patient's usual care compared with a placebo being added to a patient's usual care resulted in a non-inferior risk of composite major cardiovascular events) yielded non-inferior results. The CAROLINA study, a randomized controlled trial on linagliptin and glimepiride, also reported that the risk of cardiovascular events with DPP-4 inhibitors was non-inferior [20]. Meanwhile, the analyses of the Food and Drug Administration (FDA) and the Adverse Event Reporting System (FAERS), a spontaneous reporting system, suggested a mildly increased risk of cardiovascular events associated with the use of DPP-4 inhibitors [21,22]. Recently, with the increasingly widespread use of DPP-4 inhibitors, uncertainty regarding the risk of cardiovascular events associated with DPP-4 inhibitors has received increased attention given their clinical significance.

In this study, the effect of DPP-4 inhibitors on the prevention of cardiovascular events in consideration of the actual prescription of antidiabetic drugs in Japan was investigated. The Japanese Adverse Drug Event Report (JADER) database, a spontaneous reporting system in Japan, and the JMDC Claims Database, a database of health insurance claims and medical examinations in Japan, were used to conduct the analyses.

2. Materials and Methods

2.1. Disproportionality Analysis

2.1.1. Data Source

This study used 565,454 registered cases from the JADER database, which was released in October 2019. Generally, only cases of reported AEs, and not of all patients using the drug, are registered in the spontaneous reporting system. Because of this, it was not possible to calculate the incidence of an AE in the JADER case data. Therefore, signal detection using disproportionality analysis was performed.

2.1.2. Definitions of Suspected Drugs and Adverse Events

The suspect drugs were metformin and DPP-4 inhibitors (alogliptin, anagliptin, linagliptin, omarigliptin, saxagliptin, sitagliptin, teneligliptin, trelagliptin, and vildagliptin). However, combination drugs were excluded. The preferred term (PT) used in the Medical Terminology for Regulatory Activities/Japanese version (MedDRA/J) was used to identify adverse events, and PTs related to major cardiovascular events (defined as myocardial infarction and a stroke) and heart failure were included in this study.

2.1.3. Statistical Analysis

Although several algorithms were available for signal detection [23], in this study, the Bayesian Confidence Propagation Neural Network (BCPNN), which is also used by the World Health Organization-Uppsala Monitoring Center (WHO-UMC), was used [24]. The signal indicator is the information component (IC), and the detection criterion is the lower limit of the 95% credible interval of the IC; $IC_{025} > 0$ (Appendix A: Table A1, Equations (A1)–(A4)).

2.2. Real-World Evidence Study

2.2.1. Data Source

This study used the Japanese Medical Data Center (JMDC) Claims Database (JMDC Inc., Tokyo, Japan), which contains anonymous data provided by the employer's health insurance organizations. The subscriber information, which included sex, date of birth, and diagnoses, was recorded based on International Classification of Diseases, Tenth Edition (ICD-10) codes.

2.2.2. Patients

Patients aged <75 years who were new users of DPP-4 inhibitors or metformin from April 2017 to June 2017 were included in the study. New use was defined as the initiation of any drug by a patient who had not used any drug in the previous 3 months. The exclusion criteria (Table S1) were patients who had a major cardiovascular event within the past 3 months and those who had taken a controlled drug within 12 months of the start of the study (Figure 1).

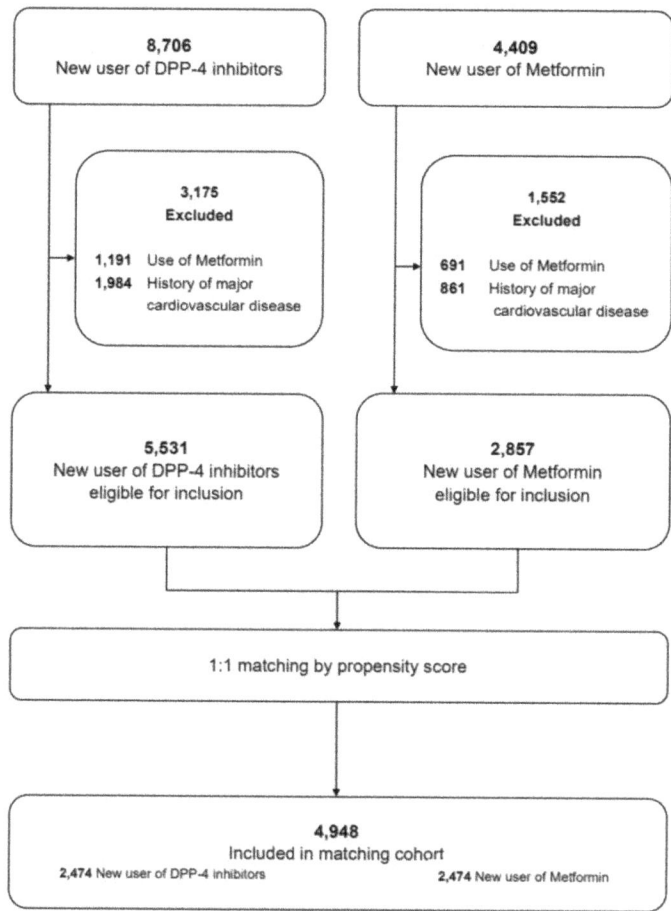

Figure 1. Flowchart of patient inclusion in the study cohort of the new user of dipeptidyl Peptidase-4 (DPP-4) inhibitors and metformin.

2.2.3. Confounder Control and Matching

The propensity score method controlled 42 potential confounders, including demographic factors, comorbidities, and drug treatment (Table S2). Propensity scores were estimated using logistic regression analysis. They were then matched in a 1:1 ratio using the nearest neighbor matching algorithm (caliper is 0.2 times the standard deviation of the logit score).

2.2.4. Outcomes

Major cardiovascular events (defined as myocardial infarction and a stroke) and heart failure were set as the endpoints of the study. Cardiovascular event outcomes were identified from the primary diagnosis assigned at admission (ICD-10 codes in Table S3), as captured by the JMDC Claims Database.

2.2.5. Statistical Analysis

Patients were followed from the start of medication to the outcome event, unless they migrated, died, or reached 75 years of age, or until the study's termination. The primary aim was to establish the non-inferiority of DPP-4 inhibitors compared with metformin over time for each cardiovascular event, defined by the upper limit of the 2-sided 95% confidence interval (CI) for the hazard ratio (HR) of DPP-4 inhibitors relative to metformin being less than 1.3 [25]. This margin (i.e., an upper limit of the 2-sided 95% CI < 1.3) was the same as in previous studies of DPP-4 inhibitors versus a placebo [15] and was deemed able to demonstrate a reassuring point estimate of the overall cardiovascular risk between study groups in the context of a non-inferiority assessment by the FDA [16]. Cox proportional hazards regression was used from the start of the treatment and the time axis was used to estimate the HR. Statistical analysis was performed using IBM SPSS Statistics 24.0 J (Armonk, New York, NY, USA).

3. Results

3.1. Disproportionality Analysis

The signals of disproportionate reporting (SDRs) for DPP-4 inhibitors were detected in major cardiovascular events (IC: 0.22, 95% credible interval: 0.03–0.40), and in the AEs of myocardial infarction (IC: 1.21, 95% credible interval: 0.87–1.55), and heart failure (IC: 0.40, 95% credible interval: 0.17–0.63). In contrast, an SDR was detected only in the AE of myocardial infarction (IC: 0.73, 95% credible interval: 0.004–1.46) with metformin treatment (Table 1).

Table 1. Number and signal score of adverse events.

Adverse Event	Drug Class/Drug	N_{11}	IC (95% Credible Interval)
Major cardiovascular events	DPP-4 inhibitors	249	0.22 (0.03–0.40)
	Metformin	40	−0.53 (−0.98–−0.07)
Myocardial infarction	DPP-4 inhibitors	162	1.21 (0.87–1.55)
	Metformin	19	0.73 (0.004–1.46)
Heart failure	DPP-4 inhibitors	75	0.40 (0.17–0.63)
	Metformin	15	−0.78 (−1.43–−0.13)
Stroke	DPP-4 inhibitors	174	−0.07 (−0.30–0.15)
	Metformin	25	−0.96 (−1.53–−0.39)

DPP-4: dipeptidyl peptidase-4, IC: information component, N_{11}: number of reports (refer to Appendix A; Table A1).

3.2. Real-World Evidence Study

3.2.1. Cohort

During the study period, 5531 new DPP-4 inhibitor users and 2857 new metformin users were identified (Table S4), among which a cohort of 2474 DPP-4 inhibitor users and 2474 metformin users were discovered using 1:1 propensity score matching (Table S5). The cohort was balanced for all measured covariates, with a mean age of 52.2 ± 9.74 years (mean ± standard deviation) and containing 3499 males (70.3%). The overall follow-up period was 33.1 ± 11.3 months, 32.6 ± 11.7 months in the DPP-4 inhibitor group and 33.6 ± 10.9 months in the metformin group.

3.2.2. Outcomes

During the follow-up period, 239 (9.7%) DPP-4 inhibitor users and 244 (9.9%) metformin users developed major cardiovascular events. Additionally, 288 (11.6%) DPP-4 inhibitor users and 270 (10.9%) metformin users developed heart failure. Other myocardial infarctions occurred in 99 (4.0%) DPP-4 inhibitor users and in 114 (4.6%) metformin users. Moreover, strokes occurred in 161 (6.5%) DPP-4 inhibitor users and in 149 (6.0%) metformin users (Table 2).

The cumulative incidence of cardiovascular events is shown in Figure 2.

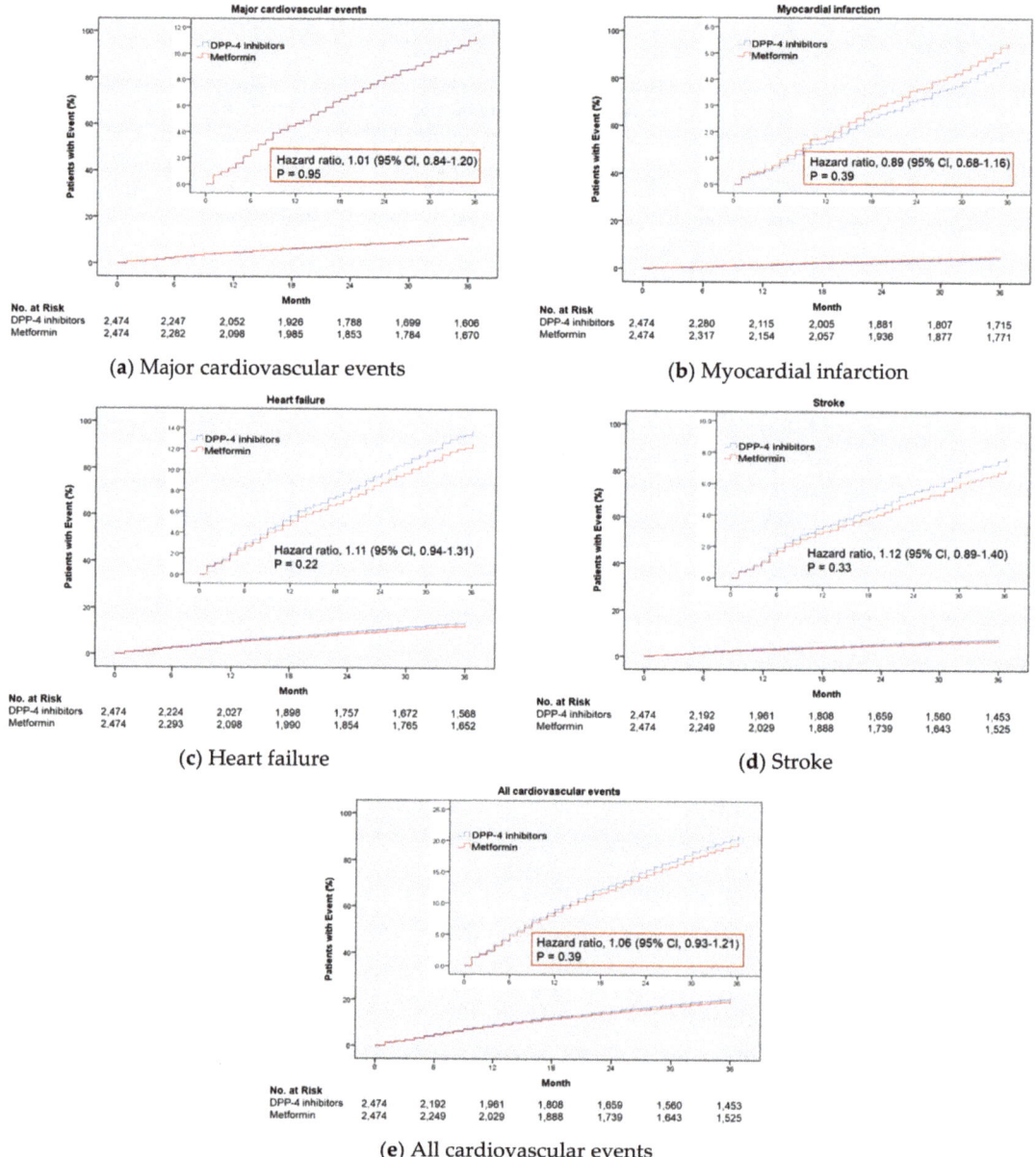

Figure 2. Cumulative incidence of cardiovascular events associated with use of dipeptidyl Peptidase-4 (DPP-4) inhibitors, compared with use of metformin.

Table 2. Number and incidence of adverse events.

Adverse Event	DPP-4 Inhibitors (%) Total: n = 2424	Metformin (%) Total: n = 2424
Major cardiovascular events	239 (9.7)	244 (9.9)
Myocardial infarction	99 (4.0)	114 (4.6)
Heart failure	288 (11.6)	270 (10.9)
Stroke	161 (6.5)	149 (6.0)

DPP-4: dipeptidyl peptidase-4.

The HRs for DPP-4 inhibitors vs. metformin were 1.01 (95% CI: 0.84–1.20) for major cardiovascular events, 0.89 (95% CI: 0.68–1.16) for myocardial infarction, 1.11 (95% CI: 0.94–1.31) for heart failure, 1.12 (95% CI: 0.89–1.40) for a stroke, and 1.06 (95% CI: 0.93–1.21) for all cardiovascular events (Figure 3).

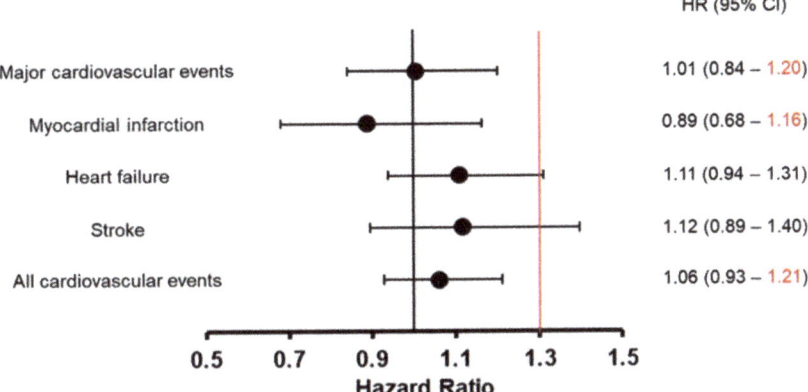

Figure 3. The hazard ratio of dipeptidyl Peptidase-4 (DPP-4) inhibitor use vs. metformin use.

4. Discussion

DPP-4 inhibitors are the most commonly prescribed first-line drugs for patients with type 2 diabetes in Japan. The prescribing pattern for type 2 diabetes in Japan differs from the pattern in the United States and in Europe. Therefore, this study investigated the effect of DPP-4 inhibitors on the prevention of cardiovascular events in Japanese patients using two different databases: the JADER, a spontaneous reporting system in Japan, and the JMDC Claims Database, a database of health insurance claims and medical examinations.

The first part of this study examined the association of DPP-4 inhibitors and metformin with cardiovascular events using the JADER. No SDR was detected for metformin with any cardiovascular events except for myocardial infarction. In contrast, SDRs were detected with DPP-4 inhibitors in all cardiovascular events except for a stroke. These results are similar to those of previous studies that used the FAERS [21], although the definition of cardiovascular events differs between this study and previous ones. However, since the publication of several clinical trials, including the SAVOR-TIMI trial [12–16], clinicians have reported episodes of cardiovascular events in patients taking DPP-4 inhibitors, a situation known as "stimulated reporting" [18]. This situation can also occur naturally in Japan.

The second part of the research was a non-inferiority study of DPP-4 inhibitors and metformin on the occurrence of cardiovascular events using real-world Japanese data from the JMDC Claims Database. The results demonstrate non-inferiority in main cardiovascular events, myocardial infarction, and all cardiovascular events for DPP-4 inhibitors versus metformin. This study reaffirms clinical recommendations for antidiabetic drugs in Japan.

Several meta-analyses designed to assess the risk of major adverse cardiovascular events in type 2 diabetic patients treated with DPP-4 inhibitors have been conducted. These results suggest that DPP-4 inhibitors reduce the risk of major adverse cardiovascular events compared to diabetes drugs (with the exception of SGLT2 inhibitors which can also be used to treat chronic heart failure) and placebo [26–28]. Some observational studies using the Taiwan National Health Insurance Research Database [29] and the IBM MarketScan Commercial Claims and Encounters Database [30,31] also showed similar results. Thus, our results regarding the risk of cardiovascular events, taking into account antidiabetic prescribing status in Japan, are generally consistent with the results of previous studies.

There are several possible reasons for the extremely high rate of DPP-4 inhibitor prescriptions in Japan despite the availability of metformin, which is less expensive and non-inferior in cardiovascular risk [15]. The genetic background of diabetes development differs between Japanese and European people [10], and Japanese patients with type 2 diabetes are less likely to have impaired insulin secretion and are less likely to be obese than Europeans [11,12]. DPP-4 inhibitors can lower glycated hemoglobin (HbA1C) levels more effectively in Japanese people than in Europeans [11,32]. Furthermore, the risk of severe hypoglycemia is extremely low when DPP-4 inhibitors are administered alone [15]. Torii et al. reported that the risk of intensified treatment for untreated type 2 diabetes patients and the risk of developing levels of HbA1C > 7% in these patients were lower with DPP-4 inhibitors than with biguanides [33]. Furthermore, the JDS attaches great importance to the safety of antidiabetic drugs, and the proper use of biguanides and SGLT2 inhibitors is noted in its recommendations, including consideration for the elderly [15,34]. Therefore, the information revealed in this study regarding the non-inferiority of DPP-4 inhibitors to metformin with respect to cardiovascular risk may have important implications for the use of DPP-4 inhibitors in Japan.

This study had several strengths and limitations. Of the two databases used in this study, the JADER is based on spontaneous reports. This study using the JADER also has limitations similar to studies using other spontaneous reporting systems [23]. However, most of those reporting to the JADER were physicians (77.3%), followed by pharmacists (6.3%), and then lawyers (less than 0.01%) [23]. There are fewer reports from patients; therefore, the accuracy of the information in the JADER database may be higher than that of other spontaneous reporting systems.

The total number of patients using the drug cannot be obtained using the JADER database; therefore, the incidence rate cannot be calculated. Furthermore, registered cases are affected by various reporting biases [23]. This is because both physicians and patients tend not to report all cases, resulting in an underestimation of events [23].

On the contrary, the JMDC Claims Database is based on health insurance claims and medical examinations and is one of the real-world datasets in Japan. Therefore, incidence rates and HRs that cannot be calculated by the JADER can be calculated by the JMDC Claims Database. However, the JMDC Claims Database uses health insurance societies as data sources, which covers private sector employees and their families, and thus has an overwhelmingly small number of elderly people (those aged 75 and older are not included because they are part of the late-stage elderly healthcare system) [35]. Furthermore, because this study is based on secondary use of claims data, the accuracy of diagnosis depends on the accuracy of the database records, which may affect internal validity. In calculating propensity scores from the database to adjust for confounders, this study followed previous studies, but may not have included all important confounders. For example, body mass index and smoking status are important confounders of cardiovascular events but could not be considered in this study. However, analysis of these two different types of databases revealed that the risk of major cardiovascular disease with DPP-4 inhibitors, while undeniable, does not differ from the risk associated with metformin.

As a class, DPP-4 inhibitors are not associated with any increase or reduction in major cardiovascular events, all-cause mortality, or heart failure. Saxagliptin seems to be associated with an increased risk of hospitalization for heart failure [36]. Future studies will need to investigate the differential effects of individual DPP-4 inhibitors on cardiovascular events.

5. Conclusions

A comprehensive analysis using two different databases in Japan, the JADER and the JMDC Claims Database, showed that DPP-4 inhibitors, which are widely used in Japan, have a non-inferior risk of cardiovascular events compared to metformin, which is used as the first-line drug in the United States and Europe.

Supplementary Materials: The following supporting information can be downloaded at: https://www.mdpi.com/article/10.3390/jcm11174988/s1, Table S1: Exclusion criteria.; Table S2: Variables included in propensity score, with definitions.; Table S3: ICD-10 codes for outcome definitions., Table S4: Baseline characteristics of new users of SGLT2 inhibitors and DPP-4 inhibitors matched by propensity score (before matching).; Table S5: Baseline characteristics of new users of SGLT2 inhibitors and DPP-4 inhibitors matched by propensity score (after matching).

Author Contributions: Conceptualization, Y.N. and H.T.; methodology, Y.N. and S.Y.; investigation, S.Y.; writing—original draft preparation, Y.N. and S.Y.; writing—review and editing, Y.N., T.T. and H.T.; project administration, Y.N. and H.T.; funding acquisition, Y.N. All authors have read and agreed to the published version of the manuscript.

Funding: This research was funded by JSPS KAKENHI grant number 22K12890.

Institutional Review Board Statement: The study was conducted in accordance with the Declaration of Helsinki and Good Clinical Practice guidelines. This study was approved by the ethics committees of Gifu Pharmaceutical University (approval number: 2-39, approved on 10 March 2021).

Informed Consent Statement: The Ethics Committee approved the waiver of informed consent because this study used data that had already been anonymized and recorded.

Data Availability Statement: Of the two datasets used in this study, the JADER is not permitted to be shared. However, the raw data of JADER (in Japanese only) can be accessed directly here: http://www.info.pmda.go.jp/fukusayoudb/CsvDownload.jsp (accessed on 1 August 2022). The JMDC Claims Database is available from JMDC, but is used under license in this study and is not available to the public.

Conflicts of Interest: The authors declare no conflict of interest.

Appendix A

The IC and 95% credible interval (IC_{025}) are calculated using Table A1 and Equations (A1)–(A4).

Table A1. The 2 × 2 contingency table for signal detection.

	Target AE	Other AEs	Total
Target drug	N_{11}	N_{10}	N_{1+}
Other drugs	N_{01}	N_{00}	N_{0+}
Total	N_{+1}	N_{+0}	N_{++}

N: the number of reports; AE: adverse event.

$$E(IC_{11}) = log_2 \frac{(N_{11} + \gamma_{11})(N_{++} + \alpha)(N_{++} + \beta)}{(N_{++} + \gamma)(N_{1+} + \alpha_1)(N_{+1} + \beta_1)} \tag{A1}$$

$$V(IC_{11}) = \left(\frac{1}{log2}\right)^2 \left[\frac{N_{++} - N_{11} + \gamma - \gamma_{11}}{(N_{11} + \gamma_{11})(1 + N_{++} + \gamma)} + \frac{N_{++} - N_{1+} + \alpha - \alpha_1}{(N_{1+} + \alpha_1)(1 + N_{++} + \alpha)} + \frac{N_{++} - N_{+1} + \beta - \beta_1}{(N_{+1} + \beta_1)(1 + N_{++} + \beta)}\right] \tag{A2}$$

$$\gamma = \gamma_{11} \frac{(N_{++} + \alpha)(N_{++} + \beta)}{(N_{1+} + \alpha_1)(N_{+1} + \beta_1)}, \; \gamma_{11} = 1, \; \alpha_1 = \beta_1 = 1, \; \alpha = \beta = 2 \tag{A3}$$

$$IC \text{ (95\% confidence interval)} = E\left(IC_{11} \pm 2\sqrt{V(IC_{11})}\right) \tag{A4}$$

References

1. Peyrot, M.; Rubin, R.R.; Lauritzen, T.; Snoek, F.J.; Matthews, D.R.; Skovlund, S.E. Psychosocial problems and barriers to improved diabetes management: Results of the Cross-National Diabetes Attitudes, Wishes and Needs (DAWN) Study. *Diabet. Med.* **2005**, *22*, 1379–1385. [CrossRef] [PubMed]
2. American Diabetes Association. Economic costs of diabetes in the U.S. in 2012. *Diabetes Care* **2013**, *36*, 1033–1046. [CrossRef] [PubMed]
3. Davies, M.J.; D'Alessio, D.A.; Fradkin, J.; Kernan, W.N.; Mathieu, C.; Mingrone, G.; Rossing, P.; Tsapas, A.; Wexler, D.J.; Buse, J.B. Management of hyperglycaemia in type 2 diabetes, 2018. A consensus report by the American Diabetes Association (ADA) and the European Association for the Study of Diabetes (EASD). *Diabetologia* **2018**, *61*, 2461–2498. [CrossRef]
4. Davies, M.J.; D'Alessio, D.A.; Fradkin, J.; Kernan, W.N.; Mathieu, C.; Mingrone, G.; Rossing, P.; Tsapas, A.; Wexler, D.J.; Buse, J.B. Management of Hyperglycemia in Type 2 Diabetes, 2018. A Consensus Report by the American Diabetes Association (ADA) and the European Association for the Study of Diabetes (EASD). *Diabetes Care* **2018**, *41*, 2669–2701. [CrossRef] [PubMed]
5. Holman, R.R.; Paul, S.K.; Bethel, M.A.; Matthews, D.R.; Neil, H.A. 10-year follow-up of intensive glucose control in type 2 diabetes. *N. Engl. J. Med.* **2008**, *359*, 1577–1589. [CrossRef] [PubMed]
6. UK Prospective Diabetes Study (UKPDS) Group. Effect of intensive blood-glucose control with metformin on complications in overweight patients with type 2 diabetes (UKPDS 34). *Lancet* **1998**, *352*, 854–865. [CrossRef]
7. Roussel, R.; Travert, F.; Pasquet, B.; Wilson, P.W.; Smith, S.C., Jr.; Goto, S.; Ravaud, P.; Marre, M.; Porath, A.; Bhatt, D.L.; et al. Metformin use and mortality among patients with diabetes and atherothrombosis. *Arch. Intern. Med.* **2010**, *170*, 1892–1899. [CrossRef]
8. Hong, J.; Zhang, Y.; Lai, S.; Lv, A.; Su, Q.; Dong, Y.; Zhou, Z.; Tang, W.; Zhao, J.; Cui, L.; et al. Effects of metformin versus glipizide on cardiovascular outcomes in patients with type 2 diabetes and coronary artery disease. *Diabetes Care* **2013**, *36*, 1304–1311. [CrossRef]
9. Cheng, Y.Y.; Leu, H.B.; Chen, T.J.; Chen, C.L.; Kuo, C.H.; Lee, S.D.; Kao, C.L. Metformin-inclusive therapy reduces the risk of stroke in patients with diabetes: A 4-year follow-up study. *J. Stroke Cereb. Dis.* **2014**, *23*, e99–e105. [CrossRef]
10. Suzuki, K.; Akiyama, M.; Ishigaki, K.; Kanai, M.; Hosoe, J.; Shojima, N.; Hozawa, A.; Kadota, A.; Kuriki, K.; Naito, M.; et al. Identification of 28 new susceptibility loci for type 2 diabetes in the Japanese population. *Nat. Genet.* **2019**, *51*, 379–386. [CrossRef]
11. Ma, R.C.; Chan, J.C. Type 2 diabetes in East Asians: Similarities and differences with populations in Europe and the United States. *Ann. N. Y. Acad. Sci.* **2013**, *1281*, 64–91. [CrossRef]
12. Huxley, R.; James, W.P.; Barzi, F.; Patel, J.V.; Lear, S.A.; Suriyawongpaisal, P.; Janus, E.; Caterson, I.; Zimmet, P.; Prabhakaran, D.; et al. Obesity in Asia Collaboration. Ethnic comparisons of the cross-sectional relationships between measures of body size with diabetes and hypertension. *Obes. Rev.* **2008**, *9* (Suppl. S1), 53–61. [CrossRef]
13. Haneda, M.; Noda, M.; Origasa, H.; Noto, H.; Yabe, D.; Fujita, Y.; Goto, A.; Kondo, T.; Araki, E. Japanese Clinical Practice Guideline for Diabetes 2016. *Diabetol. Int.* **2018**, *9*, 1–45. [CrossRef]
14. Ihana-Sugiyama, N.; Sugiyama, T.; Tanaka, H.; Ueki, K.; Kobayashi, Y.; Ohsugi, M. Comparison of effectiveness and drug cost between dipeptidyl peptidase-4 inhibitor and biguanide as the first-line anti-hyperglycaemic medication among Japanese working generation with type 2 diabetes. *J. Eval. Clin. Pract.* **2020**, *26*, 299–307. [CrossRef]
15. Bouchi, R.; Sugiyama, T.; Goto, A.; Imai, K.; Ihana-Sugiyama, N.; Ohsugi, M.; Yamauchi, T.; Kadowaki, T.; Ueki, K. Retrospective nationwide study on the trends in first-line antidiabetic medication for patients with type 2 diabetes in Japan. *J. Diabetes Investig.* **2021**, *13*, 280–291. [CrossRef]
16. Scirica, B.M.; Bhatt, D.L.; Braunwald, E.; Steg, P.G.; Davidson, J.; Hirshberg, B.; Ohman, P.; Frederich, R.; Wiviott, S.D.; Hoffman, E.B.; et al. SAVOR-TIMI 53 Steering Committee and Investigators. Saxagliptin and cardiovascular outcomes in patients with type 2 diabetes mellitus. *N. Engl. J. Med.* **2013**, *369*, 1317–1326. [CrossRef]
17. Green, J.B.; Bethel, M.A.; Armstrong, P.W.; Buse, J.B.; Engel, S.S.; Garg, J.; Josse, R.; Kaufman, K.D.; Koglin, J.; Korn, S.; et al. Effect of Sitagliptin on Cardiovascular Outcomes in Type 2 Diabetes. *N. Engl. J. Med.* **2015**, *373*, 232–242. [CrossRef]
18. White, W.B.; Cannon, C.P.; Heller, S.R.; Nissen, S.E.; Bergenstal, R.M.; Bakris, G.L.; Perez, A.T.; Fleck, P.R.; Mehta, C.R.; Kupfer, S.; et al. Alogliptin after acute coronary syndrome in patients with type 2 diabetes. *N. Engl. J. Med.* **2013**, *369*, 1327–1335. [CrossRef]
19. Rosenstock, J.; Perkovic, V.; Johansen, O.E.; Cooper, M.E.; Kahn, S.E.; Marx, N.; Alexander, J.H.; Pencina, M.; Toto, R.D.; Wanner, C.; et al. Effect of Linagliptin vs. Placebo on Major Cardiovascular Events in Adults with Type 2 Diabetes and High Cardiovascular and Renal Risk: The CARMELINA Randomized Clinical Trial. *JAMA* **2019**, *321*, 69–79. [CrossRef]
20. Rosenstock, J.; Kahn, S.E.; Johansen, O.E.; Zinman, B.; Espeland, M.A.; Woerle, H.J.; Pfarr, E.; Keller, A.; Mattheus, M.; Baanstra, D.; et al. Effect of Linagliptin vs. Glimepiride on Major Adverse Cardiovascular Outcomes in Patients with Type 2 Diabetes: The CAROLINA Randomized Clinical Trial. *JAMA* **2019**, *322*, 1155–1166. [CrossRef]
21. Raschi, E.; Poluzzi, E.; Koci, A.; Antonazzo, I.C.; de Ponti, F. Dipeptidyl peptidase-4 inhibitors and heart failure: Analysis of spontaneous reports submitted to the FDA adverse event reporting system. *Nutr. Metab. Cardiovasc. Dis.* **2016**, *26*, 380–386. [CrossRef] [PubMed]
22. Fadini, G.P.; Sarangdhar, M.; Avogaro, A. Pharmacovigilance Evaluation of the Association between DPP-4 Inhibitors and Heart Failure: Stimulated Reporting and Moderation by Drug Interactions. *Diabetes Ther.* **2018**, *9*, 851–861. [CrossRef] [PubMed]
23. Noguchi, Y.; Tachi, T.; Teramachi, H. Detection algorithms and attentive points of safety signal using spontaneous reporting systems as a clinical data source. *Brief Bioinform.* **2021**, *22*, bbab347. [CrossRef] [PubMed]

24. The UMC Measures of Disproportionate Reporting—A Brief Guide to Their Interpretation. Available online: https://who-umc.org/media/164041/measures-of-disproportionate-reporting_2016.pdf (accessed on 10 August 2022).
25. Center for Drug Evaluation and Research. Meeting expectations to exclude a CV risk margin of 1.3. In Application Number 204042Orig1s000Summary Review; p. 20. Available online: https://www.accessdata.fda.gov/drugsatfda_docs/nda/2013/204042Orig1s000SumR.pdf (accessed on 10 August 2022).
26. Kaneko, M.; Narukawa, M. Meta-analysis of dipeptidyl peptidase-4 inhibitors use and cardiovascular risk in patients with type 2 diabetes mellitus. *Diabetes Res. Clin. Pract.* **2016**, *116*, 171–182. [CrossRef]
27. Zheng, S.L.; Roddick, A.J.; Aghar-Jaffar, R.; Shun-Shin, M.J.; Francis, D.; Oliver, N.; Meeran, K. Association Between Use of Sodium-Glucose Cotransporter 2 Inhibitors, Glucagon-like Peptide 1 Agonists, and Dipeptidyl Peptidase 4 Inhibitors with All-Cause Mortality in Patients with Type 2 Diabetes: A Systematic Review and Meta-analysis. *JAMA* **2018**, *319*, 1580–1591. [CrossRef]
28. Giugliano, D.; Longo, M.; Signoriello, S.; Maiorino, M.I.; Solerte, B.; Chiodini, P.; Esposito, K. The effect of DPP-4 inhibitors, GLP-1 receptor agonists and SGLT-2 inhibitors on cardiorenal outcomes: A network meta-analysis of 23 CVOTs. *Cardiovasc. Diabetol.* **2022**, *21*, 42. [CrossRef]
29. Ou, S.M.; Shih, C.J.; Chao, P.W.; Chu, H.; Kuo, S.C.; Lee, Y.J.; Wang, S.J.; Yang, C.Y.; Lin, C.C.; Chen, T.J.; et al. Effects on Clinical Outcomes of Adding Dipeptidyl Peptidase-4 Inhibitors Versus Sulfonylureas to Metformin Therapy in Patients with Type 2 Diabetes Mellitus. *Ann. Intern. Med.* **2015**, *163*, 663–672. [CrossRef]
30. Baksh, S.N.; Segal, J.B.; McAdams-DeMarco, M.; Kalyani, R.R.; Alexander, G.C.; Ehrhardt, S. Dipeptidyl peptidase-4 inhibitors and cardiovascular events in patients with type 2 diabetes, without cardiovascular or renal disease. *PLoS ONE* **2020**, *15*, e0240141. [CrossRef]
31. Baksh, S.; Wen, J.; Mansour, O.; Chang, H.Y.; McAdams-DeMarco, M.; Segal, J.B.; Ehrhardt, S.; Alexander, G.C. Dipeptidyl peptidase-4 inhibitor cardiovascular safety in patients with type 2 diabetes, with cardiovascular and renal disease: A retrospective cohort study. *Sci. Rep.* **2021**, *11*, 16637. [CrossRef]
32. Seino, Y.; Kuwata, H.; Yabe, D. Incretin-based drugs for type 2 diabetes: Focus on East Asian perspectives. *J. Diabetes Investig.* **2016**, *7* (Suppl. S1), 102–109. [CrossRef]
33. Horii, T.; Iwasawa, M.; Shimizu, J.; Atsuda, K. Comparing treatment intensification and clinical outcomes of metformin and dipeptidyl peptidase-4 inhibitors in treatment-naïve patients with type 2 diabetes in Japan. *J. Diabetes Investig.* **2020**, *11*, 96–100. [CrossRef]
34. Committee on the Proper Use of SGLT2 Inhibitors. Recommendations on the proper use of SGLT2 inhibitors. *Diabetol. Int.* **2019**, *11*, 1–5. [CrossRef]
35. Takekuma, Y.; Imai, S.; Sugawara, M. Clinical Research Using the Large Health Insurance Claims Database. *YAKUGAKU ZASSHI* **2022**, *142*, 331–336. [CrossRef]
36. Mannucci, E.; Nreu, B.; Montereggi, C.; Ragghianti, B.; Gallo, M.; Giaccari, A.; Monami, M.; SID-AMD Joint Panel for Italian Guidelines on Treatment of Type 2 Diabetes. Cardiovascular events and all-cause mortality in patients with type 2 diabetes treated with dipeptidyl peptidase-4 inhibitors: An extensive meta-analysis of randomized controlled trials. *Nutr. Metab. Cardiovasc. Dis.* **2021**, *31*, 2745–2755. [CrossRef]

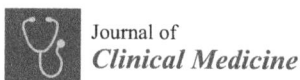 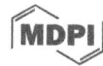

Article

Did the COVID-19 Pandemic Affect Contrast Media-Induced Adverse Drug Reaction's Reporting? A Pharmacovigilance Study in Southern Italy

Claudia Rossi [1,†], Rosanna Ruggiero [2,3,*,†], Liberata Sportiello [2,3], Ciro Pentella [2,3], Mario Gaio [2,3], Antonio Pinto [1] and Concetta Rafaniello [2,3]

1. Department of Radiology, CTO Hospital, Azienda Ospedaliera dei Colli, 80131 Naples, Italy
2. Department of Experimental Medicine, University of Campania "L. Vanvitelli", 80138 Naples, Italy
3. Campania Regional Centre for Pharmacovigilance and Pharmacoepidemiology, 80138 Naples, Italy
* Correspondence: rosanna.ruggiero@unicampania.it
† These authors contributed equally to this work and share the first authorship.

Abstract: Medical imaging is required for a complete clinical evaluation to identify lung involvement or pulmonary embolism during SARS-CoV-2 infection or pulmonary and cardiovascular sequelae. Contrast media (CM) have undoubtedly been useful in clinical practice due to their ability to improve medical imaging in COVID-19 patients. Considering their important use, especially in hospitalized COVID-19 patients, and that increased use of a medical tool could also be associated with its deeper knowledge, we chose to explore if new information emerged regarding CM safety profiles. We analyzed all Individual Case Safety Reports (ICSRs) validated by Campania Pharmacovigilance Regional Centre from 1 January 2018 to 31 December 2021 and reported a CM (ATC code V08) as a suspected drug. We compared CM-related reporting between 2 years before (period 1) and 2 years during (period 2) the COVID-19 pandemic. From our analysis, it emerged that, during the COVID-19 pandemic, CM-related ADR reporting decreased, but a significant increase in reporting of serious cases emerged. Serious ADRs were mainly related to iodinated CM (V08A ATC) compared to magnetic resonance imaging CM (V08C ATC). Cutaneous and respiratory disorders were the most frequently reported in both periods. No new or unknown ADRs were reported in the overall study period.

Keywords: contrast media; safety; spontaneous reporting; COVID-19

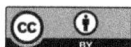

1. Introduction

Since the outbreak of unknown pneumonia in Wuhan (China) at the end of 2019, the new coronavirus, identified as severe acute respiratory syndrome coronavirus 2 (SARS-CoV-2), has required global attention [1,2]. SARS-CoV-2 succeeds in entering the human cells through the spike protein present on its envelope surface, binding the angiotensin-converting enzyme 2 (ACE2) receptors and subsequentially using the serine protease TMPRSS2 for spike protein priming [3]. Once in the cell, its transcription and replication start exploiting the host cellular structures, causing an infection termed coronavirus disease 2019 (COVID-19) [1]. COVID-19 has posed an extraordinary threat to global public health [4]. The major impact on health systems was due to the increased hospitalization rates required for severely affected patients, especially in the first pandemic phases related to the more pathogenic SARS-CoV-2 variants (alpha and delta). According to the latest data, as of 23 May 2022, there have been 522,783,196 confirmed COVID-19 cases, including 6,276,210 deaths, reported to the WHO since the beginning of the pandemic [5]. Interstitial pneumonia represents the predominant clinical manifestation of mild and severe COVID-19 forms. Thromboembolic complications, including pulmonary embolism (PE) [6–8], are very frequent in COVID-19 patients [9–11]. Computed tomography (CT) has represented the reference standard for identifying lung involvement due to SARS-CoV-2 infection [12]. CT angiography is the key technique used for confirming pulmonary embolism [13]. In addition to respiratory complications, COVID-19 can also have implications on the cardiovascular system [14]. These include myocardial edema, fibrosis, and impaired right ventricle function, as revealed by cardiovascular magnetic resonance (CMR) [15,16]. Moreover, several long-term manifestations related to SARS-CoV-2 infection should not be excluded or underestimated. Long COVID-19 syndrome is characterized by several complications and sequelae, including pulmonary and cardiovascular ones, which require medical imaging for their clinical evaluation [17,18]. Therefore, contrast media (CM) have undoubtedly been clinically useful in the pandemic context due to their ability to improve medical imaging in COVID-19 patients [19]. Newer contrast agents, characterized by lower ionic concentrations and lower osmolarity, are better tolerated [20]. However, CM, like all medicines, is not risk-free [21], with possible negative effects, for example, on kidney function, especially in previously nephropathic patients when exposed to iodine-based agents [13]. CM-induced nephropathy has been the object of several studies that aimed to identify possible risk factors or biomarkers and evaluate procedures to prevent it [21]. Moreover, non-renal complications can also emerge following CM exposure, including anaphylactoid reactions (Krause et al., 2020). Post-marketing surveillance had an important role in identifying some CM-induced adverse drug reactions (ADRs), especially in some sub-populations with less evidence available due to their typical exclusion from clinical trials [19]. Considering the important use of CM for clinical imaging evaluations during the COVID-19 pandemic, especially in hospitalized patients, and that increased use of a medical tool could also be associated with its deeper knowledge, we wanted to explore if new information emerged regarding their safety profiles. For these reasons, we decided to investigate the effects of the COVID-19 pandemic on reporting suspected ADRs related to CM agents to the Italian National Pharmacovigilance Network (Rete Nazionale di Farmacovigilanza, RNF).

2. Materials and Methods

2.1. Data Source

For our study, we analyzed the individual case safety reports (ICSRs) related to CM and recorded them in the Campania Region (Southern Italy). Regional safety data were obtained from the RNF, the Italian Pharmacovigilance Database, coordinated by the Italian Medicines Agency (AIFA) since 2001. It allows for collecting Italian reports of suspected ADR and AEFI sent by physicians, other healthcare professionals and patients/citizens. ADR reporting is carried out through a standardized reporting form to describe details of the patient who experienced an adverse event (age, sex, medical history, etc.), the suspected ADR(s)/AEFI(s) (signs and symptoms or diagnosis, seriousness, outcome, etc.), the suspected and any concomitant drug(s)/vaccine(s) as well as previous or current patient medical conditions. In each Italian regional territory, Pharmacovigilance Regional Centers validate the information of each ICSR and perform the causality assessment for each adverse event–drug couple.

2.2. Study Design

We compared the CM-related reporting before and during the COVID-19 pandemic for our analysis. Therefore, we selected all ICSRs validated by the Campania Pharmacovigilance Regional Center from 1 January 2018 to 31 December 2021 and reported a contrast media (Anatomical Therapeutic Chemical classification code, ATC code V08) as a suspected drug. This reference period was chosen to compare the main features of ADRs' reports entry into RNF during the 2 years before and during the COVID-19 pandemic (period 1: 1 January 2018 to 31 December 2019; period 2: 1 January 2020 to 31 December 2021).

2.3. Data Analysis

We performed a descriptive analysis of selected ICSRs, comparing and stratifying the two study periods by suspected contrast media, mean age, sex, and seriousness criteria according to the International Conference on Harmonization E2D guidelines principles (death; hospitalization or its prolongation; severe or permanent disability; life threat; congenital abnormalities/birth deficits; clinically relevant; not serious), outcome (favorable: completely resolved or improved; unfavorable: resolved with sequelae or unchanged), system organ class (SOC), High-Level Group Term (HLGT) MedDRA, source of the report, and causality assessment. We used MedDRA version 25.0. We evaluated the CM-related reporting trend stratifying by three-month/year.

Chi-squared analysis with Yates' continuity correction or Fisher's exact test, where appropriate, and t-test were employed to examine differences in the rate of the ADR's report between the two periods. A 5% significance level was considered for analysis. Data were analyzed using the software SPSS version 21.

3. Results

From 1 January 2018 to 31 December 2021, a total of 144 ICSRs, describing 246 ADRs induced by CM, were sent to the Campania Pharmacovigilance Regional Center. All ICSRs were sent by a healthcare professional (Table 1).

Table 1. Main features of 144 ICSRs related to contrast media in the Campania region comparing the 2018–2019 (period 1) and 2020–2021 (period 2).

Variables	Levels	Total ICSR $n = 144$	Contrast Media ICSRs During Period 1 $n = 105\ n\ (\%)$	Contrast Media ICSRs During Period 2 $n = 39\ n\ (\%)$	p-Value (<0.05)
Age	Mean age (SD)	55 (±16.1)	54 (±16.9)	57 (±13.4)	0.26
Sex	Female n (%)	77 (53.5)	52 (49.5)	25 (64.1)	0.17
	Male n (%)	65 (45.1)	51 (48.6)	14 (35.9)	0.24
	Not Reported n (%)	2 (1.4)	2 (1.9)	-	-
Seriousness of ADRs' reports	Serious n (%)	30 (20.8)	17 (16.2)	13 (33.3)	0.04
	Not Serious n (%)	109 (75.7)	83 (79.0)	26 (66.7)	0.18
	Not available	5 (3.5)	5 (4.8)	-	-
Outcome of ADRs' reports	Favorable n (%)	125 (86.8)	87 (82.9)	38 (97.4)	0.04
	Unfavorable n (%)	1 (0.7)	1 (0.9)	-	-
	Not Available n (%)	18 (12.5)	17 (16.2)	1 (2.6)	0.05
Source of ADRs' reports	Healthcare professional n (%)	144 (100)	105 (100)	39 (100)	-
	Suspected drug				
V08A	Iomeprol n (%)	32 (22.2)	23 (21.9)	9 (23.1)	0.94
	Iopamidol n (%)	63 (43.8)	46 (43.8)	17 (43.6)	0.86
	Iopromide n (%)	11 (7.6)	5 (4.8)	6 (15.4)	0.07
	Ioexol n (%)	1 (0.7)	1 (0.9)	-	-
	Iodixanol n (%)	7 (4.9)	7 (6.7)	-	-
	Iobitridol n (%)	6 (4.2)	6 (5.7)	-	-
	TOTAL	121 (84.0)	88 (84.8)	32 (82.1)	0.99
V08C	Gadoteric acid n (%)	11 (7.6)	9 (8.6)	2 (5.1)	0.73
	Gadoteridol n (%)	9 (6.3)	6 (5.7)	3 (7.7)	0.96
	Gadobutrol n (%)	1 (0.7)	1 (0.9)	-	-
	Gadoxetic acid n (%)	1 (0.7)	1 (0.9)	-	-
	Gadobenic acid n (%)	2 (1.3)	-	2 (5.1)	-
	TOTAL	24 (16.0)	17 (15.2)	7 (17.9)	0.99

Table 1. Cont.

Variables	Levels	Total ICSR $n = 144$	Contrast Media ICSRs During Period 1 $n = 105\ n\ (\%)$	Contrast Media ICSRs During Period 2 $n = 39\ n\ (\%)$	p-Value (<0.05)
	Other suspect drugs				
	Clorexidine n (%)	1 (0.7)	1 (0.9)	-	-
	Mepivacaine n (%)	1 (0.7)	1 (0.9)	-	-

V08A: X-ray contrast media, iodinated; V08C: magnetic resonance imaging contrast media.

As reported in Figure 1, we found a substantial decrease in CM-related reporting trends during the COVID-19 pandemic (105 ICSRS for period 1 vs. 39 ICSRs for period 2).

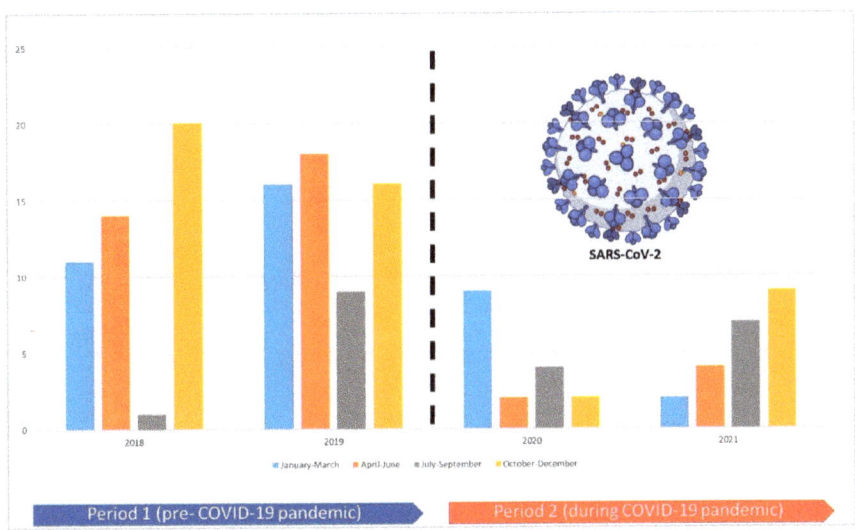

Figure 1. Before and during the COVID-19 pandemic, reporting trends stratified by three months/year.

Overall, the mean age of patients who experienced ADRs was 55 years old (±16.1), and 53.5% were female (Table 1). These variable trends persist in both periods, even if the mean age was slightly higher in period 2, and the female sex is slightly less predominant in period 1. No significant differences in terms of age and sex between ICSRs sent to the RNF during periods 1 and 2 were found (Table 1). Considering the whole study period, the most commonly suspected drugs were iodinated X-ray CM (V08A ATC), reported in 84% of ICSRs. Among these, iopamidol ($n = 63$; 43.8%) and iomeprol ($n = 32$; 22.2%) were the most frequently reported. This distribution also persisted in both considered periods, before and during the COVID-19 emergency. Magnetic resonance imaging CM (ATC V08C), in particular gadoteric acid and gadoteridol, were the other CM class reported as suspected drugs in the retrieved ICSRs. Among CM belonging to V08C ATC, comparing the two periods, the most frequently reported were gadoteric acid in period 1 ($n = 9$; 8.6%) and gadoteridol in period 2 ($n = 3$; 7.7%). Moreover, we found 2 ICSRs sent during period 1 reporting other suspect drugs, in particular chlorhexidine and mepivacaine (Table 1). CM was mainly used for the CAT scan (data not shown). Regarding the outcome of ADRs' reports, overall, 86.8% of collected ICSRs had a favorable outcome. Comparing the two periods, we found an increase in the number of ICSRs with favorable outcomes (82.9% in period 1 vs. 97.4% in period 2). This difference was statistically significant ($p = 0.04$) (Table 1). Overall, a seriousness degree was available for 139 reports: 75.7% of cases were classified as not serious, while only about 21% were classified as serious. Stratifying results by reference periods, the percentage of serious ICSRs increased in period 2 (16.2% in period 1 vs. 33.3% in period 2) (Table 1). Additionally, this difference was statistically significant ($p = 0.04$) (Table 1). Since each ICSR can report more than 1 ADR, overall, 77 serious ADRs were described in 30 ICSRs sent to Campania Regional Centre (17 in period 1 vs. 13 in period 2) (Table 2). Among those 77 serious ADRs, 90% were related to iodinated CM (V08A ATC), while the remaining 10% were related to magnetic resonance imaging CM (V08C ATC) (Table 2).

Table 2. Distribution of serious ADRs associated with individual contrast-media categorized for 3rd level ATC.

	Number of Serious Suspected ADR in Total Contrast Media's Reports $n = 77$	Number of Suspected Serious ADRs in Contrast Media's Reports During Period 1 $n = 41$	Number of Suspected Serious ADRs in Contrast Media's Reports During Period 2 $n = 36$	p-Value
V08A	70 (90)	40 (97.5)	30 (83.3)	0.07
Iomeprol	18 (23.4)	11 (26.8)	7 (19.4)	0.62
Iopamidol	29 (37.7)	13 (31.7)	16 (44.4)	0.36
Iopromide	11 (14.3)	4 (9.8)	7 (19.4)	0.37
Ioexol	2 (2.6)	2 (4.9)	0	0
Iodixanol	6 (7.8)	6 (14.6)	0	0
Iobitridol	4 (5.2)	4 (9.8)	0	0
V08C	7 (10)	1 (2.4)	6 (16.7)	0.07
Gadobenic acid	5 (6.5)	0	5 (13.9)	0
Gadoteric acid	1 (1.3)	0	1 (2.8)	0
Gadoteridol	1 (1.3)	1 (2.4)	0	0

V08A: X-ray contrast media, iodinated; V08C: magnetic resonance imaging contrast media. The total number of ADRs reported for each contrast media exceeds the total number of ICSRs since a single report might include more than one suspected ADR. Database from the Campania Region, Southern Italy.

Comparing the two-reference period, this distribution, with the major involvement of V08C in the occurrence of serious ADRs, was confirmed. Iopamidol (37.7%) and iomeprol (23.4%) persisted as the more frequently iodinated CM involved in serious cases (V08A ATC). Regarding V08C CM, we found a few serious cases related to gadobenic ($n = 5$) and gadoteric ($n = 1$) acids reported only in period 2, while the only serious ICSR related to gadoteridol was reported in period 1. As reported in Table 2, no statistically significant difference emerged.

The distribution of ADRs by SOC and HLGTs in two reference periods is shown in Figure 2 and Table 3, respectively.

"Skin and subcutaneous tissue disorders" (61.8% in period 1 vs. 38.3% in period 2) and "respiratory, thoracic and mediastinal disorders" (9.1% in period 1 vs. 16% in period 2) were the first two SOCs more frequently reported in both periods. Moreover, gastrointestinal (7.9% in period 1 vs. 12.3% in period 2) and general disorders (6.1% in period 1 vs. 3.7% in period 2) were commonly reported, even if less frequently in period 2, as per the general trend. Vascular disorders represented 6.1% of reported ADRs in period 1 and 8.6% of those reported in period 2. Otherwise, we found a more frequent reporting of ADRs belonging to "nervous system disorders" SOC in period 2 (1.2% vs. 4.9%). Regarding CM renal toxicity, ADRs belonging to "renal and urinary disorders" SOC were reported only in a few ICSRs in both periods, representing 1.2% vs. 2.5% of reported ADRs in the two reference periods, respectively (Figure 2). Comparing two reference periods, statistically significant differences emerged for "epidermal and dermal conditions" and "oral soft tissue conditions" HLGTs (Table 3). CM belonging to V08A ATC was always the most involved category in reporting ADRs per all SOCs (data not shown).

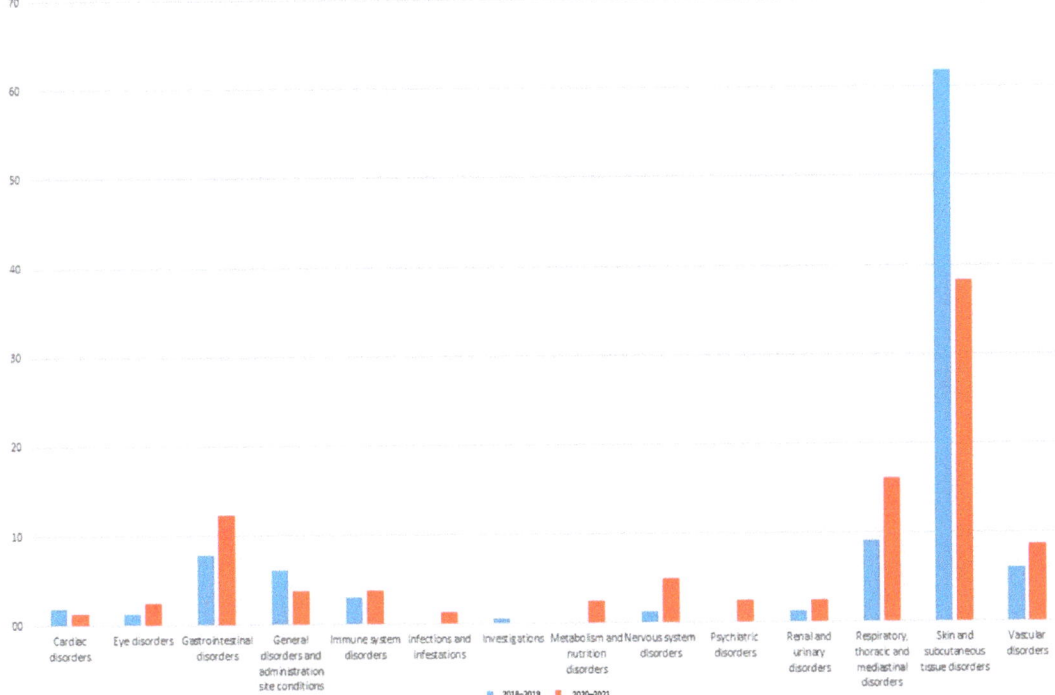

Figure 2. ADR distributions by system organ class in ICSRs reporting contrast media as suspected drugs and collected in the Campania Region. Comparison between pre-COVID-19 pandemic (period 1 = 2018–2019; blue color) and during the COVID-19 pandemic (period 2 = 2020–2021; red color).

Table 3. ADR distributions by high-level group terms (HLGTs) in ICSRs reporting contrast media as suspected drugs and collected in the Campania Region. Comparison between pre-COVID-19 pandemic (period 1: 2018–2019) and during the COVID-19 pandemic (period 2: 2020–2021).

	Period 1		Period 2		p-Value
High-Level Group Terms	N	%	N	%	p
Acid-base disorders	-	-	1	1.2	-
Allergic conditions	5	3.0	3	3.7	0.8
Angioedema and urticaria	27	16.4	10	12.3	0.4
Arteriosclerosis, stenosis, vascular insufficiency and necrosis	-	-	2	2.5	-
Body temperature conditions	1	0.6	-	-	-
Bronchial disorders (excl neoplasms)	1	0.6	1	1.2	-
Cardiac and vascular investigations (excluding enzyme tests)	-	-	1	1.2	-
Cardiac arrhythmias	3	1.8	1	1.2	0.7
Central nervous system vascular disorders	-	-	2	2.5	-
Decreased and nonspecific blood pressure disorders and shock	4	2.4	1	1.2	0.5
Deliria (including confusion)	-	-	1	1.2	-
Dental and gingival conditions	1	0.6	-	-	-
Electrolyte and fluid balance conditions	-	-	1	1.2	-

Table 3. Cont.

High-Level Group Terms	Period 1		Period 2		p-Value
	N	%	N	%	p
Epidermal and dermal conditions	73	44.2	18	22.2	0.0007
Eye disorders NEC	-	-	1	1.2	-
Gastrointestinal haemorrhages NEC	1	0.6	-	-	-
Gastrointestinal motility and defaecation conditions	-	-	1	1.2	-
Gastrointestinal signs and symptoms	10	6.1	5	6.2	0.9
General system disorders NEC	9	5.5	3	3.7	0.5
Infections—pathogen unspecified	1	0.6	-	-	-
Lower respiratory tract disorders (excluding obstruction and infection)	-	-	8	9.9	-
Nephropathies	2	1.2	-	-	-
Neurological disorders NEC	2	1.2	1	1.2	0.9
Neuromuscular disorders	-	-	1	1.2	-
Ocular infections, irritations and inflammations	2	1.2	1	1.2	0.9
Oral soft tissue conditions	1	0.6	4	4.9	0.02
Renal disorders (excluding nephropathies)	-	-	2	2.5	-
Respiratory disorders NEC	7	4.2	3	3.7	0.8
Respiratory tract signs and symptoms	6	3.6	-	-	-
Skin appendage conditions	1	0.6	3	3.7	0.07
Skin vascular abnormalities	1	0.6	-	-	-
Sleep disorders and disturbances	-	-	1	1.2	-
Upper respiratory tract disorders (excluding infections)	1	0.6	1	1.2	0.6
Vascular disorders NEC	6	3.6	3	3.7	0.9
Vascular hypertensive disorders	-	-	1	1.2	-

Considering serious ADRs, allergic or anaphylactic reactions were the more frequent ones reported during period 1, which required/prolonged patient hospitalization or represented life-threatening. These ADRs included mild manifestations such as allergic purpura or gum and mouth swelling and important systemic adverse events like anaphylactic shock. In the same period, flushing, erythematous skin rash, and hives are some examples of not serious ADRs that were more frequently reported. In particular, iopamidol was involved in 3 cases of anaphylactoid reaction reported in period 1 and 2 cases of reversible ischaemic neurological deficit reported in period 2. The remaining serious ADR reports were mainly related to hypotension or hypertensive crisis, cardiac rhythm disorders (including tachycardia and bradycardia and a case of cardiac arrest). Moreover, only one case reported in period 2 described toxic renal events that occurred in a 60-year-old female treated with iopromide for abdominal CAT, who experienced dependent edema, hyperkalaemia, acidosis metabolic, oliguria and renal failure, which required patient hospitalization. Finally, following Naranjo's algorithm computation, the causality assessment was shown to be probable (61%) for the majority of period 1 ICSRs, while the remaining 39% were evaluated as possible. Regarding period 2, the causality assessment resulted in possible, probable or doubtful assessments in 46.2%, 51.3% and 2.6% of cases, respectively (Figure 3). Distributions of cases by causality assessment in the two reference periods are reported in Figure 3, in which CM is categorized for III levels of ATC classes (V08A and V08C).

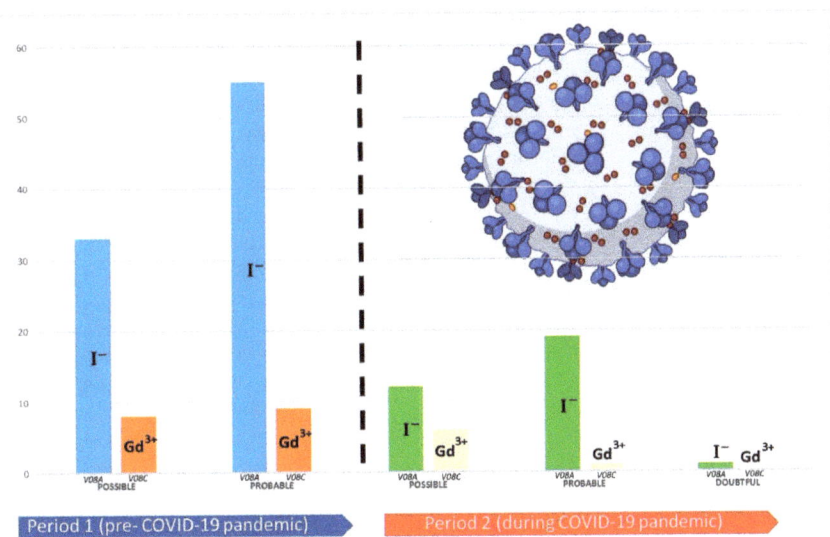

Figure 3. Distribution by causality assessment of ICSRs reporting contrast media as suspected drugs and collected in the Campania Region from 1 January 2018 to 31 December 2021. Comparison between pre-COVID-19 pandemic (period 1 = 2018–2019) and during the COVID-19 pandemic (period 2 = 2020–2021). Contrast media are categorized for III levels of ATC classes. V08A: X-ray contrast media, iodinated; V08C: magnetic resonance imaging contrast media.

4. Discussion

The COVID-19 pandemic has had several impacts on society, influencing various aspects related to drugs, such as pharmacovigilance and spontaneous reporting. Safety assessment and issues related to anti-COVID-19 vaccines have turned the spotlight on pharmacovigilance systems and mechanisms. Due to the media and civil attention focused on COVID-19 vaccines, the reporting by citizens has considerably increased during the pandemic. Nevertheless, from our analysis, the reporting of ADR induced by CM has not been the object of interest for patients and citizens. In fact, healthcare professionals sent all CM-related ICSRs in our study period. Generally, the COVID-19 pandemic has negatively influenced CM-related ADR reporting. Several reasons can justify this result. Firstly, the observed substantial decrease in the CM-related reporting trend is in line with reporting national trends registered during the COVID-19 pandemic. According to the 2020 Vaccine Report published by the Italian Medicines Agency, the reporting rate for all vaccines (excluding COVID-19 vaccines) showed a sharp decline compared with recent years [22]. Primary sources, limited access, and attention focused on global emergencies can certainly be involved in the generally reduced reporting, including CM-related ones.

Generally, doctors, followed by nurses and other health workers, represent the primary sources of spontaneous reports, especially in South Italy [23–31]. Several initiatives have been implemented, and others are still necessary to implement a pharmacovigilance culture among all healthcare professionals and the general population [32–37]. The pressure to which healthcare personnel have been subjected during the COVID-19 emergency is well known. This was especially noted for those working in departments/wards dedicated to treating COVID-19 patients, for which medical imaging using CM was required for a complete clinical evaluation. Moreover, radiology departments were widely involved in the pandemic context since the key role of clinical imaging in diagnosing and managing COVID-19 patients [38]. In light of this, the observed reduction in reporting trends can be easily understood and expected. Moreover, the public health emergency has monopolized attention and energy in all fields, including pharmaco- and vaccine vigilance. In fact, even if these activities were implemented during the pandemic, they were strongly focused on vaccines and drugs repositioned against SARS-CoV-2 infection [39]. Finally, the decreased trend is likely attributed to lower patient access to non-emergency or essential health services, including diagnostic investigation [40]. Patients' fear and the health pressure on hospitals and medical centers, as well as the limitations imposed by lockdowns and quarantines, have certainly been involved in this last aspect. However, if their wide use for clinical evaluation of hospitalized COVID-19 patients is considered, the reduced CM-related reporting during the pandemic should be in contrast with what is expected. Even if the COVID-19 pandemic was characterized by a decrease in elective diagnostic imaging procedures and clinical imaging, radiology departments played an essential part in detecting and following up on patients with COVID-19 during the pandemic [41,42]. Diagnostic procedures, such as CT, resulted in the fundamental disease course and severity assessment tools. Their usefulness in clinical management orienting was also confirmed during the COVID-19 pandemic. In fact, imaging techniques are included as part of the integrated approach necessary for diagnosis, monitoring and identification of the most appropriate therapy in COVID-19 patients, especially when hospitalized [41,42]. Compared to previous viral pandemics, imaging modalities played an essential role in the respiratory tract, cardiovascular, neurologic, and gastrointestinal evaluation of COVID-19 patients [41]. However, according to national data published by AIFA, a decrease in consumption and expenditure of CM has been registered in 2020. This decrease was probably due to a lower number of diagnostic tests carried out for chronic diseases during the first year of the COVID-19 pandemic [43]. Data related to Italian consumption and expenditure in 2021 are still not available. According to our results, iodinated CM, particularly iomeprol and iopamidol, were the most frequently involved in spontaneous reporting. Especially during period 2, they were mainly used for CAT scans. Instead, no ICSR reported angiograph coronary as their therapeutic indication. However, CT coronary angiography use increased during the COVID-19 pandemic since it was associated with a significantly reduced length of hospitalization both pre-COVID-19 and post-COVID-19 lockdown [44]. The strong effort of health care professionals engaged on the COVID-19 front can also be related to the increased reporting of serious ADRs emerging in period 2, with statistical significance. To emphasize this aspect, reporting attention was limited to the most severe adverse events. However, any new adverse events emerged during the two periods. Considering the event's notoriety, all the ADRs reported in the overall study period were known and reported in the Summaries of Products Characteristics (SmPCs). In line with Sessa et al.'s results (Sessa et al., 2015a), our results also revealed that skin and respiratory disorders continued to be the more frequently reported ADRs in patients who received CM. As expected, the main reported ADRs were angioedema, urticaria and epidermal phenomena. Even if decreased in our study period, spontaneous reporting confirmed general toxicity more frequently related to iodinated CM compared to gadolinium-based CM. In fact, from our results, iodinated CM was more frequently involved in a major number of ICSRs, and serious ADRs, resulting in a more probable relationship with drug-adverse events according to the applied Naranjo algorithm. In the last years, attention has been given to CM nephrotoxicity among organ-specific adverse reactions, probably caused by induced endothelial dysfunction and renal cell apoptosis [21,45]. However, in our period study, renal disorders did not emerge as frequently, and only a few cases reported nephropathies or renal disorders. These were all related to iodine-based agents. In particular, a case of renal failure with oliguria associated with acidosis metabolic and hyperkaliemia, requiring hospitalization but favorably evolving, was reported in period 2. Considering CM-related organ-specific toxicity, cardiovascular is another important aspect that emerged, together with anaphylactic shock, among the most frequently reported fatal CM-related ADRs in the Campania Region [46]. According to our results, cardiac arrhythmias, including tachycardia and cardiac arrest, were other rarely reported ADRs that need close monitoring since they represent life-threatening for patients. Malignant arrhythmogenesis is not an uncommon complication of some imaging techniques, such as invasive coronary angiography [47].

Often, the main cause can be related to technical procedural issues. Following the trigger of such arrhythmic events can be the CM administration since iodine-based effects are influenced not only by their osmolarity but also by their sodium concentration and calcium-binding properties. It is well known that administering CM makes patients more susceptible to ventricular fibrillation or sustained ventricular [47]. Finally, neurotoxicity represents another CM-related organ-specific issue that recently emerged. A recent safety review of EMA confirmed in 2018 the possible accumulation of small amounts of gadolinium in the cerebral tissues following the use of linear gadolinium-based CM more than macrocyclic ones. Since the long-term risks associated with this phenomenon were unknown, the EMA was suspended in the EU gadolinium containing linear CM with the exception of gadoxetic acid and gadobenic acid, available exclusively for use in hepatic scans [48]. In line with these use restrictions, only a few cases related to these two CM agents emerged from our results. No cases of long-term nervous adverse events were reported.

In light of our results, the adopted measures against COVID-19 are likely to have an important impact on spontaneous reporting related to other medicine not specifically indicated to COVID-19 treatment, such as CM. Whilst our results could be reassuring regarding the safety profile of CM as drugs well-known and long been used in clinical practice, on the other hand, the pandemic was likely to be a missed opportunity to deepen the safety of drugs so important for the evaluation of patients and the course of COVID-19 and many other diseases.

5. Strengths and Limitations

Our study presents the well-known limitations related to the spontaneous reporting system, including possible under-reporting and inaccurate, incomplete or lack of clinical data [49,50]. Unavailable/not reported data can have an important impact on the results of pharmacovigilance studies, such as ours. Moreover, since we have decided to perform our pharmacovigilance analysis during 4 years of observation in one single Italian region, we have extracted a very limited number of reports, which should not be considered representative of the other Italian regions. Despite these limitations, we present a comprehensive evaluation of safety data related to CM in the Campania region during the COVID-19 pandemic and compare them with those emerging from the previous two years using the Italian spontaneous reporting system. Although the spontaneous reporting system has an intrinsic limitation, it is largely accepted that it represents a simple and inexpensive tool to detect rare and serious ADRs that have not emerged during premarketing clinical phases. Furthermore, this method allows for generating safety hypotheses on medicines that shall be confirmed or refuted by other ad hoc studies.

6. Conclusions

During the COVID-19 pandemic, the imaging techniques with CM achieved a better clinical evaluation of patients affected with COVID-19, especially if hospitalized, allowing an integrated approach to diagnosing, monitoring, and managing SARS-CoV-2 infection. Despite the wide use of CM during the COVID-19 pandemic, there was a decrease in ADR reporting. In our opinion, reasons for this are undoubtedly various, including the strong effort of health care professionals engaged on the COVID-19 front, with less time to spend in spontaneous ADR reporting and attention focused on the global emergency. Pharmacovigilance activities were more focused on vaccines or repurposed drugs used for COVID-19 treatment. Despite those effects on ADRs' reporting, there is no doubt about the usefulness of the CM in imaging for a greater assessment of acute and chronic complications related to COVID, reducing the length of hospitalization. Although the pandemic was likely to be a missed opportunity to deepen CM safety, the continuous monitoring of CM safety and the full implementation of pharmacovigilance activities will play a key role in achieving optimal clinical imaging.

Author Contributions: Conceptualization, all the authors; Data curation, C.R. (Claudia Rossi), M.G. and R.R.; Supervision, L.S. and C.R. (Concetta Rafaniello); Validation, C.P. and A.P.; Writing—original draft, C.R. (Claudia Rossi) and R.R.; Writing—review & editing, M.G., L.S. and C.R. (Concetta Rafaniello). All authors have read and agreed to the published version of the manuscript.

Funding: This research received no external funding.

Institutional Review Board Statement: Not applicable.

Informed Consent Statement: Not applicable.

Data Availability Statement: Data supporting reported results can be found in the National Pharmacovigilance Network, but their availability is limited to Regional Pharmacovigilance Centers and the Italian Medicine Agency.

Conflicts of Interest: The authors declare no conflict of interest.

References

1. Chang, L.; Yan, Y.; Wang, L. Coronavirus Disease 2019: Coronaviruses and Blood Safety. *Transfus. Med. Rev.* **2020**, *34*, 75–80. [CrossRef]
2. Romano, M.; Ruggiero, A.; Squeglia, F.; Maga, G.; Berisio, R. A Structural View of SARS-CoV-2 RNA Replication Machinery: RNA Synthesis, Proofreading and Final Capping. *Cells* **2020**, *9*, 1267. [CrossRef]
3. Hoffmann, M.; Kleine-Weber, H.; Schroeder, S.; Krüger, N.; Herrler, T.; Erichsen, S.; Schiergens, T.S.; Herrler, G.; Wu, N.H.; Nitsche, A.; et al. SARS-CoV-2 Cell Entry Depends on ACE2 and TMPRSS2 and Is Blocked by a Clinically Proven Protease Inhibitor. *Cell* **2020**, *181*, 271–280.e8. [CrossRef]
4. Hu, B.; Guo, H.; Zhou, P.; Shi, Z.L. Characteristics of SARS-CoV-2 and COVID-19. *Nat. Rev. Microbiol.* **2021**, *19*, 1. [CrossRef]
5. World Health Organization. WHO Coronavirus (COVID-19) Dashboard | WHO Coronavirus (COVID-19) Dashboard With Vaccination Data. Available online: https://covid19.who.int/ (accessed on 14 March 2022).
6. Suh, Y.J.; Hong, H.; Ohana, M.; Bompard, F.; Revel, M.P.; Valle, C.; Gervaise, A.; Poissy, J.; Susen, S.; Hékimian, G.; et al. Pulmonary Embolism and Deep Vein Thrombosis in COVID-19: A Systematic Review and Meta-Analysis. *Radiology* **2021**, *298*, E70–E80. [CrossRef]
7. Faggiano, P.; Bonelli, A.; Paris, S.; Milesi, G.; Bisegna, S.; Bernardi, N.; Curnis, A.; Agricola, E.; Maroldi, R. Acute Pulmonary Embolism in COVID-19 Disease: Preliminary Report on Seven Patients. *Int. J. Cardiol.* **2020**, *313*, 129–131. [CrossRef]
8. Bompard, F.; Monnier, H.; Saab, I.; Tordjman, M.; Abdoul, H.; Fournier, L.; Sanchez, O.; Lorut, C.; Chassagnon, G.; Revel, M.P. Pulmonary Embolism in Patients with COVID-19 Pneumonia. *Eur. Respir. J.* **2020**, *56*, 2001365. [CrossRef]
9. Connors, J.M.; Levy, J.H. COVID-19 and Its Implications for Thrombosis and Anticoagulation. *Blood* **2020**, *135*, 2033–2040. [CrossRef]
10. Ali, M.A.M.; Spinler, S.A. COVID-19 and Thrombosis: From Bench to Bedside. *Trends Cardiovasc. Med.* **2021**, *31*, 143–160. [CrossRef]
11. Müller, S.; Beyer-Westendorf, J. Thromboembolic Complications in COVID-19. *Dtsch. Med. Wochenschr.* **2020**, *145*, 1728–1734. [CrossRef]
12. Soldati, G.; Giannasi, G.; Smargiassi, A.; Inchingolo, R.; Demi, L. Contrast-Enhanced Ultrasound in Patients With COVID-19: Pneumonia, Acute Respiratory Distress Syndrome, or Something Else? *J. Ultrasound Med.* **2020**, *39*, 2483–2489. [CrossRef] [PubMed]
13. Kistner, A.; Tamm, C.; Svensson, A.M.; Beckman, M.O.; Strand, F.; Sköld, M.; Nyrén, S. Negative Effects of Iodine-Based Contrast Agent on Renal Function in Patients with Moderate Reduced Renal Function Hospitalized for COVID-19. *BMC Nephrol.* **2021**, *22*, 1–10. [CrossRef] [PubMed]
14. Mascolo, A.; Scavone, C.; Rafaniello, C.; Ferrajolo, C.; Racagni, G.; Berrino, L.; Paolisso, G.; Rossi, F.; Capuano, A. Renin-Angiotensin System and Coronavirus Disease 2019: A Narrative Review. *Front. Cardiovasc. Med.* **2020**, *7*, 143. [CrossRef]
15. Puntmann, V.O.; Carerj, M.L.; Wieters, I.; Fahim, M.; Arendt, C.; Hoffmann, J.; Shchendrygina, A.; Escher, F.; Vasa-Nicotera, M.; Zeiher, A.M.; et al. Outcomes of Cardiovascular Magnetic Resonance Imaging in Patients Recently Recovered from Coronavirus Disease 2019 (COVID-19). *JAMA Cardiol.* **2020**, *5*, 1265. [CrossRef] [PubMed]
16. Huang, L.; Zhao, P.; Tang, D.; Zhu, T.; Han, R.; Zhan, C.; Liu, W.; Zeng, H.; Tao, Q.; Xia, L. Cardiac Involvement in Patients Recovered from COVID-2019 Identified Using Magnetic Resonance Imaging. *JACC Cardiovasc. Imaging* **2020**, *13*, 2330–2339. [CrossRef]
17. Desai, A.D.; Lavelle, M.; Boursiquot, B.C.; Wan, E.Y. Long-Term Complications of COVID-19. *Am. J. Physiol. Cell Physiol.* **2022**, *322*, C1. [CrossRef]
18. Sudre, C.H.; Murray, B.; Varsavsky, T.; Graham, M.S.; Penfold, R.S.; Bowyer, R.C.; Pujol, J.C.; Klaser, K.; Antonelli, M.; Canas, L.S.; et al. Attributes and Predictors of Long COVID. *Nat. Med.* **2021**, *27*, 626–631. [CrossRef]

19. Sessa, M.; Rossi, C.; Mascolo, A.; Scafuro, A.; Ruggiero, R.; di Mauro, G.; Cappabianca, S.; Grassi, R.; Sportiello, L.; Rafaniello, C. Contribution of Italian Clinical Research for Contrast Media-Induced Nonrenal Adverse Drug Reactions over the Last Three Decades: A Systematic Review. *J. Pharmacol. Pharmacother.* **2018**, *9*, 131–146. [CrossRef]
20. Krause, D.; Marycz, D.; Ziada, K.M. Nonrenal Complications of Contrast Media. *Interv. Cardiol. Clin.* **2020**, *9*, 311–319. [CrossRef]
21. Sessa, M.; Rossi, C.; Mascolo, A.; Scavone, C.; di Mauro, G.; Grassi, R.; Sportiello, L.; Cappabianca, S.; Rafaniello, C. Contrast Media-Induced Nephropathy: How Has Italy Contributed in the Past 30 Years? A Systematic Review. *Ther. Clin. Risk Manag.* **2017**, *13*, 1463–1478. [CrossRef]
22. Italian Medicines Agency. Rapporto Vaccini 2020. Available online: https://www.aifa.gov.it/en/-/rapporto-vaccini-2020 (accessed on 26 May 2022).
23. Ferrajolo, C.; Capuano, A.; Trifirò, G.; Moretti, U.; Rossi, F.; Santuccio, C. Pediatric drug safety surveillance in Italian pharmacovigilance network: An overview of adverse drug reactions in the years 2001–2012. *Expert Opin. Drug Saf.* **2014**, *13* (Suppl. 1), 9–20. [CrossRef] [PubMed]
24. Rafaniello, C.; Ferrajolo, C.; Sullo, M.G.; Sessa, M.; Sportiello, L.; Balzano, A.; Manguso, F.; Aiezza, M.L.; Rossi, F.; Scarpignato, C.; et al. Risk of gastrointestinal complications associated to NSAIDs, low-dose aspirin and their combinations: Results of a pharmacovigilance reporting system. *Pharmacol. Res.* **2016**, *104*, 108–114. [CrossRef]
25. Scavone, C.; Sessa, M.; Clementi, E.; Corrao, G.; Leone, R.; Mugelli, A.; Rossi, F.; Spina, E.; Capuano, A. Real World Data on the Utilization Pattern and Safety Profile of Infliximab Originator Versus Biosimilars in Italy: A Multiregional Study. *BioDrugs* **2018**, *32*, 607–617. [CrossRef] [PubMed]
26. Scavone, C.; Di Mauro, C.; Brusco, S.; Bertini, M.; di Mauro, G.; Rafaniello, C.; Sportiello, L.; Rossi, F.; Capuano, A. Surveillance of adverse events following immunization related to human papillomavirus vaccines: 12 years of vaccinovigilance in Southern Italy. *Expert Opin. Drug Saf.* **2019**, *18*, 427–433. [CrossRef] [PubMed]
27. Scavone, C.; Di Mauro, C.; Ruggiero, R.; Bernardi, F.F.; Trama, U.; Aiezza, M.L.; Rafaniello, C.; Capuano, A. Severe Cutaneous Adverse Drug Reactions Associated with Allopurinol: An Analysis of Spontaneous Reporting System in Southern Italy. *Drugs-Real World Outcomes* **2020**, *7*, 41. [CrossRef]
28. Scavone, C.; Mascolo, A.; Ruggiero, R.; Sportiello, L.; Rafaniello, C.; Berrino, L.; Capuano, A. Quinolones-Induced Musculoskeletal, Neurological, and Psychiatric ADRs: A Pharmacovigilance Study Based on Data From the Italian Spontaneous Reporting System. *Front. Pharmacol.* **2020**, *11*, 428. [CrossRef]
29. Sultana, J.; Moretti, U.; Addis, A.; Caduff, P.; Capuano, A.; Kant, A.; Laporte, J.R.; Lindquist, M.; Raine, J.; Sartori, D.; et al. Workshop on the Italian Pharmacovigilance System in the International Context: Critical Issues and Perspectives. *Drug Saf.* **2018**, *42*, 683–687. [CrossRef]
30. Mascolo, A.; Ruggiero, R.; Sessa, M.; Scavone, C.; Sportiello, L.; Rafaniello, C.; Rossi, F.; Capuano, A. Preventable cases of oral anticoagulant-induced bleeding: Data from the spontaneous reporting system. *Front. Pharmacol.* **2019**, *10*, 425. [CrossRef]
31. Pagani, S.; Lombardi, N.; Crescioli, G.; Vighi, G.V.; Spada, G.; Romoli, I.; Andreetta, P.; Capuano, A.; Marrazzo, E.; Marra, A.; et al. Analysis of fatal adverse drug events recorded in several Italian emergency departments (the MEREAFaPS study). *Intern. Emerg. Med.* **2021**, *16*, 741–748. [CrossRef]
32. Ruggiero, S.; Rafaniello, C.; Bravaccio, C.; Grimaldi, G.; Granato, R.; Pascotto, A.; Sportiello, L.; Parretta, E.; Rinaldi, B.; Panei, P.; et al. Safety of attention-deficit/hyperactivity disorder medications in children: An intensive pharmacosurveillance monitoring study. *J. Child. Adolesc. Psychopharmacol.* **2012**, *22*, 415–422. [CrossRef]
33. Parretta, E.; Rafaniello, C.; Magro, L.; Coggiola Pittoni, A.; Sportiello, L.; Ferrajolo, C.; Mascolo, A.; Sessa, M.; Rossi, F.; Capuano, A. Improvement of patient adverse drug reaction reporting through a community pharmacist-based intervention in the Campania region of Italy. *Expert Opin. Drug Saf.* **2014**, *13* (Suppl. 1), 21–29. [CrossRef] [PubMed]
34. Sessa, M.; Bernardi, F.F.; Vitale, A.; Schiavone, B.; Gritti, G.; Mascolo, A.; Bertini, M.; Scavone, C.; Sportiello, L.; Rossi, F.; et al. Adverse drug reactions during hepatitis C treatment with direct-acting antivirals: The role of medication errors, their impact on treatment discontinuation and their preventability. New insights from the Campania Region (Italy) spontaneous reporting system. *J. Clin. Pharm. Ther.* **2018**, *43*, 867–876. [CrossRef] [PubMed]
35. Sessa, M.; Rafaniello, C.; Sportiello, L.; Mascolo, A.; Scavone, C.; Maccariello, A.; Iannaccone, T.; Fabrazzo, M.; Berrino, L.; Rossi, F.; et al. Campania Region (Italy) spontaneous reporting system and preventability assessment through a case-by-case approach: A pilot study on psychotropic drugs. *Expert Opin. Drug Saf.* **2016**, *15*, 9–15. [CrossRef]
36. Scavone, C.; Sportiello, L.; Sullo, M.G.; Ferrajolo, C.; Ruggiero, R.; Sessa, M.; Berrino, P.M.; di Mauro, G.; Berrino, L.; Rossi, F.; et al. Safety Profile of Anticancer and Immune-Modulating Biotech Drugs Used in a Real World Setting in Campania Region (Italy): BIO-Cam Observational Study. *Front. Pharmacol.* **2017**, *8*, 607. [CrossRef]
37. Maniscalco, G.T.; Scavone, C.; Moreggia, O.; Di Giulio Cesare, D.; Aiezza, M.L.; Guglielmi, G.; Longo, G.; Maiolo, M.; Raiola, E.; Russo, G.; et al. Flu vaccination in multiple sclerosis patients: A monocentric prospective vaccine-vigilance study. *Expert Opin. Drug Saf.* **2022**, 1–6. [CrossRef]
38. Alhasan, M.; Hasaneen, M. The Role and Challenges of Clinical Imaging During COVID-19 Outbreak. *J. Diagn. Med. Sonogr.* **2022**, *38*, 72–84. [CrossRef]
39. Rafaniello, C.; Ferrajolo, C.; Sullo, M.G.; Gaio, M.; Zinzi, A.; Scavone, C.; Gargano, F.; Coscioni, E.; Rossi, F.; Capuano, A. Cardiac Events Potentially Associated to Remdesivir: An Analysis from the European Spontaneous Adverse Event Reporting System. *Pharmaceuticals* **2021**, *14*, 611. [CrossRef]

40. Bucciarelli-Ducci, C.; Ajmone-Marsan, N.; Di Carli, M.; Nicol, E. The year in cardiovascular medicine 2021: Imaging. *Eur. Heart J.* **2022**, *43*, 1288–1295. [CrossRef]
41. Sotoudeh, H.; Gity, M. The Role of Medical Imaging in COVID-19. *Adv. Exp. Med. Biol.* **2021**, *1318*, 413–434. [CrossRef] [PubMed]
42. Varadarajan, V.; Shabani, M.; Venkatesh, B.A.; Lima, J.A. Role of Imaging in Diagnosis andManagement of COVID-19: A Multiorgan Multimodality Imaging Review. *Front. Med.* **2021**, *8*, 765975. [CrossRef]
43. OsMed 2020 National Report on Medicines Use in Italy. 2020. Available online: https://www.aifa.gov.it/en/-/rapporto-nazionale-osmed-2020-sull-uso-dei-farmaci-in-italia (accessed on 26 May 2022).
44. Cronin, M.; Wheen, P.; Armstrong, R.; Kumar, R.; McMahon, A.; White, M.; Sheehy, N.; McMahon, G.; Murphy, R.T.; Daly, C. CT coronary angiography and COVID-19: Inpatient use in acute chest pain service. *Open Heart* **2021**, *8*, e001548. [CrossRef] [PubMed]
45. Macdonald, D.B.; Hurrell, C.D.; Costa, A.F.; McInnes, M.D.F.; O'Malley, M.; Barrett, B.J.; Brown, P.A.; Clark, E.G.; Hadjivassiliou, A.; Kirkpatrick, I.D.C.; et al. Canadian Association of Radiologists Guidance on Contrast-Associated Acute Kidney Injury. *Can J Kidney Health Dis.* **2022**, *9*, 7455. [CrossRef]
46. Sessa, M.; Rossi, C.; Mascolo, A.; Grassi, E.; Fiorentino, S.; Scavone, C.; Reginelli, A.; Rotondo, A.; Sportiello, L. Suspected adverse reactions to contrast media in Campania Region (Italy): Results from 14 years of post-marketing surveillance. *Expert Opin. Drug Saf.* **2015**, *14*, 1341–1351. [CrossRef]
47. Kariki, O.; Kontonika, M.; Miliopoulos, D.; Bazoukis, G.; Vlachos, K.; Dragasis, S.; Gouziouta, A.; Letsas, K.P.; Efremidis, M.; Voudris, V. CASE PRESENTATION Contrast-induced early repolarization pattern and ventricular fibrillation. *Clin. Case Rep.* **2021**, *9*, 4630. [CrossRef] [PubMed]
48. European Medicines Agency. EMA's Final Opinion Confirms Restrictions on Use of Linear Gadolinium Agents in Body Scans. Available online: https://www.ema.europa.eu/en/news/emas-final-opinion-confirms-restrictions-use-linear-gadolinium-agents-body-scans (accessed on 19 August 2022).
49. Noguchi, Y.; Tachi, T.; Teramachi, H. Detection algorithms and attentive points of safety signal using spontaneous reporting systems as a clinical data source. *Brief. Bioinform.* **2021**, *22*, bbab347. [CrossRef]
50. Montastruc, J.L.; Sommet, A.; Bagheri, H.; Lapeyre-Mestre, M. Benefits and strengths of the disproportionality analysis for identification of adverse drug reactions in a pharmacovigilance database. *Br. J. Clin. Pharmacol.* **2011**, *72*, 905–908. [CrossRef]

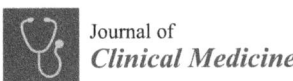

Article

COVID-19 Vaccines Adverse Reactions Reported to the Pharmacovigilance Unit of Beira Interior in Portugal

Carina Amaro [1], Cristina Monteiro [2,*] and Ana Paula Duarte [2,3,*]

1 Health Science Faculty, University of Beira Interior, 6201-001 Covilhã, Portugal
2 UFBI-Pharmacovigilance Unit of Beira Interior, University of Beira Interior, 6201-001 Covilhã, Portugal
3 CICS-UBI-Health Sciences Research Centre, University of Beira Interior, 6201-001 Covilhã, Portugal
* Correspondence: csjmonteiro79@gmail.com (C.M.); apcd@ubi.pt (A.P.D.)

Abstract: Coronavirus disease 2019 is an acute respiratory disease caused by the severe acute respiratory syndrome coronavirus 2. As the virus spreads rapidly, it has become a major public health emergency, which has led to rapid vaccines development. However, vaccines can present harmful and unintended responses, which must be notified to the National Pharmacovigilance System. The aim of this study is to characterize the adverse drug reactions (ADRs) of these vaccines notified in the region covered by the Regional Pharmacovigilance Unit (RPU) of Beira Interior, in Portugal, between 1 and 31 December 2020. During this period, 4 vaccines were administered: Comirnaty®, Spikevax®, Vaxzevria® and Jcovden®. The RPU of Beira Interior received 2134 notifications corresponding to 5685 ADRs, of which 20.34% (n = 434) of the notifications were considered serious reactions. Of these, 9.52% (n = 42) resulted in hospitalization and 0.45% (n = 2) resulted in death. Among the ADRs notified, reactions at or around the injection site, myalgia, headaches and pyrexia were the most commonly notified. Most ADRs were resolved within a few hours or days without sequelae. These ADRs are in accordance with clinical trials, the summary of product characteristics (SmPC) of each vaccine and ADR notifications from other countries. However, further studies are needed to confirm these results.

Keywords: adverse drug reactions; COVID-19 vaccines; mRNA vaccines; vaccines with a viral vector; pharmacovigilance; immunization; safety

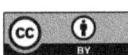

1. Introduction

Coronavirus Disease 2019 (COVID-19) is an acute respiratory disease caused by the severe acute respiratory syndrome coronavirus 2 (SARS-CoV-2), which first emerged in Wuhan in December 2019. Its transmission occurs by droplets, respiratory secretions and direct contact [1,2].

As the virus has a rapid spread, it has become a serious public health emergency [2]. Given that vaccination can be used to prevent infections or reduce the seriousness of a disease, some strategies were studied to generate vaccines against the new coronavirus, including vaccines based on DNA and RNA [3,4].

Nucleic acid vaccines consist of mRNA with information against coronavirus-specific structural proteins and do not contain any viral proteins capable of causing disease. The mRNA is taken up by cells and translated into a viral antigen, the spike protein. When recognized by the immune system as something foreign, antibodies are produced, and T cells are activated to attack the protein. If the vaccinated person later comes into contact with coronavirus, their immune system will recognize the spike protein and be ready to defend itself [5–9]. In the European Union (EU), during the study period, 2 mRNA-based vaccines were authorized by the European Medicines Agency (EMA): Comirnaty® and Spikevax® [7–9].

In addition to mRNA vaccines, there is another type of vaccine approved for immunization against COVID-19: vaccines with a viral vector without the ability to replicate. This type of vaccine is produced from another virus (e.g., adenovirus) that has been modified to contain information regarding the virus of interest, which will be delivered to human cells. The viral vector is a harmless virus and different from coronavirus, so it does not cause the disease. It enters human cells and releases the gene that encodes the spike protein present in SARS-CoV-2. It then uses the cell's machinery to produce this glycoprotein which, when recognized by the immune system, leads to the production of antibodies and activation of T cells, as is in nucleic acid vaccines [10–13]. In the EU, during the study period, two vaccines based on viral vectors were authorized by the EMA: Vaxzevria® and Jcovden® [7,12,13].

Although medicines are essential elements in the treatment of pathologies, diagnosis and prevention, they also have risks. Thus, due to the fact that there is a limited knowledge of the therapeutic profile of some drugs, it is important to continue to monitor their safety after marketing, through several available methodologies, one of which is the notification of adverse drug reactions (ADRs) to the National Systems of Pharmacovigilance (NPS), present around the world, and created in order to monitor the safety of medicines. The NPS cover all information related to ADRs and guarantee the safety of users who have contact with medicines, especially medicines recently introduced on the market. This is the case of vaccines used to immunize against COVID-19 [14,15].

In 1992, the SNF was created in Portugal, currently coordinated by INFARMED, I.P. In the early 2000s, the SNF was decentralized into 4 Regional Pharmacovigilance Units (RPU)- Norte, Centro, Sul and Açores-, with the aim of publicizing the system and promoting notification, bringing the system closer to health professionals and promote the involvement of university centres. Since 2017, the number of RPUs in the SNF increased, and there are currently 10 covering different areas in the country. The RPU of Beira Interior is placed at the University of Beira Interior, in the interior of Portugal, covers the districts of Castelo Branco, Viseu and Guarda and involves some under reporting [16,17].

When the appearance of ADRs is suspected, the process of spontaneous notification through an online or paper form or by telephone becomes important. Spontaneous reporting is a voluntary pharmacovigilance methodology, which consists of reporting an ADR associated with a particular drug and a patient, which can be by the patient, a family member or a healthcare professional. Spontaneous reporting makes it possible to detect ADRs that occur rarely or unexpectedly, generating an alert signal for subsequent epidemiological studies [16].

Therefore, pharmacovigilance, a science involved in the detection, evaluation and prevention of ADRs, through the methodology of spontaneous reporting is an essential step to assess the safety of vaccines used in the immunization against COVID-19 [17–20].

Thus, this study had two objectives. The first objective was to characterize the ADRs associated with vaccines used in the immunization against COVID-19, notified in the region covered by the Regional Pharmacovigilance Unit of Beira Interior, in Portugal. The second objective was to compare the results obtained with the safety data from studies carried out in other countries around the world. This period was the subject of study since it was the initial period in which the vaccines authorized in the EU began to be administered to the Portuguese population.

2. Materials and Methods

This work is a retrospective observational study. The data under analysis were collected through spontaneous notifications sent to the Portuguese NPS by healthcare professionals, patients or family member. The Portuguese database is "Portal RAM" which is coordinated by the National Authority of Medicines and Health Products, I.P. (INFARMED). The search was carried out in this database taking into account the International Common Denomination of each vaccine (Comirnaty®, Vaxzevria®, Spikevax® and Jcovden®), study period (1–31 December 2021) and the area covered by the RPU of Beira Interior, in Portugal.

Statistical analysis of the data obtained was performed using the Microsoft Office Excel 365 tool. In this tool, the data were organized according to the variables under study and were later represented in tables and appropriate graphics.

It is important to note that each notification concerns a single patient. However, more than one ADR and seriousness criteria may be associated with each notification. Of the 2145 notifications received, only 2134 were studied because of the lack of information in 11 notifications.

It is also important to mention that this work did not require prior authorization from the Ethics Committee, since the patients' personal information was not used.

2.1. Population

The study population comprised only cases of suspected ADR associated with vaccines used in the immunization against COVID-19, notified to the Regional Pharmacovigilance Unit of Beira Interior, and no age restriction was imposed.

2.2. Variables

2.2.1. Characterization of the Notification Source

Notifier Characterization

ADRs can be notified by professionals in the pharmaceutical industry, patients, family members or healthcare professionals. The healthcare professionals considered are classified as physicians, pharmacists, nurses or other healthcare professionals. These professionals play a crucial role in reporting ADRs, with the aim of reducing the negative outcomes associated with them. Bearing in mind that this study only focuses on a regional unit, there are no notifications from the pharmaceutical industry, since these professionals notify directly to the RAM portal, and no specific region is assigned to them.

District of Origin

For the study, only the RPU of Beira Interior was considered, which covers 3 districts: Castelo Branco, Guarda and Viseu. This area corresponds to about 700,000 inhabitants and about 8000 healthcare professionals (doctors, nurses and pharmacists). Thus, the notifications were analyzed according to the district of origin.

2.2.2. Demographic Characterization of the Population

The analysis was carried out by characterizing the notifications by age and gender. In terms of age, 8 age groups were considered: 5 to 11 years old; 12 to 17 years old; 18 to 24 years old; 25 to 49 years old; 50 to 64 years old; 65 to 79 years old; $\geq$80 years; and unknown. Gender was classified as male, female or unknown.

2.2.3. Characterization of Adverse Drug Reactionss

Characterization by Administered Vaccine

Notified ADRs were classified based on the associated vaccine. Only 4 vaccines were considered: Comirnaty, Spikevax, Vaxzevria, and Janssen as they were the vaccines authorized for administration in Portugal during the study period.

Analysis of ADRs

The description of each ADR is performed by the notifier, which is later coded according to the Medical Dictionary for Regulatory Activities (MedDRA) terminology. MedDRA is an international medical terminology developed in 1994 by the International Conference on Harmonization (ICH). Prior to the creation of this dictionary, there was no international medical terminology, so the existence of multiple terminologies created several problems in the analysis of data related to pharmaceutical products. In this way, there was a need to create an international medical terminology, in order to facilitate communication between the various health professionals, and the crossing of data regarding pharmaceutical products [21].

MedDRA terms are hierarchically organized into: system organ class (SOC); high level group term (HLGT); high level terms (HLT); preferred term (PT) and lowest level term

(LLT), with the SOC level being the widest and most comprehensive and the LLT level being the most specific [21].

Thus, the ADRs were initially grouped according to the SOC group, and finally, they were organized according to the PT term.

Description in the Summary of Drug Characteristics (SmPC)

In order to verify the previous descriptions of the ADRs under study associated with the vaccines, the SmPC of each vaccine was used, grouping the data into 2 categories: "Described in the SmPC" and "Not described in the SmPC".

Regarding ADRs not described, they were grouped into 2 parameters: "Degree of Causality Studied" and "Degree of Causality not studied". Causality is attributed by an expert from the regulatory authority or the pharmaceutical company, in ADRs considered serious, and from the information provided during the notification.

Subsequently, the ADRs for which the degree of causality was studied were grouped into 6 categories: Definitive, Probable, Possible, Unlikely, Conditional, Unclassifiable [22].

Seriousness and Seriousness Criteria

Regarding the seriousness, notifications were grouped into serious and non-serious based on the notifier's assessment and/or Regional Pharmacovigilance. Subsequently, serious ADRs were grouped by seriousness criteria.

There was also the characterization of ADRs associated with the seriousness criteria "Hospitalization", "Life Risk" and "Death", according to age and associated vaccine brand.

An ADR is considered serious if it "results in temporary or permanent disability, causes a congenital abnormality, results in hospitalization or prolongation of hospitalization, causes death or is life-threatening, or fulfills another clinically important condition" [23].

Evolution of ADRs

Data were grouped into the following categories: Cure, Cure with collateral damage, in recovery, Death and Unknown, based on the information provided by the notifier.

Characterization of Notifications with the Outcome "Death" with Terms Belonging to the IME List

Finally, the characterization of the notifications that culminated in death was carried out, taking into account the presence of terms belonging to the Important Medical Events (IME) list.

In order to facilitate the classification of ADRs, as well as assist in the analysis of notifications submitted to the National Pharmacovigilance Systems, Eudravigilance created a list of medical terms considered important, called the IME list, based on the definitions adopted by the ICH. Important Medical Events are events that may not immediately lead to death or hospitalization but compromise the individual's life or require medical or surgical intervention in order to avoid the outcomes listed in the definition of seriousness ADR [24].

3. Results

As mentioned above, the number of notifications to be analyzed, after the duplicate and annulled notifications have been withdrawn, was 2134.

3.1. Characterization of the Notification Source

3.1.1. Notifier Characterization

In this study, the type of notifier who submitted the notification was analyzed. Through Figure 1, it is possible to observe that most notifications were submitted by the pharmacist (82.15%, n = 1753), followed by the user or other non-healthcare professional (6.47%, n = 138) and later the physician (6.09%, n = 130). Nurses had a notification rate of 4.87% (n = 104), and finally, other healthcare professionals submitted only 0.42% (n = 9) of the notifications.

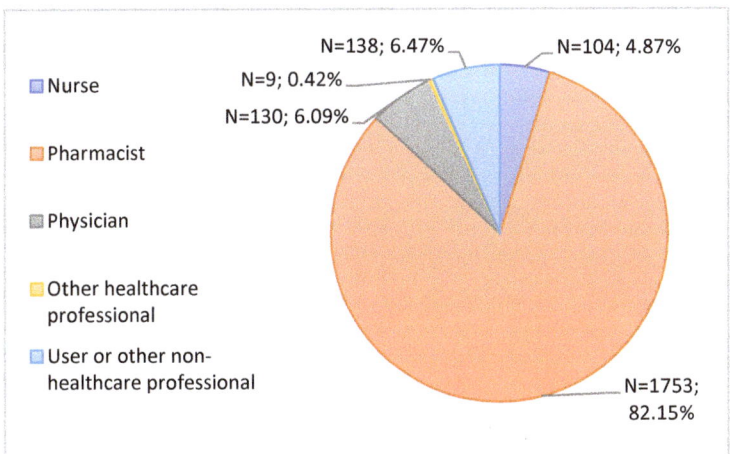

Figure 1. Characterization of notifications by type of notifier.

3.1.2. District of Origin

For the study, only the RPU of Beira Interior was considered. Through Figure 2, it is possible to observe that most notifications presented Castelo Branco as the district of origin (86.36%, n = 1843), followed by Viseu (9.18%, n = 196) and finally Guarda (4.45%, n = 95).

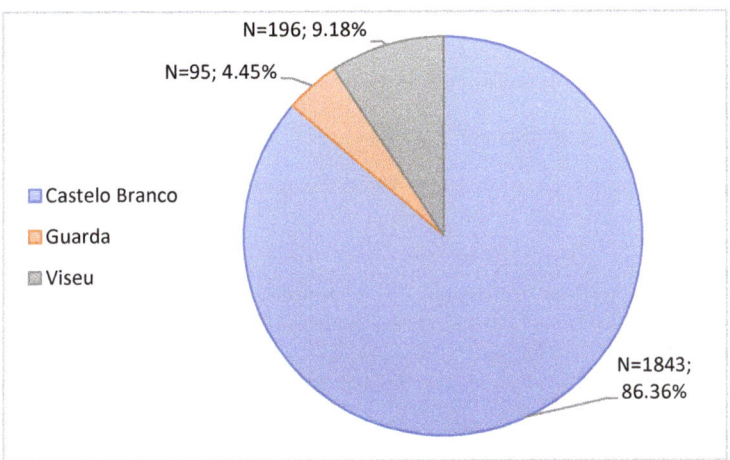

Figure 2. Characterization of notifications by District of Origin of notification.

3.2. Demographic Characterization of the Population

The notifications were characterized as to the age and gender of the patients, as can be seen in Table 1 and Figure 3, respectively.

Analyzing Table 1, it is possible to verify that most notifications were associated with patients aged between 25 and 49 years (57.64%, n = 1230), followed by patients aged between 50 and 64 years. (26.90%, n = 574).

Regarding gender, notifications were grouped into female, male and unknown. The female gender presented the most notifications, accounting for 1534 (71.88%) out of 2134 total notifications.

Table 1. Distribution of notifications by age group.

Age Groups	Frequency	Percentage (%)
(5–11)	0	0.0
(12–17)	7	0.33
(18–24)	108	5.06
(25–49)	1230	57.64
(50–64)	574	26.90
(65–79)	97	4.55
≥80	66	3.09
Unknown	52	2.44
Total	2134	100.00

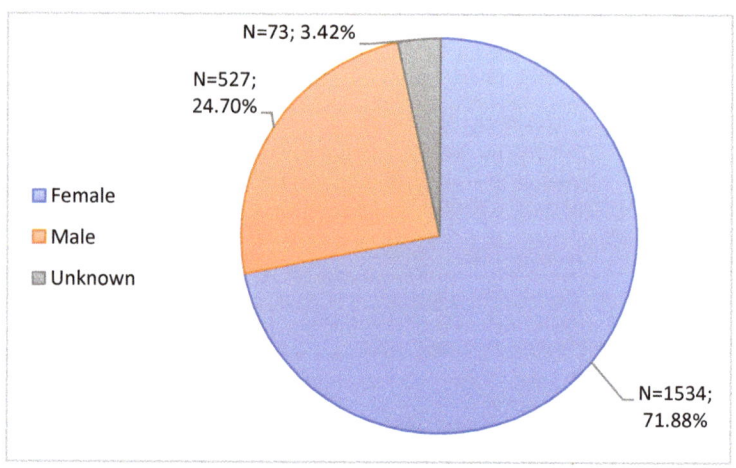

Figure 3. Characterization of notifications according to Gender.

3.3. Characterization of Adverse Drug Reactions

3.3.1. Characterization by Administered Vaccine

During the study period, only 2 types of vaccines were administered–mRNA vaccines and non-replicating viral vector vaccines. It is important to note that each notification concerns a single vaccine. According to Figure 4, mRNA vaccines were highlighted (82.52%, n = 1761). In turn, vaccines with a non-replicating viral vector had a notification rate of 17.48% (n = 373).

Subsequently, the ADRs were organized into 4 classes, according to the brand name of the administered vaccine. Analyzing Figure 5, it is possible to observe that most of the notifications submitted were associated with the Comirnaty vaccine (79.29%, n = 1692), followed by the Vaxzevria vaccine with 325 notifications (15.23%). The Spikevax vaccine had a notification rate of 3.23% (n = 69), and finally, the Jcovden vaccine was associated with 2.25% (n = 48) of the notifications submitted.

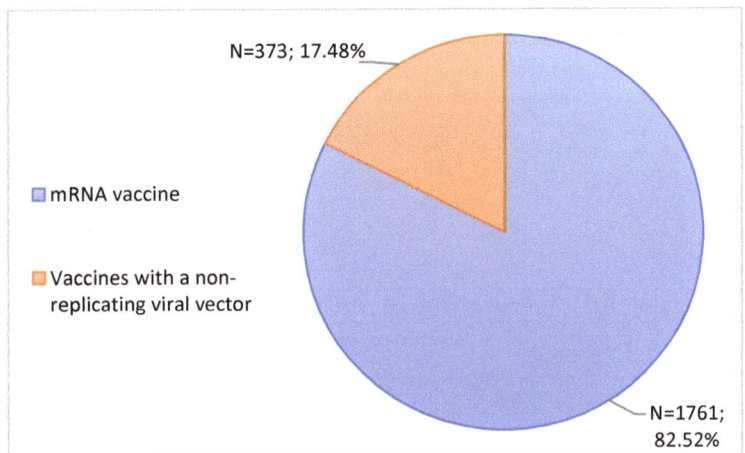

Figure 4. Characterization of notifications according to the type of vaccine.

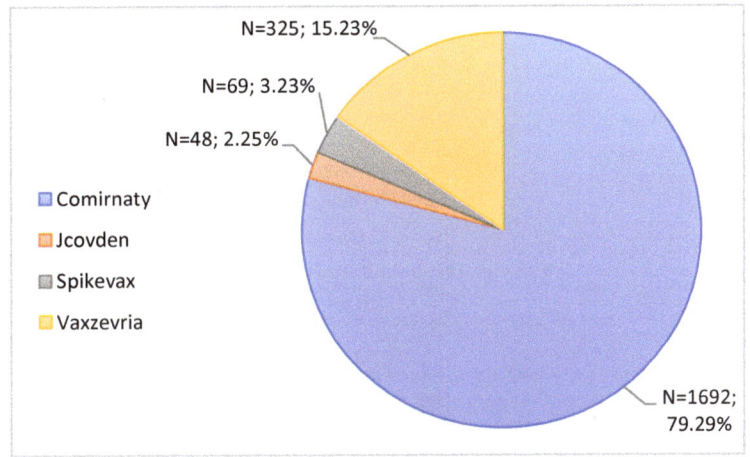

Figure 5. Characterization of notifications according to the brand name of the vaccine.

3.3.2. Analysis of Adverse Drug Reactions

In this study, the notifications sent to the Regional Pharmacovigilance Unit of Beira Interior were initially characterized according to the SOC classification of the MedDRA dictionary. The 2134 notifications were organized into 5685 SOC reactions, meaning that there were, on average, approximately 3 SOC reactions for each notification.

Through Table 2, it is possible to conclude that the three SOC groups most frequently notified were "General disorders and administration site conditions", "Nervous system disorders", and "Musculoskeletal and connective tissue disorders", presenting the following frequencies 2454 (43.17%), 1048 (18.43%) and 1015 (17.85%), respectively. The least notified SOC groups were "Pregnancy, puerperium and perinatal conditions", constituting 0.02% (n = 1) of the notifications, and "Social Circumstances", with 0.04% (n = 2).

Table 2. Characterization of Adverse Drug Reactions by System Organ Class groups.

System Organ Class Groups	Frequency	Percentage (%)
General disorders and administration site conditions	2454	43.17
Nervous system disorders	1048	18.43
Musculoskeletal and connective tissue disorders	1015	17.85
Gastrointestinal disorders	464	8.16
Blood and lymphatic system disorders	147	2.59
Skin and subcutaneous tissue disorders	144	2.53
Respiratory, thoracic and mediastinal disorders	115	2.02
Infections and infestations	65	1.14
Vascular disorders	62	1.09
Cardiac disorders	42	0.74
Psychiatric disorders	22	0.39
Injury, poisoning and procedural complications	21	0.37
Ear and labyrinth disorders	19	0.33
Eye disorders	16	0.28
Metabolism and nutrition disorders	13	0.23
Investigations	11	0.19
Reproductive system and breast disorders	10	0.18
Immune system disorders	8	0.14
Renal and urinary disorders	6	0.11
Social Circumstances	2	0.04
Pregnancy, puerperium and perinatal conditions	1	0.02
Total	5685	100.00

After the analysis by SOC groups, the ADRs notified to the URF of Beira Interior were classified according to the PT terms. The results are shown in Table 3. The "Other reactions" category encompassed adverse reactions with a notification rate ≤1%.

Table 3. Characterization of Adverse Drug Reactions according to the Preferred Term.

Adverse Drug Reaction	Frequency	Percentage (%)
Reaction at or around the site of administration	1147	20.18
Myalgia	751	13.21
Headache	608	10.69
Pyrexia	499	8.78
Chills	222	3.91
Nauseas	219	3.85
Fatigue	214	3.76
Somnolence	178	3.13
Arthralgia	160	2.81
General Pain and Malaise	156	2.74
Lymphadenopathy	141	2.48

Table 3. Cont.

Adverse Drug Reaction	Frequency	Percentage (%)
Asthenia	106	1.86
Diarrhoea	98	1.72
Dizziness	92	1.62
Vomiting	91	1.60
Pain in extremity	68	1.20
Rash	65	1.14
Change in body temperature	65	1.14
Influenza	63	1.11
Other reactions *	742	13.05
Total	5685	100.00

* The "Other reactions" category encompasses adverse reactions with a notification rate ≤1%.

Through Table 3, it is possible to conclude that the 3 ADRs most frequently notified were "Reaction at or around the site of administration", "Myalgias", and "Headache", with the following frequencies 1147 (20.18%), 751 (13.21%) and 608 (10.69%), respectively.

Regarding the "Other reactions" category, it included ADRs with a low reporting rate, such as miscarriage, anaphylactic shock, seizures, respiratory distress and syncope.

3.3.3. Description in the Summary of Drug Characteristics (SmPC)

The ADRs were analyzed in terms of their prior knowledge. Thus, the SmPC of the respective vaccines under study was used for further characterization in: "Described in the SmPC" and "Not described in the SmPC" [25–28].

Through Figure 6, it is possible to verify that 5299 ADRs were described in the SmPC (93.21%), among which it is possible to highlight "Reaction at or around the administration site", "Myalgias", "Arthralgias", "Pyrexia" and "Headaches". 386 ADRs were not described in the SmPC (6.79%).

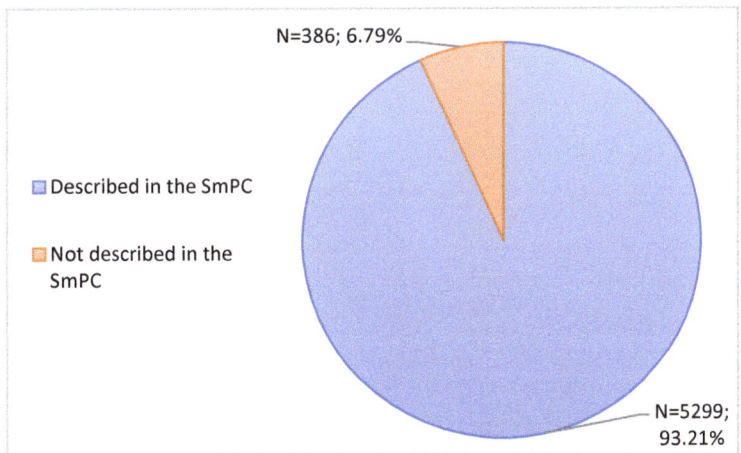

Figure 6. Characterization of Adverse Drug Reactions according to the description in the SmPC.

ADRs not described in the SmPC were grouped according to 2 categories: "Degree of Causality Studied" and "Degree of Causality not studied". The category of "Degree of Causality Studied" obtained the most prominence (61.66%; n = 238) (Figure 7).

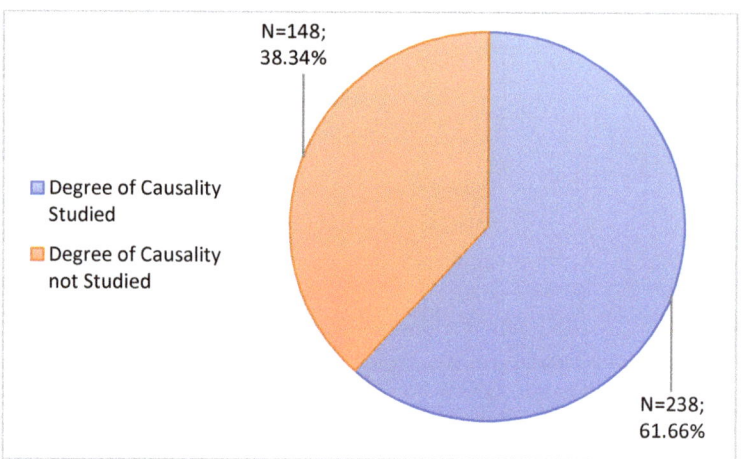

Figure 7. Study of Causality.

The ADRs for which the degree of causality was studied were grouped into 6 categories: "Definitive", "Probable", "Possible", "Unlikely", "Conditional", and "Unclassifiable". According to Table 4, it is possible to observe that most ADRs were classified as "Possible" (n = 118, 49.58%). 100 ADRs (42.02%) have a "Probable" degree of causality and 18 (7.56%) were classified as "Unlikely". The degree of causality that was less prominent was the "Unclassifiable" (n = 2; 0.84%). The "Definite" and "Conditional" degrees of causality were not assigned to ADRs notified.

Table 4. Characterization of Adverse Drug Reactions according to the degree of causality attributed.

Causality	Frequency	Percentage (%)
Definitive	0	0.00
Probable	100	42.02
Possible	118	49.58
Unlikely	18	7.56
Conditional	0	0.00
Unclassifiable	2	0.84
Total	238	100.00

3.3.4. Seriousness and Seriousness Criteria
Seriousness

In this study, the 2134 notifications were further characterized according to seriousness. Among these notifications, 1700 notifications were considered non-serious (79.66%) as they did not fulfill any of the criteria mentioned in Seriousness and Seriousness Criteria section. In turn, 434 notifications were considered serious, representing 20.34%, as can be seen in Figure 8.

Subsequently, the 434 notifications considered serious were organized according to the brand of vaccine administered. Figure 9 shows that most ADRs considered serious belonged to the Comirnaty vaccine (70.51%, n = 306), followed by the Vaxzevria vaccine with 60 serious ADRs (13.82%). The Jcovden vaccine had 35 serious notifications (8.06%) followed by Spikevax with 33 notifications (7.60%).

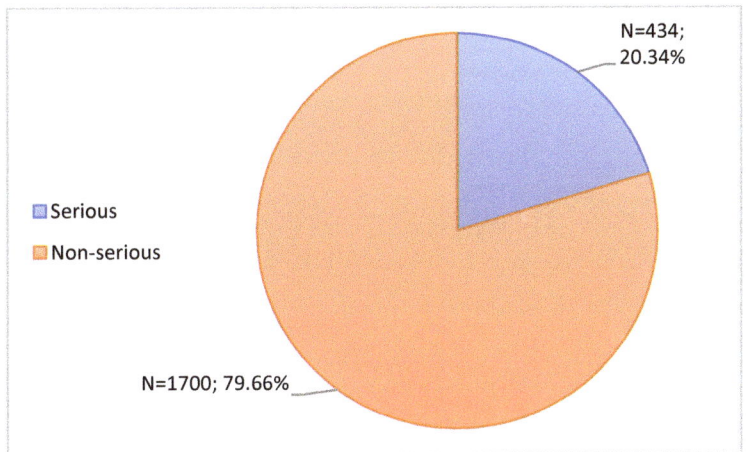

Figure 8. Characterization of notifications according to seriousness.

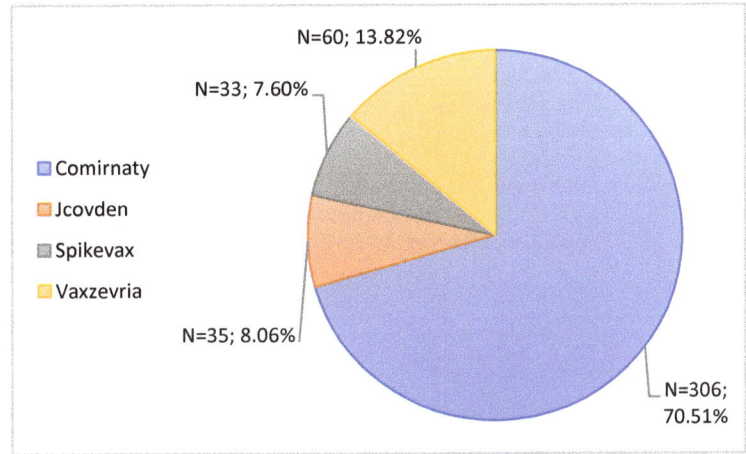

Figure 9. Characterization of serious notifications according to the brand name of the vaccine administered.

Seriousness Criteria

ADRs considered severe were grouped by seriousness into 5 criteria: "Clinically important", "Disability", "Hospitalization", "Life Risk" and "Death". Some serious notifications had more than one seriousness criteria, with a total of 441 seriousness criteria notified for 434 serious notifications.

The seriousness criteria "Clinically important" had great prominence, with a percentage of 64.63% (n = 285), followed by "Disability" (24.04%, n = 106). Then came the criteria "Hospitalization" with 9.52% of serious notifications, which corresponds to 42 notifications. Finally, the criteria "Life Risk" and "Death" appeared with 6 and 2 notifications (1.36% and 0.45%), respectively, as can be seen in Figure 10.

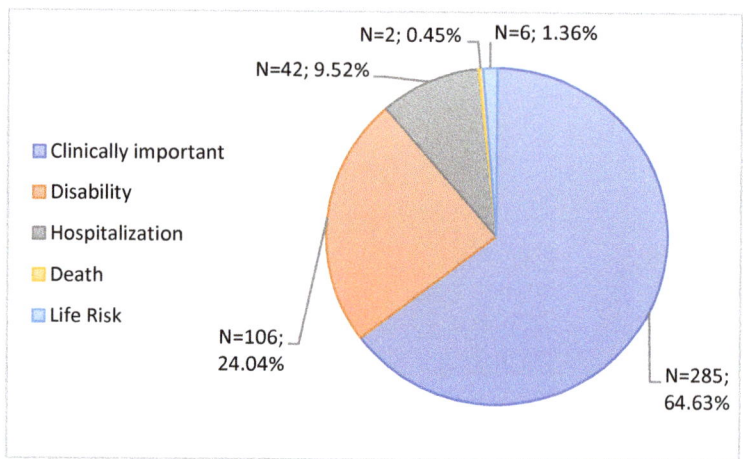

Figure 10. Characterization of serious notifications according to the seriousness criteria.

Then, the ADRs with seriousness criteria "Hospitalization", "Life Risk" and "Death", were characterized according to patient's age and associated vaccine brand.

Initially, there was a characterization of the 42 notifications with the seriousness criteria "Hospitalization" according to the brand of vaccine administered and age, and the results can be found in Figure 11 and Table 5, respectively. Regarding the brand of the associated vaccine, the Comirnaty vaccine was responsible for most hospitalizations (45.24%, n = 19), followed by Vaxzevria responsible for 35.71% (n = 15). The Jcovden vaccine was associated with 14.29% (n = 6) of notifications with the seriousness criteria Hospitalization, and finally, Spikevax originated 4.76% (n = 2) of hospitalizations.

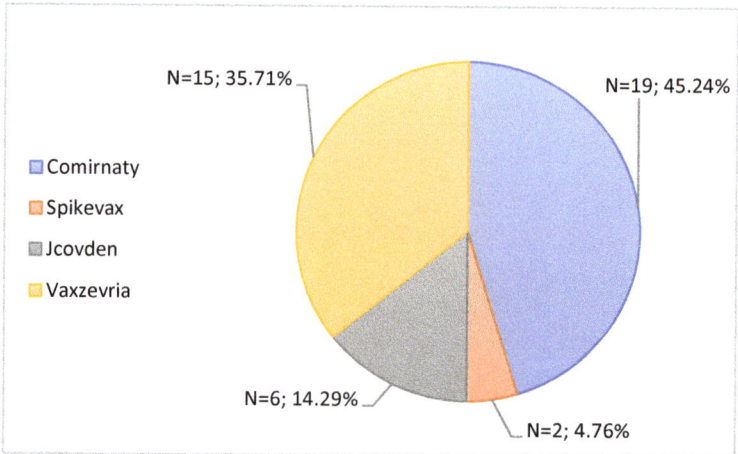

Figure 11. Characterization of serious notifications with the seriousness criteria "Hospitalization", according to the brand of vaccine administered.

Table 5. Characterization of serious notifications with the seriousness criteria "Hospitalization", according to the associated age.

Age Group	Frequency	Percentage (%)
(5–11)	0	0.00
(12–17)	0	0.00
(18–24)	2	4.76
(25–49)	13	30.95
(50–64)	7	16.67
(65–79)	12	28.57
≥80	7	16.67
Unknown	1	2.38
Total	42	100.00

Analyzing Table 6, most hospitalizations were associated with patients aged between 25 and 49 years (30.95%, n = 13), followed by patients aged between 65 and 79 years (28.57%, n = 12).

Table 6. Characterization of serious notifications with the seriousness criterion "Life Risk", according to the associated age.

Age Group	Frequency	Percentage (%)
(5–11)	0	0.00
(12–17)	0	0.00
(18–24)	1	16.67
(25–49)	3	50.00
(50–64)	1	16.67
(65–79)	0	0.00
≥80	1	16.67
Unknown	0	0.00
Total	6	100.00

Subsequently, the 6 notifications with the seriousness criteria "Life Risk" were characterized, and the results are found in Figure 12 and Table 7. In Figure 12 it is possible to observe that the vaccines responsible for this seriousness criteria were the Comirnaty vaccine, the Spikevax vaccine and the Jcovden vaccine, each responsible for three, two and one case, respectively. In fact, the most prominent vaccine was Comirnaty, the most administered vaccine in Portugal [29].

Regarding the age groups associated with the seriousness criteria "Life Risk", it's possible to observe through the Table 6 that the age group with the most cases was the group from 25 to 49 years old (50.00%, n = 3). The age groups from 18 to 24 years old, 50 to 64 years old and ≥80 years old were associated with a single case of "Life Risk".

Finally, the 2 notifications associated with the seriousness criteria "Death" were characterized. In Figure 13 it's possible to observe that the vaccines responsible for this seriousness criteria were the Comirnaty and the Vaxzevria vaccine, each responsible for one case. These patients were 76 and 84 years old, respectively.

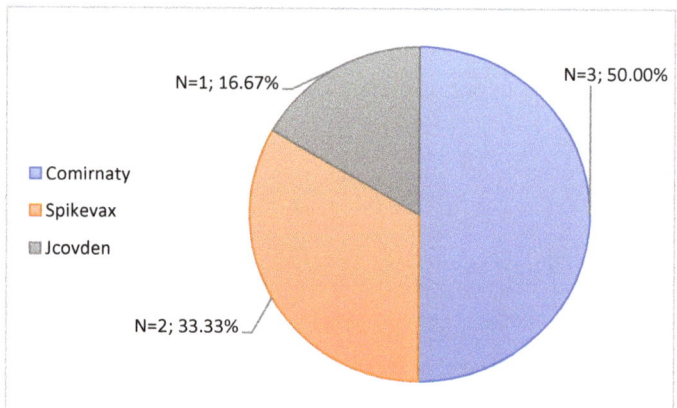

Figure 12. Characterization of serious notifications with the seriousness criteria "Life Risk", according to the brand of vaccine administered.

Table 7. Evolution of Adverse Drug Reactions associated with vaccines used in immunization against COVID-19.

Evolution of Adverse Drug Reactions	Frequency	Percentage (%)
Cure	5361	94.30
Cure with collateral damage	9	0.16
In recovery	6	0.11
Death	6	0.11
Unknown	303	5.33
Total	5685	100.00

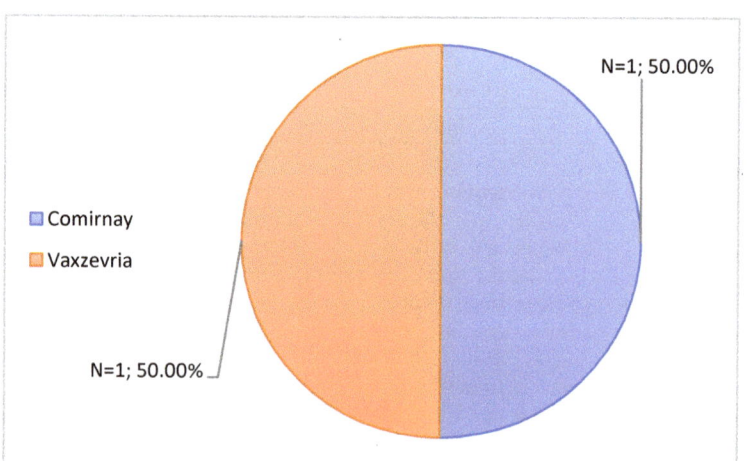

Figure 13. Characterization of serious notifications with the seriousness criteria "Death", according to the brand of vaccine administered.

3.3.5. Evolution of Adverse Drug Reactions

Another important parameter to be evaluated is the evolution of the patient's clinical condition, whose data allow us to understand the possible risks to the patient's life after the administration of the drug in humans (Table 7).

Of the 5685 ADRs notified, 5361 (94.30%) resolved within a few hours or days without the appearance of collateral damage, 9 (0.16%) led to the appearance of collateral damage, 6 (0.11%) ADRs patients were in recovery at the time of reporting and in 6 (0.11%) ADRs the result was death. In 5.33% of the ADRs (n = 303), it was not possible to obtain information regarding the outcome of the reaction.

3.3.6. Characterization of Notifications with the Outcome "Death" with Terms Belonging to the Important Medical Events List

In total, 2 notifications were obtained that culminated in death, corresponding to a total of 6 ADRs, of which 5 were on the IME list. Through Table 8, it is possible to see that the 6 ADRs associated with the outcome "Death" belonged to 3 SOC groups, among which the "Cardiac disorders" group was more prominent.

Table 8. Relationship between the Adverse Drug Reactions of the notifications that progressed to death with the terms belonging to the Import Medical Event (IME) list.

System Organ Class Group	IME List Terms
Cardiac disorders (3)	Acute myocardial infarction (2); Cardiogenic shock (1)
Renal and urinary disorders (1)	Acute kidney injury (1)
Metabolism and nutrition disorders (1)	Hyperkalaemia (1)

These 2 cases obtained a causality study by the regulatory authority, with a conclusion of an unlikely causal relationship, i.e., there was no causal relationship between ADR and the associated vaccine.

4. Discussion

This study allowed the characterization of the notifications of ADRs associated with vaccines used in the immunization against COVID-19, notified to the Pharmacovigilance Unit of Beira Interior, in Portugal, in the time period between December 2020 and December 2021.

Initially, the type of notifier who submitted the notification was analyzed. Through data analysis, it was found that pharmacists had the highest notification rate. The user or other non-healthcare professional also contributed to improving the safety profile of vaccines, followed later by physicians. According to the graph "Evolution of ADR Notifications received in the SNF, by origin, 1992–2021", made available by INFARMED, over the years, the biggest notifier of ADRs has been the pharmaceutical industry [30]. In the year 2021, the industry was the biggest notifier, followed by physicians and later by pharmacists. The results obtained in this study are not in accordance with the INFARMED graph, presenting the pharmacist as the greatest notifier of ADRs associated with vaccines used in the immunization against COVID-19. This is related to the fact that the pharmaceutical services of 2 hospital centers established pharmacovigilance protocols and were later involved in collecting information from patients after the administration of these vaccines, thus increasing the notification rate obtained by pharmacists. However, in general, the results obtained in the study support the fact that healthcare professionals are increasingly aware of the need to notify suspected ADRs, in order to improve the safety profile of medicines. As mentioned in the Notifier Characterization section, the fact that this study focused only on a regional unit explains why we did not obtain ADRs notified by the pharmaceutical industry, as these professionals notify them directly on the ADR portal, with no specific region being assigned to them.

Regarding the district of origin of the notification, it was found that most notifications presented Castelo Branco as the district of origin, followed by Viseu and finally Guarda.

Among the analyzed data, the age group with the highest notification rate, among the groups considered, was the group from 25 to 49 years old, followed by patients aged between 50 and 64 years old. These data are in accordance with the document "Pharmacovigilance Report: Monitoring the safety of vaccines against COVID-19 in Portugal. Data received until 01/31/2022.", which indicates that the age groups 25 to 49 years old and 50 to 64 years old had the highest number of ADR notifications at the national level [29]. This fact may be due to the greater number of vaccines being administered in these two age groups, in addition to being age groups with greater ability to recognize an ADR. It is also important to point out that, according to the data referring to the resident population in Portugal by age group, these are the age groups with the largest population [31]. Regarding gender, the population was mostly female, and these data are supported by the aforementioned document [29]. Generally, the female gender is the one that most notified to any drug, due to the greater susceptibility to develop ADRs, compared to the male gender, probably due to the physiological differences between both sexes. Additionally, it may be related to women's greater attention to their health and signals developed by their body [29,32,33]. International studies also confirm the aforementioned data regarding the age groups and gender with the highest notification rates of vaccine-associated ADRs [34,35].

Subsequently, ADRs were analyzed according to the type and brand of the vaccine administered. In this study, during the analysis period, mRNA vaccines were the most notified. Most of the notifications submitted were associated with the Comirnaty vaccine, followed by the Vaxzevria vaccine. In fact, these data were in agreement with the INFARMED Pharmacovigilance Report, which indicates that the majority of ADRs notified in Portugal correspond to mRNA vaccines [29]. It should be noted that these results may be due to the fact that these were the most administered vaccines in Portugal as well as in the EU and the United States [36,37]. The same report mentions that the vaccine with the highest number of ADR notifications was Comirnaty, followed by the Vaxzevria vaccine, which reinforces the data in Figure 5 available in Section 3.3.1. of the results [29]. These data are corroborated by EMA data, which indicate that these were also the most ADR vaccines reported in Europe [38]. According to data from the Centers for Disease Control and Prevention, the Comirnaty vaccine was the vaccine with the most ADRs reported in the United States [39].

The three most frequently notified SOC groups were "General disorders and administration site conditions", "Nervous system disorders", and "Musculoskeletal and connective tissue disorders". Thus, with regard to "General disorders and administration site changes", it is easy to see why they represented the most frequent SOC group, given that this group encompassed non-specific symptoms that affect various sites in the body, such as general malaise or fatigue, as well as ADRs frequently associated with the administration of any vaccine, such as pain, swelling, itching or bruising at the injection site. These signs are usually mild and transient. As for the second group, "Nervous System Diseases", they included symptoms such as headaches, migraines and convulsions. The third most notified group was "Musculoskeletal and connective tissue disorders", which included myalgias, arthralgias and pain in the extremities. It is easy to understand why it was among the three most notified groups, as SARS-CoV-2 binds to host cells through the spike glycoprotein, through the ACE2 receptor [40]. This receptor is found in the epithelial cells of the pulmonary alveoli and in the enterocytes of the small intestine, as well as in the skeletal muscle and central nervous system, which may be related to myalgias. Additionally, another phenomenon associated with myalgias is the "cytokine storm", in which interleukin-6 plays a key role in inducing the production of prostaglandin E2, associated with inflammation and pain [40]. The vaccines used to immunize against COVID-19, despite not containing the virus in their constitution, have information that encodes the spike protein, recognized by the immune system, and capable of causing an inflammatory response, through a large production of pro-inflammatory cytokines, which leads to the appearance of myalgias and other musculoskeletal symptoms [41,42]. These data are in accordance with the aforementioned Pharmacovigilance Report [29]. According to the document "Rapporto sulla Sorveglianza dei vaccini anti-COVID-19", issued by the Agenzia italiana del farmaco, the three most frequently notified SOC groups were the "General disorders and administration site conditions", "Nervous system disorders", and "Musculoskeletal and connective tissue disorders" which are in accordance with the results obtained through this study [43].

Following the analysis by SOC groups, the ADRs were classified according to the PT terms. The three most frequently notified ADRs were "Reaction at or around the injection site", "Myalgias", and "Headache". These data are in agreement with the data from the most frequently notified SOC groups referred to in the previous paragraph ("General disorders and administration site disorders", "Nervous System Disorders", and "Musculoskeletal and connective tissue disorders"). The explanation for the ADR "Reaction at or around the injection site" being among the three most frequently reported ADRs is related to the way in which the vaccines are administered. This group belongs to the SOC group "General disorders and administration site conditions", referred in the previous paragraph. "Headache" is among the three most reported ADRs, however the mechanism by which it occurs remains unclear. Some authors suggest that "Headache" may be due to a direct activation of the trigeminal vascular system, which consists of nerve fibers originating from the trigeminal nerve that innervate cerebral blood vessels. Additionally, another phenomenon possibly associated with "Headaches" is the "cytokine storm", associated with inflammation and pain [44]. These data are in agreement with the INFARMED Pharmacovigilance Report, which mentions "Headache", "Myalgias" and "Pain at the injection site" among the most frequently notified ADRs. This report also mentions that "Pyrexia" is the most prominent ADR, something that was not verified through the data under study [29]. However, this is a term that also has a high notification rate, ranking 4th in Table 3 of Section 3.3.2. It is easy to understand why it had a high notification rate, taking into account that it is characterized by an immune system response to a foreign body introduced into our system, as is the case with the vaccine [39,40]. These data are also corroborated by studies carried out in other countries, which indicate that "Reaction at or around the injection site", "Myalgias", "Pyrexia" and "Headache" are among the ADRs most commonly associated with vaccines [45–47]. During the study period, several countries suspended or restricted the use of vaccines to certain populations due to the emergence of rare adverse reactions [48–50].

The notified ADRs were compared with the SmPCs of the respective vaccines, showing that most RAMs were already described. Regarding the degree of causality, most ADRs were classified as "Possible" or "Probable", followed by the degree "Unlikely" and the degree "Unclassifiable". Although ADRs not described in the SmPCs represent a low percentage, it is crucial that they receive a degree of importance, especially in those in which it was possible to conclude the degree of causality as "Possible" and "Probable", since they allow updating the safety profile of each vaccine and consequently its SmPCs, thus reinforcing the importance of reporting ADRs.

Regarding seriousness, 20.34% of ADRs were considered serious ADRs, most of which were associated with the Comirnaty vaccine. In fact, these data are in agreement with the INFARMED Pharmacovigilance Report, which indicates that the majority of ADRs associated with vaccines used in the immunization against COVID-19 correspond to non-serious ADRs [29]. According to the document "Rapporto sulla Sorveglianza dei vaccini anti-COVID-19", most ADRs were classified as non-serious, which corroborates the results obtained in this study. However, this document indicates that the vaccine most associated with serious reactions was Spikevax, which is not in agreement with the results obtained in this study [43]. Our results may be due to the fact that Comirnaty was the most administered vaccine in Portugal [29]. Even so, there is a large percentage of serious notifications, which again reinforces the importance of healthcare professionals and users to carry out the notifications of ADRs.

The seriousness criteria with the highest rate were the "Clinically important" criteria, followed by the seriousness criteria "Disability", "Hospitalization", "Life risk" and "Death". It is important to note that there were notifications in which the notifier had selected more than one seriousness criterion. These data are in accordance with the documents "Pharmacovigilance Report: Monitoring the safety of vaccines against COVID-19 in Portugal.

Data received until 01/31/2022" and "Rapporto sulla Sorveglianza dei vaccini anti-COVID-19", which indicates that the seriousness criteria that stands out the most is "Clinically important", with the criteria "Life Risk" and "Death" being less prominent [29,43]. The Comirnaty vaccine was responsible for the most hospitalizations as well as for half of the cases associated with the "Life Risk". In fact, these results may be due to the fact that this was the most administered vaccine in Portugal as well as in the EU and in the United States [36,37]. Regarding the seriousness criteria "Death", the associated vaccines were Comirnaty and Vaxzevria, with patients aged 86 and 74 years, respectively, both of whom had a history of acute myocardial infarction.

Most of the ADRs notified progressed to cure. In total, there were 2 notifications that progressed to death, of which 5 terms were on the IME list, most of the terms referred to "Cardiac disorders". These 2 notifications corresponded to patients aged 74 and 86 years, with a history of acute myocardial infarction as well as in the presence of cardiovascular risk factors, among which diabetes mellitus, arterial hypertension, obesity and dyslipidemia stand out. Regarding the notified ADRs, the regulatory authority classified them with a degree of causality "Improbable", based on the history that the patients had, which meant that the vaccines were not the cause of death for both patients. These data are in agreement with several studies that indicated that the cases of death that occurred in patients after vaccination against COVID-19 were not related to the vaccines administered, being nothing more than mere coincidence [51].

4.1. Limitations

This study had some limitations, among which we can highlight the rate of under reporting of suspected ADRs, i.e., not all ADRs that occurred were notified to the National Pharmacovigilance System, which may have occurred, for example, due to lack of time or ignorance regarding the existence of the "Portal RAM" [16,17]. Another limitation is related to the fact that some notifications presented a lack of information, making their study difficult. Additionally, the fact that the Comirnaty vaccine is the most administered vaccine in Portugal, leading to the majority of ADRs reported being associated with this vaccine, may have biased the results obtained, since the vaccines under study were not administered in the same number of patients, making it more difficult to compare the results.

4.2. Strengths of Study

The strengths of our study included a large sample size in which it was possible to characterize several parameters associated with the reported ADRs. Additionally, it was the first study carried out in Portugal, to our knowledge, over a long period involving data corresponding to the first, second and third doses.

5. Conclusions

The notification of suspected ADRs was mainly related to common and non-serious reactions (e.g., pyrexia, fatigue, myalgia and reaction at or around the injection site), which is in accordance with clinical trials, in the vaccine SmPCs and in ADR notifications of vaccines from other countries. In general, ADRs resolved within a few hours/days without any consequences, which confirms a favorable safety profile of the COVID-19 vaccines. Despite the results obtained, further studies are needed to confirm these data.

Author Contributions: C.M. supervised collection of data and interaction with INFARMED. C.A. collected the data, organised the results. C.M. and A.P.D. supervised writing of the manuscript. C.A. wrote the first draft. All authors made substantial contributions, approved the final version of the manuscript and agreed to be accountable for all aspects of the work. All authors have read and agreed to the published version of the manuscript.

Funding: This work was supported by INFARMED—National Authority of Medicines and Health Products, I.P. through the Pharmacovigilance Unit of Beira Interior and by the CICS-UBI projects UIDB/00709/2020 and UIDP/00709/2020, financed by national funds through the Portuguese Foundation for Science and Technology/MCTES.

Institutional Review Board Statement: Not applicable.

Informed Consent Statement: Patient consent was waived because this is an observational study and data was reported voluntarily by participants anonymously.

Data Availability Statement: The raw data used in this research are available to the authors, depending on INFARMED's authorization.

Acknowledgments: The data presented in our work belong to the Portuguese Pharmacovigilance System. The authors would like to thank the National Authority of Medicines and Health Products, I.P. (INFARMED).

Conflicts of Interest: The authors declare no conflict of interest.

References

1. Lotfi, M.; Hamblin, M.R.; Rezaei, N. COVID-19: Transmission, prevention, and potential therapeutic opportunities. *Clin. Chim. Acta* **2020**, *508*, 254–266. [CrossRef] [PubMed]
2. Guo, Y.-R.; Cao, Q.-D.; Hong, Z.-S.; Tan, Y.-Y.; Chen, S.-D.; Jin, H.-J.; Tan, K.-S.; Wang, D.-Y.; Yan, Y. The origin, transmission and clinical therapies on coronavirus disease 2019 (COVID-19) outbreak—An update on the status. *Mil. Med. Res.* **2020**, *7*, 11. [CrossRef] [PubMed]
3. Liu, X.; Liu, C.; Liu, G.; Luo, W.; Xia, N. COVID-19: Progress in diagnostics, therapy and vaccination. *Theranostics* **2020**, *10*, 7821–7835. [CrossRef] [PubMed]
4. Izda, V.; Jeffries, M.A.; Sawalha, A.H. COVID-19: A review of therapeutic strategies and vaccine candidates. *Clin. Immunol.* **2021**, *222*, 108634. [CrossRef]
5. Dai, L.; Gao, G.F. Viral targets for vaccines against COVID-19. *Nat. Rev. Immunol.* **2021**, *21*, 73–82. [CrossRef]
6. Centers for Disease Control and Prevention. Understanding mRNA COVID-19 Vaccines. 2022. Available online: https://www.cdc.gov/coronavirus/2019-ncov/vaccines/different-vaccines/mrna.html (accessed on 5 August 2022).
7. European Medicines Agency. COVID-19 Vaccines. Available online: https://www.ema.europa.eu/en/human-regulatory/overview/public-health-threats/coronavirus-disease-covid-19/treatments-vaccines/covid-19-vaccines (accessed on 5 August 2022).
8. European Medicines Agency. Comirnaty. 2020. Available online: https://www.ema.europa.eu/en/medicines/human/EPAR/comirnaty (accessed on 5 August 2022).
9. European Medicines Agency. Spikevax (Previously COVID-19 Vaccine Moderna). 2021. Available online: https://www.ema.europa.eu/en/medicines/human/EPAR/spikevax (accessed on 5 August 2022).
10. Centers for Disease Control and Prevention. Understanding Viral Vector COVID-19 Vaccines. 2022. Available online: https://www.cdc.gov/coronavirus/2019-ncov/vaccines/different-vaccines/viralvector.html (accessed on 5 August 2022).
11. Malik, J.A.; Mulla, A.H.; Farooqi, T.; Pottoo, F.H.; Anwar, S.; Rengasamy, K.R.R. Targets and strategies for vaccine development against SARS-CoV-2. *Biomed. Pharmacother.* **2021**, *137*, 111254. [CrossRef]
12. European Medicines Agency. Vaxzevria (Previously COVID-19 Vaccine Astrazeneca). 2021. Available online: https://www.ema.europa.eu/en/medicines/human/EPAR/vaxzevria-previously-covid-19-vaccine-astrazeneca (accessed on 5 August 2022).
13. European Medicines Agency. Jcovden (Previously COVID-19 Vaccine Janssen). 2021. Available online: https://www.ema.europa.eu/en/medicines/human/EPAR/jcovden-previously-covid-19-vaccine-janssen (accessed on 5 August 2022).
14. Ferreira-da-Silva, R.; Ribeiro-Vaz, I.; Morato, M.; Silva, A.M.; Junqueira Polónia, J. The Role of Pharmacovigilance in the context of the COVID-19 Pandemic. *Acta Med. Port.* **2021**, *34*, 173–175. [CrossRef]
15. INFARMED, I.P. Why Should I Report an Adverse Reaction? *Boletim de Farmacovigilância* **2017**, *21*, 10. Available online: https://www.infarmed.pt/documents/15786/1983294/Boletim%2bde%2bFarmacovigil%ff%ffncia%2c%2bVolume%2b21%2c%2bn%ff%ff10%2c%2boutubro%2bde%2b2017/06e28ef9-09a0-4f04-87a2-9da68719e61e?version=1.0 (accessed on 5 August 2022).
16. Herdeiro, M.T.; Ferreira, M.; Ribeiro-Vaz, I.; Junqueira Polónia, J.; Costa-Pereira, A. The Portuguese Pharmacovigilance System. *Acta Med. Port.* **2012**, *25*, 241–249.
17. INFARMED, I.P. Farmacovigilância/Portal RAM, Common Questions. Available online: https://www.infarmed.pt/web/infarmed/institucional/documentacao/informacao/publicacoes?p_p_id=101&p_p_lifecycle=0&p_p_state=maximized&p_p_mode=view&_101_struts_action=%2Fasset_publisher%2Fview_content&_101_assetEntryId=2326140&_101_type=content&_101_urlTi (accessed on 5 August 2022).
18. Shrestha, S.; Khatri, J.; Shakya, S.; Danekhu, K.; Khatiwada, A.P.; Sah, R.; Kc, B.; Paudyal, V.; Khanal, S.; Rodriguez-Morales, A.J. Adverse events related to COVID-19 vaccines: The need to strengthen pharmacovigilance monitoring systems. *Drugs Ther. Perspect.* **2021**, *37*, 376–382. [CrossRef]

19. Khan, Z.; Karataş, Y.; Rahman, H.; Qayum, M.; Alzahrani, K.J.; Kashif, S.M. COVID-19 treatments and associated adverse reactions: The need for effective strategies to strengthen pharmacovigilance system in Lower- and middle-income countries. *Le Pharm. Clin.* **2022**, *57*, 77–80. [CrossRef]
20. De Oliveira, M.M.M.; Wagner, G.A.; Gattás, V.L.; Arruda, L.S.; Taminato, M. Pharmacovigilance quality system for vaccine monitoring (COVID-19) using quality indicators: A scoping review. *Int. J. Infect. Control* **2021**, *17*. [CrossRef]
21. International Conference on Harmonization. Introductory Guide MedDRA Version 25.0. 2022. Available online: https://www.meddra.org/how-to-use/support-documentation/english (accessed on 7 August 2022).
22. The Uppsala Monitoring Centre. The Use of the WHO-UMC System for Standardized Case Causality Assessment. 2018. Available online: https://who-umc.org/media/164200/who-umc-causality-assessment_new-logo.pdf (accessed on 7 August 2022).
23. European Medicines Agency. Guideline on Good Pharmacovigilance Practices (GVP). Module VI—Collection, Management and Submission of Reports of Suspected Adverse Reactions to Medicinal Product. 2017. Available online: https://www.ema.europa.eu/en/human-regulatory/post-authorisation/pharmacovigilance/good-pharmacovigilance-practices (accessed on 7 August 2022).
24. European Medicines Agency. EudraVigilance System Overview. 2018. Available online: https://www.ema.europa.eu/en/human-regulatory/research-development/pharmacovigilance/eudravigilance/eudravigilance-system-overview (accessed on 7 August 2022).
25. European Medicines Agency. Summary of Product Characteristics—Comirnaty. 2021. Available online: https://www.ema.europa.eu/en/documents/product-information/comirnaty-epar-product-information_en.pdf (accessed on 8 August 2022).
26. European Medicines Agency. Summary of product Characteristics—Spikevax. 2021. Available online: https://www.ema.europa.eu/en/documents/product-information/spikevax-previously-covid-19-vaccine-moderna-epar-product-information_en.pdf (accessed on 8 August 2022).
27. European Medicines Agency. Summary of Product Characteristics—Vaxzevria. 2021. Available online: https://www.ema.europa.eu/en/documents/product-information/vaxzevria-previously-covid-19-vaccine-astrazeneca-epar-product-information_en.pdf (accessed on 8 August 2022).
28. European Medicines Agency. Summary of Product Characteristics—Jcovden. 2021. Available online: https://www.ema.europa.eu/en/documents/product-information/jcovden-previously-covid-19-vaccine-janssen-epar-product-information_en.pdf (accessed on 8 August 2022).
29. Pharmacovigilance Report: Monitoring the Safety of Vaccines against COVID-19 in Portugal. Data received until 01/31/2022. NFARMED I.P. 2022. Available online: https://www.infarmed.pt/documents/15786/4268692/Relat%C3%B3rio+de+Farmacovigil%C3%A2ncia.+Monitoriza%C3%A7%C3%A3o+da+seguran%C3%A7a+das+vacinas+contra+a+COVID+19+em+Portugal+atualizado+31+de+mar%C3%A7o+de+%C2%A0+2022/709e77f5-ab06-092d-338b-44c99586f796 (accessed on 8 August 2022).
30. INFARMED, I.P. Evolution of ADR Notifications Received in the SNF, by Origin, 1992–2021. Available online: https://www.infarmed.pt/web/infarmed/institucional/documentacao_e_informacao/campanhas/qualidade_medicamento?p_p_id=101&p_p_lifecycle=0&p_p_state=maximized&p_p_mode=view&_101_struts_action=%2Fasset_publisher%2Fview_content&_101_assetEntryId=2297488&_101_t (accessed on 8 August 2022).
31. Resident Population, Annual Average: Total and by Age Group. PORDATA—Statistics about Portugal and Europe. Available online: https://www.pordata.pt/Portugal/Popula%C3%A7%C3%A3o+residente++m%C3%A9dia+anual+total+e+por+grupo+et%C3%A1rio-10 (accessed on 9 August 2022).
32. Brabete, A.C.; Greaves, L.; Maximos, M.; Huber, E.; Li, A.; Lê, M.-L. A sex- and gender-based analysis of adverse drug reactions: A scoping review of pharmacovigilance databases. *Pharmaceuticals* **2022**, *15*, 298. [CrossRef]
33. Rademaker, M. Do women have more adverse drug reactions? *Am. J. Clin. Dermatol.* **2001**, *2*, 349–351. [CrossRef] [PubMed]
34. Xiong, X.; Yuan, J.; Li, M.; Jiang, B.; Lu, Z.K. Age and gender disparities in adverse events following COVID-19 vaccination: Real-world evidence based on big data for risk management. *Front. Med.* **2021**, *8*, 700014. [CrossRef] [PubMed]
35. Swissmedic. Reports of Suspected Adverse Reactions to COVID-19 Vaccines in Switzerland. 2022. Available online: https://www.swissmedic.ch/swissmedic/en/home/news/coronavirus-covid-19/covid-19-vaccines-safety-update-11.html (accessed on 9 August 2022).
36. Ritchie, H.; Mathieu, E.; Rodés-Guirao, L.; Appel, C.; Giattino, C.; Ortiz-Ospina, E.; Hasell, J.; Macdonald, B.; Beltekian, D.; Roser, M. Coronavirus Pandemic (COVID-19). 2020. Available online: https://ourworldindata.org/covid-vaccinations (accessed on 11 August 2022).
37. COVID-19 Vaccinations Administered Number by Manufacturer U.S. Statista. 2022. Available online: https://www.statista.com/statistics/1198516/covid-19-vaccinations-administered-us-by-company/ (accessed on 11 August 2022).
38. European Medicines Agency. Safety of COVID-19 Vaccines. 2022. Available online: https://www.ema.europa.eu/en/human-regulatory/overview/public-health-threats/coronavirus-disease-covid-19/treatments-vaccines/vaccines-covid-19/safety-covid-19-vaccines (accessed on 11 August 2022).
39. Centers for Disease Control and Prevention. About the Vaccine Adverse Event Reporting System (VAERS). Available online: https://wonder.cdc.gov/controller/datarequest/D8 (accessed on 11 August 2022).
40. Wang, L.; Yang, N.; Yang, J.; Zhao, S.; Su, C. A review: The manifestations, mechanisms, and treatments of musculoskeletal pain in patients with COVID-19. *Frontiers Pain Res.* **2022**, *3*, 826160. [CrossRef]

41. World Health Organization. Side Effects of COVID-19 Vaccines. 2021. Available online: https://www.who.int/news-room/feature-stories/detail/side-effects-of-covid-19-vaccines (accessed on 11 August 2022).
42. Rapsinski, G.J. What Happens When the COVID-19 Vaccines Enter the Body—A Road Map for Kids and Grown-Ups. 2021. Available online: https://theconversation.com/what-happens-when-the-covid-19-vaccines-enter-the-body-a-road-map-for-kids-and-grown-ups-164624 (accessed on 11 August 2022).
43. Agenzia Italiana del Fármaco. Rapporto Sulla Sorveglianza dei Vaccini anti-COVID-19 (27/12/2020–26/06/2022). 2022. Available online: https://www.aifa.gov.it/documents/20142/1315190/Rapporto_sorveglianza_vaccini_COVID-19_12.pdf (accessed on 11 August 2022).
44. Castaldo, M.; Waliszewska-Prosół, M.; Koutsokera, M.; Robotti, M.; Straburzyński, M.; Apostolakopoulou, L.; Capizzi, M.; Çibuku, O.; Ambat, F.D.F.; Frattale, I.; et al. Headache onset after vaccination against SARS-CoV-2: A systematic literature review and meta-analysis. *J. Headache Pain* **2022**, *23*, 41. [CrossRef]
45. Tan, A.Y.; Chang, C.T.; Yu, Y.K.; Low, Y.X.; Razali, N.F.M.; Tey, S.Y.; Lee, S.W.H. Adverse events following BNT162b2 mRNA COVID-19 vaccine immunization among healthcare workers in a tertiary hospital in Johor, Malaysia. *Vaccines* **2022**, *10*, 509. [CrossRef]
46. Paczkowska, A.; Hoffmann, K.; Michalak, M.; Hans-Wytrychowska, A.; Bryl, W.; Kopciuch, D.; Zaprutko, T.; Ratajczak, P.; Nowakowska, E.; Kus, K. Safety profile of COVID-19 vaccines among healthcare workers in Poland. *Vaccines* **2022**, *10*, 434. [CrossRef]
47. Riad, A.; Pokorná, A.; Mekhemar, M.; Conrad, J.; Klugarová, J.; Koščík, M.; Klugar, M.; Attia, S. Safety of ChAdOx1 nCoV-19 vaccine: Independent evidence from two EU states. *Vaccines* **2021**, *9*, 673. [CrossRef]
48. European Medicines Agency. COVID-19 Vaccine AstraZeneca: PRAC Investigating Cases of Thromboembolic Events—Vaccine's Benefits Currently Still Outweigh Risks—Update. 2021. Available online: https://www.ema.europa.eu/en/news/covid-19-vaccine-astrazeneca-prac-investigating-cases-thromboembolic-events-vaccines-benefits (accessed on 15 September 2022).
49. US Food & Drug Administration. FDA and CDC Lift Recommended Pause on Johnson & Johnson (Janssen) COVID-19 Vaccine Use Following Thorough Safety Review. 2021. Available online: https://www.fda.gov/news-events/press-announcements/fda-and-cdc-lift-recommended-pause-johnson-johnson-janssen-covid-19-vaccine-use-following-thorough (accessed on 15 September 2022).
50. Paterlini, M. COVID-19: Sweden, Norway, and Finland suspend use of Moderna vaccine in young people "as a precaution". *BMJ* **2021**, *375*, n2477. [CrossRef] [PubMed]
51. Lamptey, E. Post-vaccination COVID-19 deaths: A review of available evidence and recommendations for the global population. *Clin. Exp. Vaccine Res.* **2021**, *10*, 264–275. [CrossRef] [PubMed]

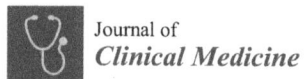 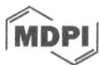

Article

Safety Surveillance of Mass Praziquantel and Albendazole Co-Administration in School Children from Southern Ethiopia: An Active Cohort Event Monitoring

Tigist Dires Gebreyesus [1,2], Eyasu Makonnen [3,4], Tafesse Tadele [5], Habtamu Gashaw [2], Workagegnew Degefe [2], Heran Gerba [2], Birkneh Tilahun Tadesse [1,5], Parthasarathi Gurumurthy [6] and Eleni Aklillu [1,*]

1. Division of Clinical Pharmacology, Department of Laboratory Medicine, Karolinska Institutet, Karolinska University Hospital Huddinge, 14186 Stockholm, Sweden
2. Ethiopian Food and Drug Authority, Addis Ababa P.O. Box 5681, Ethiopia
3. Center for Innovative Drug Development and Therapeutic Trials for Africa, College of Health Sciences, Addis Ababa University, Addis Ababa P.O. Box 9086, Ethiopia
4. Departments of Pharmacology and Clinical Pharmacy, College of Health Sciences, Addis Ababa University, Addis Ababa P.O Box 9086, Ethiopia
5. College of Medicine and Health Sciences, Hawassa University, Hawassa P.O. Box 1560, Ethiopia
6. Pharmacovigilance and Clinical Trials, Botswana Medicines Regulatory Authority, Gaborone P.O. Box 505155, Botswana
* Correspondence: eleni.aklillu@ki.se

Abstract: Preventive chemotherapy (PC) with praziquantel and albendazole co-administration to all at-risk populations is the global intervention strategy to eliminate schistosomiasis and soil-transmitted helminth (STH) from being public health problems. Due to weak pharmacovigilance systems, safety monitoring during a mass drug administration (MDA) is lacking, especially in sub-Saharan Africa. We conducted large-scale active safety surveillance to identify the incidence, types, severity, and associated risk factors of adverse events (AEs) following praziquantel and albendazole MDA in 5848 school children (5–15 years old). Before MDA, 1484 (25.4%) children were prescreened for *S. mansoni* and STH infections, of whom 71.8% were infected with at least one parasite; 34.5% (512/1484) had *S. mansoni* and 853 (57.5%) had an STH infection. After collecting the baseline socio-demographic, clinical, and medical data, including any pre-existing clinical symptoms, participants received single dose praziquantel and albendazole MDA. Treatment-associated AEs were actively monitored on days 1 and 7 of the MDA. The events reported before and after the MDA were cross-checked and verified to identify MDA-associated AEs. The cumulative incidence of experiencing at least one type of MDA-associated AE was 13.3% (95% CI = 12.5–14.2%); 85.5%, 12.4%, and 1.8% of reported AEs were mild, moderate, and severe, respectively. The proportion of experiencing one, two, or ≥ three types of AEs was 57.7%, 34.1%, and 8.2%, respectively. The cumulative incidence of AEs in *S. mansoni*- and (17.0%) and STH (14.1%)-infected children was significantly higher ($p < 0.001$, $\chi^2 = 15.0$) than in non-infected children (8.4%). Headache, abdominal pain, vomiting, dizziness, and nausea were the most common AEs. Being female, older age, having *S. mansoni* or STH infection were significant predictors of MDA-associated AEs. In summary, praziquantel and albendazole co-administration is generally safe and tolerable. MDA-associated AEs are mostly mild-to-moderately severe and transient. The finding of few severe AEs and significantly high rates of AEs in helminth-infected children underscores the need to integrate pharmacovigilance in MDA programs, especially in high schistosomiasis and STH endemic areas.

Keywords: safety surveillance; pharmacovigilance; praziquantel; albendazole; school children; preventive chemotherapy; cohort event monitoring; schistosomiasis; STH; Ethiopia; drug safety

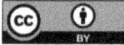

1. Introduction

In sub-Saharan Africa (SSA), soil-transmitted helminth (STH) and schistosomiasis are the first and second most prevalent neglected tropical diseases (NTDs), respectively [1]. More than 90% of the global schistosomiasis burden is from SSA. Both STH and schistosomiasis have been associated with different health complications among the chronically infected groups by causing malnutrition, anemia, a poor cognitive function, impaired childhood development, fatigue, and exercise intolerance [2–6]. In Ethiopia, intestinal schistosomiasis, which *Schistosoma mansoni* causes, is endemic in most parts of the country and remains among the main causes of morbidity in the country [6–8]. STH is endemic throughout the country.

Due to the long-term health consequences and economic burden in endemic areas, the World Health Organization (WHO) established a global program to eliminate NTDs as a public health problem. Among the interventions recommended by the WHO for schistosomiasis and STH elimination and control is preventive chemotherapy (PC), which is defined as a large scale distribution of anthelmintics at regular intervals without prior screening to all at-risk population groups [9–12]. School children are the main target for PC using praziquantel and albendazole due to their increased risk of infection [13,14]. In line with the WHO 2012–2020 strategic plan for the control and elimination of NTDs, drug donations for PC through a mass drug administration (MDA) to at-risk population groups has been escalated globally due to increased donor funds and support from pharmaceutical industries [9,15]. This large-scale donation of drugs and funds has resulted in reaching millions of at-risk populations through PC. For instance, 105 million individuals received praziquantel PC against schistosomiasis in 2019. Similarly, 613 million children received PC for the control of STH through the annual deworming program the same year [16].

The WHO has expanded the target population group with a recommendation of annual PC to people older than two years in endemic countries where the prevalence exceeds 10% [17]. The increase in the target population and frequency of PC use will increase the number of individuals who will be exposed to drugs, which will have implications for safety monitoring. Firstly, the large-scale distribution of drugs without a prior screening of individuals for the disease may expose the non-infected ones to unnecessary MDA-related adverse events [17,18]. Secondly, drugs used in PC, like for schistosomiasis and STH, are often co-administered, increasing the risk of rare and unexpected adverse events due to drug–drug interaction and/or overlapping toxicities [19]. Third, most clinical trials on drugs used in an MDA are tested in different population groups than the target population for the MDA. Thus, host-genetic and environmental variations may predispose the target population to the occurrence of rare adverse events. Finally, the drug distribution during PC implementation is mainly conducted by non-healthcare professionals with no or little knowledge of drug-related adverse events, further underscoring the need for integrating safety monitoring (pharmacovigilance) in PC programs.

Adverse events following an MDA might be associated with the disease characteristics (the intensity of infection), participant characteristics (their age and nutritional status), or other factors in the context of drug use (operational errors or coincidences) [20–22]. Therefore, the integration of safety monitoring in the NTD control program is crucial for ascertaining the cause of adverse events and taking the necessary preventive and corrective measures. Previous studies have evaluated the safety of praziquantel and/or albendazole [20–23]. However, these studies had relatively small sample sizes, and some assessed only the safety of praziquantel alone, and the follow-up period was also short. Furthermore, no active surveillance study has evaluated and compared the safety outcome of praziquantel and albendazole between helminth-infected and non-infected children. Hence, safety data on mass praziquantel and albendazole administration, especially in SSA, are scarce.

The pharmacovigilance system in most endemic countries, especially in SSA countries, is weak, and the spontaneous reporting system captures few to no adverse events during an MDA [24,25]. Furthermore, the spontaneous reporting only shows the trend of adverse events and does not help determine the incidence since the denominator (the number of populations who took the drug) is unknown. In settings where the pharmacovigilance system is weak and the implementation of passive surveillance is challenging, other robust safety surveillance mechanisms like active safety monitoring in the form of cohort event monitoring is recommended [26,27]. Therefore, with the aim of identifying the incidence, types, severity, and risk factors of the adverse events associated with mass praziquantel and albendazole co-administration, we conducted a large-scale observational prospective safety surveillance using active cohort event monitoring among school children in selected primary schools in southern Ethiopia.

2. Materials and Methods

2.1. Study Design, Area, and Population

The study observational prospective active safety surveillance of mass praziquantel and albendazole administration was conducted in six primary schools in the Hawella Tula and Wondo Gennet districts in the southern part of Ethiopia, at approximately 300 km south to Addis Ababa. The former district is located along the shore of lake Hawassa and residents rely on the lake water for their major domestic use. The Wondo Gennet district has various small water sources and most of the community members use these water sources for their consumption purpose. The study participants were school children attending six primary schools in two rural districts located in in Hawella Tula and Wondo Gennet districts. The schools involved from the Hawella Tula district were Bushulo, Kidus Pawulos, Finchawa, and Cheffe primary schools, while those involved from Wondo Gennet district were Wosha and Chukko primary schools. These districts were labeled as high schistosomiasis and STH prevalence districts by the national NTD public program based on the mapping results.

A total of 5848 school children aged 5–15 years from the six schools were enrolled in this study. The sample size for each school was calculated based on the proportion of the student population size. According to the WHO, a sample size of 10,000 gives a 95% probability (confidence) to detect at least three events at a frequency of 1 per 3333 [28,29]. Therefore, based on that estimation, our study sample size of 5848 will detect at least three events at a frequency of 1 per 1949 with a 95% confidence.

2.2. Study Enrolment and Baseline Data Collection

This study obtained ethics approval from the Institutional Review Board of the Southern Nations, Nationalities and Peoples Region Health Bureau ethical clearance committee (Ref no 902-6-19/14966) and the Ethiopian national research ethics review committee (Ref no MoSHE//RD/141/9848/20). Before the study's initiation, permission to conduct the study was obtained from the regional health and education bureaus, zonal and district health, and education offices. Orientation meetings with representatives from the district's education and health offices, healthcare professionals, schoolteachers, and the school administrator were done to give information about the study. Prior to the enrolment, participants and their parents or legal guardians received information about the study. School children whose parents/guardians gave consent and provided assent to participate (if applicable) were enrolled.

After their enrollment, the children's baseline socio-demographic data including their age, sex, and, nutritional status using anthropometric data, medical history, any comorbidities, concomitant medications, and any pre-existing clinical symptoms (pre-MDA events) were recorded from all the study participants. For measuring their nutritional status, their weight in kilograms and height in centimeters were converted to the height-for-age Z score (HAZ) and the body mass index (BMI)-for-age Z score (BAZ) using the WHO Anthro-plus software for school-age children [30]. Participants with values less than two standard deviation for both the HAZ and BAZ scores were considered as stunted and wasted, respectively.

2.3. Pre-Screening for S. mansoni and STH Infection

Two weeks prior to the MDA, 1484 (25.4%) out of the 5848 enrolled children were pre-screened for *S. mansoni* and STH infections. The number of prescreened children was proportionally distributed across the study schools and districts. The screening for a *S. mansoni* and STH infection was done using the standard Kato–Katz technique recommended by the WHO [31]. In brief, fresh stool samples from each study participant were collected and two Kato–Katz smears were prepared [32]. The egg counts from two smear readings were recorded, and the average value was taken and converted to the eggs per gram of stool using a factor of 24. The intensity of the infection was determined for each parasite as light, moderate, and heavy, based on the WHO criteria.

2.4. Mass Drug Administration and Safety Outcome Measures

The study participants received a single dose of praziquantel and albendazole, provided through the school-based MDA campaign led by the district health office of the NTD control program. The praziquantel dose was calculated according to height of the children ($\geq$94 cm dose pole, designed to deliver a dose of at least 40 mg/kg) and 400 mg of albendazole was administered following the national and WHO MDA guidelines [33]. The MDA program was organized and implemented nationwide by the national NTD public health program, and the study team had no role in the implementation of PC. After receiving the MDA, the study participants were actively monitored for any MDA-associated AEs on days 1 and 7 post-MDA. The participants were requested to record any adverse event during days 2–6. Any adverse events reported after receiving the MDA by each study participant were crosschecked and verified to differentiate MDA-associated AEs from any which were previously reported in an event pre-MDA.

The primary study outcome was the incidence of experiencing at least one type of MDA-associated AE (post-MDA AEs), defined as any event that was not reported before receiving the MDA but occurred after the drug exposure. The type and severity of the AEs were secondary outcomes. The severity grading of the treatment-associated adverse events were done using the Common Terminology Criteria for Adverse Events (CTCAE) Version 5.0 [34], as follows:

- Grade 1—Mild: asymptomatic or mild symptoms; clinical or diagnostic observations only; and intervention not indicated.
- Grade 2—Moderate: limiting age-appropriate instrumental activities of daily living (ADL). Minimal, local, or non-invasive intervention indicated.
- Grade 3—Severe: medically significant but not immediately life-threatening: disabling and limiting the self-care activities of daily living. Hospitalization or prolongation of hospitalization indicated.
- Grade 4—Life-threatening consequences: urgent intervention indicated.
- Grade 5—Death related to an AE.

2.5. Statistical Analysis

Data were entered on an open-source mobile data-based application Open Data Kit (ODK) for collecting information onto the Ethiopian Food and Drug Authority database and exported to an Excel file for cleaning. The data analysis was done by Statistical Package for Social Sciences (SPSS) version 24. Descriptive statistics was used to analyze the sociodemographic and baseline data. The Chi-square test was used to analyze the associations between the outcome variable (having any AEs or not) with the independent categorical variables. Univariate and multivariate regression analysis using binomial regression was used to determine the predictors of adverse events. Variables with a p-value ≤ 0.2 on the univariate analysis were included in the multivariate regression model. For interpretation without changing the estimations, we used a log transformation to change the coefficients into the incidence risk ratio (IRR). Probability values of less than or equal to 0.05 ($p < 0.05$) was considered to be statistically significant.

3. Results

3.1. Baseline Characteristics of Study Participants

A total of 5848 school children (50.5% were male) who were attending six primary schools in the HawellaTulla and Wondo Gennet districts were enrolled in this study. A quarter of the participants, 25.4% (1484), were prescreened for *S. mansoni* and STH infections two weeks before receiving a praziquantel and albendazole MDA. The study flow chart and MDA safety outcomes stratified by parasite infection status is presented in Figure 1.

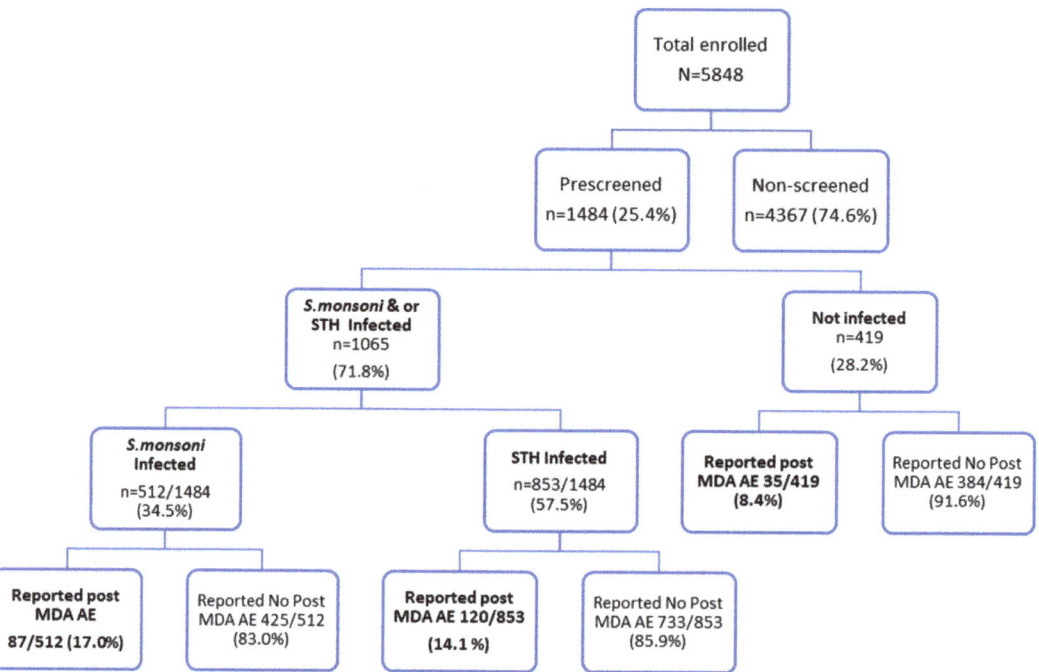

Figure 1. Study flow chart of prescreened participants for *S. mansoni* and soil-transmitted helminth (STH) infections before receiving mass drug administration (MDA) and safety outcomes after MDA stratified by infection status. AEs = adverse events.

Among the 1484 prescreened children, 1065 (71.8%) were infected with at least one type of parasite (*S. mansoni* or/and STH). Five hundred and twelve (34.5%) children were *S. mansoni* infected and 853 (57.5%) were STH infected. The baseline characteristics of the study participants are presented in Table 1. Of the total enrolled participants, 2.2% (129) reported pre-MDA events.

3.2. Cumulative Incidence of MDA-Associated AEs

Thirty-nine (0.7%) out of the 5848 study participants did not complete their day seven follow-up for safety monitoring. A total of 1187 AEs were reported by 780 participants during the seven-day follow-up period. The cumulative incidence of experiencing at least one type of MDA-associated AE during the 7 day follow-up period was 13.3% (780/5848; 95% CI = 12.5–14.2%). Among those who reported MDA-associated AEs, the proportion of individuals who experienced one, two, or three or more types of AEs were 57.7% (450), 34.1% (266), and 8.2% (64), respectively. Of the total participants who experienced at least one type of MDA-associated AE, 63.5% (495) experienced at least one type of AE on day one and the rest, 38.7% (302), experienced an AE within day 2–7 of the follow-up period.

The cumulative incidence of AEs over the seven days of the follow-up period stratified by the occurrence days during the follow-up is presented in Figure 2.

Table 1. Socio-demographic and baseline characteristics of study participants.

Variables	Category	Frequency N (%)
Sex	Male	2956 (50.5)
	Female	2892 (49.5)
Age Group	5–9 years	1046 (17.9)
	10–15 years	4802 (82.1)
Enrolment site	Hawella Tula	2306 (39.4)
	Wondo Gennet	3542 (60.6)
Types of infection (n = 1484)	Non-infected	419 (28.2)
	Schistosomiasis only	211 (14.2)
	STH only	552 (37.2)
	Schistosomiasis + STH	302 (20.4)
Stunting status	Normal	5228 (89.4)
	Stunted	620 (10.6)
Wasting status	Normal	5391 (92.2)
	Wasted	457 (7.8)
Type of food eaten Pre MDA.	Carbohydrate	5753 (98.4)
	Fatty meal	50 (0.9)
	Protein	45 (0.8)
Pre MDA-Events	Yes	129 (2.2)
	No	5719 (97.2)

STH = soil transmitted helminths; MDA = mass drug administration.

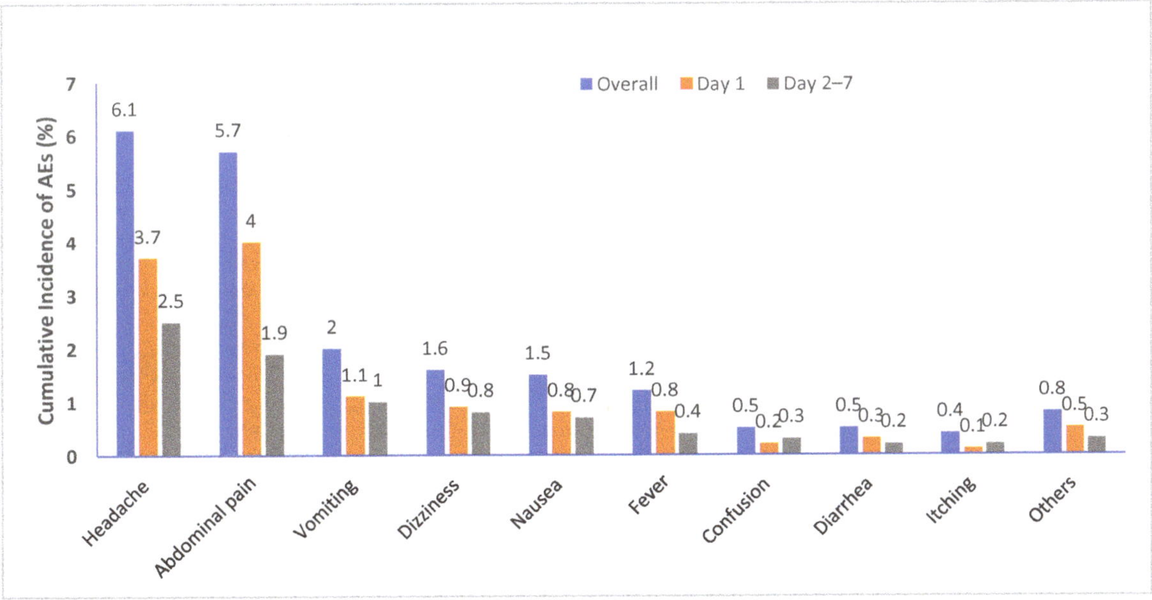

Figure 2. Cumulative incidence of AEs and stratified by days of follow-up.

3.3. Types of MDA-Associated Adverse Events

The most common MDA-associated AEs reported were headache 30.2% (n = 358), abdominal pain 28.1% (n = 334), vomiting 9.8% (n = 116), dizziness 7.8 % (n = 92), and nausea 7.5% (n = 89). The proportion of the adverse events over the seven days of the follow-up stratified by their type of AE is presented in Figure 3. On day one of the follow-up, abdominal pain, at 32.1% (233), was the most reported AE, followed by a headache at 29.5% (n = 214). On the contrary, on day 2–7 of the follow-up period, a headache was the most reported AE, with a proportion of 30.3% (n = 148), followed by abdominal pain, with a proportion of 22.5% (n = 110).

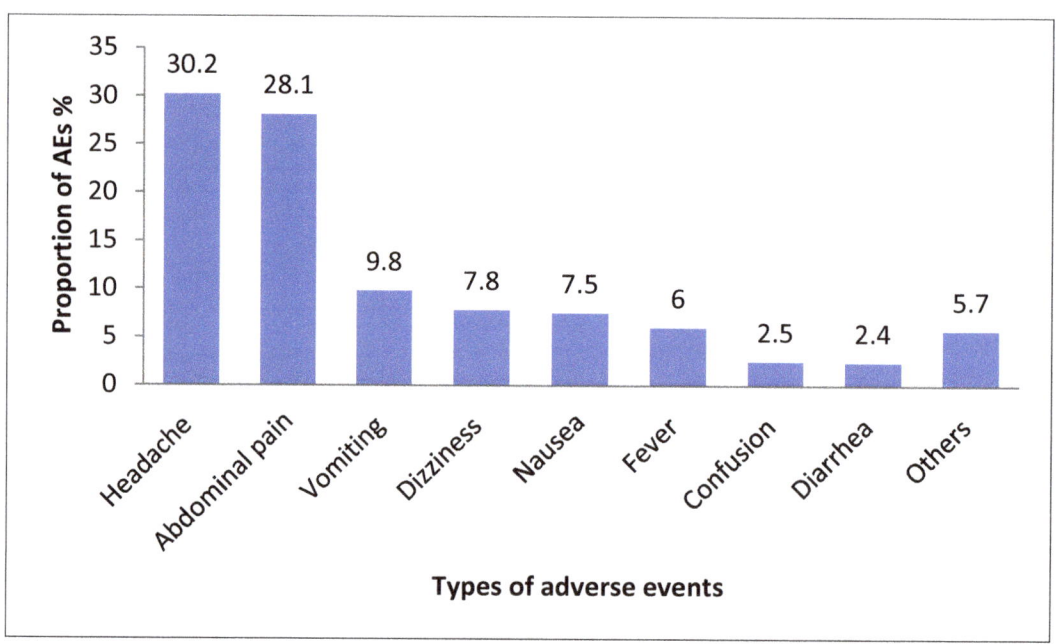

Figure 3. Proportions of AEs stratified by type of AEs.

3.4. Adverse Events by S. mansoni and STH Infection Status

Among the 1484 prescreened participants, 1065 (71.8%) were positive at least for one parasite; out of which, 512 (34.5%) were infected with intestinal schistosomiasis, and 853 (57.5%) were infected with STH. Children infected with at least one type of parasite were more likely to develop MDA-associated adverse events than the non-infected children (15.9% versus 8.4%) ($p < 0.001$). The cumulative incidence of the MDA-associated AEs stratified by the parasite infection status is presented in Figure 1. The cumulative incidence of AEs was significantly influenced by the parasite infection status ($p < 0.001$, $\chi^2 = 15.0$), with the occurrence of AEs being higher in S. mansoni-(17.0%) and STH (14.1%)-infected children than in non-infected children (8.4%). Abdominal pain with an incidence of 35.2% versus 5.5% was the most common AE reported, followed by a headache at 15.2% versus 3.6%, and vomiting at 6.7% versus 2.1% among infected and non-infected children, respectively. The types of AEs stratified by infection status are presented in Figure 4.

3.5. Severity Grading of Adverse Events

Out of the total 1187 MDA-associated AEs reported by 780 participants, 85.8% (n = 1019) were mild in their severity grading, followed by moderate at 12.4% (n = 147), and participants with severe AEs were only at an occurrence of 1.8% (n = 21). Most of the AEs were transient and resolved within 2–3 days after the drug administration. No serious AE that required hospitalization (Grade 4) was reported. The summary of the severity grading for each type of AEs is presented in Table 2.

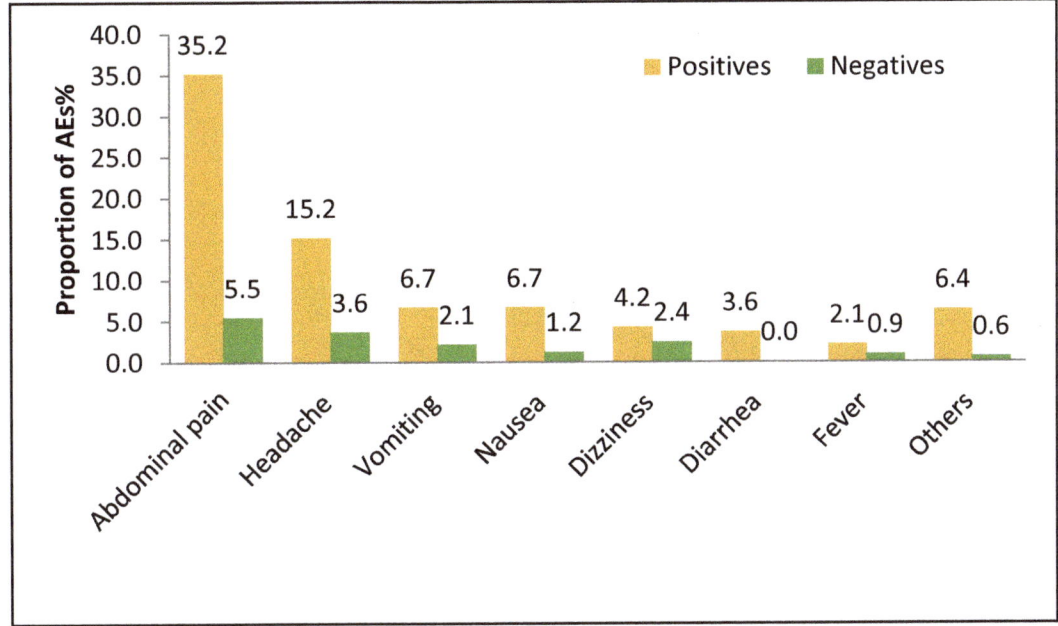

Figure 4. Proportions of AEs among the prescreened participants stratified by *S. mansoni* or STH infection status.

Table 2. Severity grading of AEs after mass praziquantel and albendazole administration.

Types of Adverse Events	Cumulative		Severity Grading		
	Number	Incidence	Mild (N/%)	Moderate (N/%)	Severe (N/%)
Headache	358	6.1	319 (89.1)	35 (9.8)	4 (1.1)
Abdominal pain	334	5.7	294 (88.0)	36 (0.8)	4 (1.2)
Vomiting	116	2.0	88 (75.9)	24 (20.7)	4 (3.4)
Dizziness	92	1.6	80 (87.0)	11 (12.0)	1 (1.1)
Nausea	89	1.5	74 (83.1)	13 (14.6)	2 (2.2)
Fever	71	1.2	58 (81.7)	12 (16.9)	1 (1.4)
Confusion	30	0.5	27 (90.0)	3 (10.0)	0
Diarrhea	29	0.5	20 (69.0)	7 (24.1)	2 (6.9)
Itching	21	0.4	21 (100)	0	0
Drowsiness	13	0.2	13 (100)	0	0
Loss of appetite	10	0.2	5 (50.0)	4 (40.0)	1 (10.0)
Rash	4	0.1	4 (100)	0	0
Difficulty Breathing	3	0.1	2 (66.7)	1 (33.3)	0
Cough	1	0	1 (100)	0	0
Other symptoms	16	0.3	13 (81.3)	1 (6.3)	2 (12.5) *
Total	1187	13.3	1019 (85.8)	147 (12.4)	21 (1.8)

* Other symptoms—tremor.

3.6. Factors Associated with MDA-Associated Adverse Events

The sex of the participants, their age group, their wasting status, and their parasite infection status were independent significant factors associated with experiencing an AE following the MDA. The cumulative incidence of AEs amongst female participants were significantly higher than amongst male participants ($p < 0.001$). Participants in the age group of 10–15 years old experienced more AEs than younger age participants (5–9 years old) ($p = 0.002$). *S. mansoni*- or STH-infected children experienced significantly higher AEs compared to non-infected participants ($p < 0.001$). Children infected with *S. mansoni* were more likely to develop AEs than participants infected with STH ($p < 0.001$). The occurrence of AEs was not associated with the stunting status or number of praziquantel tablets taken. The cumulative incidence and factor associations with the MDA-associated adverse events during the follow-up is presented in Table 3.

Table 3. Cumulative incidence AEs following mass praziquantel and albendazole administration and associated factors.

Variables	Category	Adverse Events No (N/%)	Adverse Events Yes (N/%)	χ^2	p-Value
Total		5068 (86.7)	780 (13.3)		
Sex	Male	2622 (88.7)	334 (11.3)	21.5	<0.001
	Female	2446 (84.6)	446 (15.4)		
Age group	5–9 years	938 (89.7)	108 (10.3)	10.0	0.002
	10–15 years	4130 (86.0)	672 (14.0)		
Stunting	Normal	4530 (86.6)	698 (13.4)	0.008	0.93
	Stunted	538 (86.8)	82 (13.2)		
Wasting	Normal	4653 (86.3)	738 (13.7)	7.4	0.007
	Wasted	415 (90.8)	42 (9.2)		
Enrolment district	Hawella Tula	1961 (85.0)	345 (15.0)	8.7	0.003
	WondoGennet	3107 (87.7)	435 (12.3)		
Infection status (*S.mansoni* or STH)	Infected	896 (84.1)	169 (16.0)	14.3	<0.001
	Non-infected	384 (91.6)	35 (8.4)		
Infection types	Non infected	384 (91.6)	35 (8.4)	24.5	<0.001
	Schistosomiasis only	163 (77.3)	48 (22.7)		
	STH only	470 (85.1)	82 (14.9)		
	Schistosomiasis + STH	263 (87.1)	39 (12.9)		
Number of praziquantel tablet taken	<3 tablets	2416 (87.1)	357 (12.9)	1	0.32
	≥3 tablets	2652 (86.2)	423 (13.8)		

STH = Soil-transmitted helminth.

3.7. Predictors of Adverse Events

To identify the factors predicting the occurrence of at least one type of MDA-associated AE, we conducted univariate followed by multivariate log binomial regression analysis. The sex of the participants, their age category, their enrolment site, their wasting status, and their infection types were significant predictors for developing at least one post-MDA AE in the univariate analysis. In the multivariate analysis, their sex, age category, and infection type remained significant predictors of AEs following the MDA; the female sex, participants in the age category of 10–15 years, and participants infected with schistosomiasis had the highest risk of developing AEs post-MDA (Table 4).

Table 4. Predictors of AEs following mass praziquantel and albendazole administration for school children.

Variables	Category	Univariate Analysis			Multivariate Analysis		
		cRR	95% CI	p-Value	aRR	95% CI	p-Value
Sex	Male	1					
	Female	1.4	1.2–1.6	<0.001	1.3	1.0–1.7	0.04
Age group	5–9 years	1					
	10–15 years	1.4	1.1–1.6	0.002	1.5	1.0–2.1	0.04
Stunting (HAZ)	Normal	1					
	Stunted	1.0	0.8–1.2	0.93			
Wasting (BAZ)	Normal	1					
	Wasted	0.7	0.5–0.9	0.008	1.3	0.8–2.1	0.3
Type of meal eaten before MDA.	Carbohydrate	1					
	Fatty meal	1.2	0.6–2.2	0.6			
	Protein	0.8	0.4–1.9	0.7			
S.mansoniand/or STH Infection	Non-Infected	1					
	Infected	1.8	1.3–2.6	<0.001			
Type of Infection	Negatives						
	SM only	2.6	1.8–3.9	<0.001	2.5	1.7–3.7	<0.001
	SM + STH	1.5	0.97–2.3	0.07	1.5	1.2–2.5	0.005
	STH only	1.7	1.2–2.5	0.003	1.7	0.98–2.3	0.057
Number of praziquanltel tablets	<3 tablets						
	≥3 tablets	1.1	0.9–1.6	0.32			

Due to the co-linearity of S.monsoni and/or STH infection and type of infection, the variable S.monsoni and/or STH Infection was not included in the adjusted model. cRR = crude relative risk, aRR = adjusted relative risk, CI = confidence interval. STH = soil transmitted helminths; MDA = mass drug administration; HAZ = height-for-age z- scores; BAZ = BMI-for-age z-scores.

4. Discussion

A school-based mass praziquantel and albendazole preventive chemotherapy to all at-risk populations without a prior diagnosis has been implemented in schistosomiasis and STH endemic countries for many years. Although safety monitoring in MDA programs is recommended, it is not practiced, especially in SSA countries due to the limited pharmacovigilance capacity. We conducted a large-scale active safety surveillance of AEs following a mass praziquantel and albendazole administration in school children living in high endemic districts of southern Ethiopia. Our study was well controlled to differentiate the MDA-associated adverse events from any pre-existing clinical symptoms. Most previous studies investigated treatment-associated AEs among infected children or MDA-associated AEs in the general population. To investigate whether drug safety is influenced by a helminth infection status, we prescreened one-fourth of the study participants for S. mansoni and STH infection. To our knowledge, this is the first large sample size active safety surveillance study to investigate the incidence, types, severity, and risk factors of MDA-associated AEs following praziquantel and albendazole PC considering the participants' helminth infection status.

The overall cumulative incidence of experiencing at least one type of MDA-associated AE within a week of MDA exposure was 13.3%. The incidence of developing one, two, or three or more types of AEs was 57.7%, 34.1%, and 8.2%, respectively. The most common AEs, in descending order, were a headache, abdominal pain, vomiting, dizziness, and nausea. The participants' sex, age group, enrolment site, and infection type were significant factors associated with the occurrence of AEs following the mass praziquantel and albendazole administration. Using a similar study design, a recent study from Rwanda reported that one in five child who received a praziquantel and albendazole MDA reported at least one type of MDA-associated AE [35]. The cumulative incidence of an MDA-associated AE (13.3%) in our study was slightly lower than the report from Rwanda, which could be due to variations in the prevalence of an STH or *S. mansoni* infection status of the study participants [32,36]. Using various study designs, follow-up durations, and study populations, incidences of AEs ranging from 8.6% to 83% were reported [21–23,37].

Most reported AEs were mild and moderate on the severity grading, transient, and self-limiting, which resolved within 2–3 days of the drug administration. This indicates that PC through a mass praziquantel and albendazole administration is safe and tolerable. Although few severe adverse events were reported (1.8%), none of them required hospitalization and no serious outcome was recorded. Similar observations were reported from other safety studies and meta-analyses [20,22,23,38,39]. Though few, the finding of severe AEs in our study ascertains the importance of integrating active pharmacovigilance in the routine MDA program.

The total number of AEs observed was 1187 from 780 study participants, indicating that some participants experienced more than one type of AE. The occurrence of AEs following the praziquantel and albendazole administration is associated with one's age, infection intensity, and nutritional status [20–22]. In our study, the most frequently reported AEs were headaches, abdominal pain, vomiting, dizziness, and nausea, which is in line with the previous findings [20,38]. Similar AEs were reported to the global pharmacovigilance data base at the WHO-UMC through spontaneous reporting [40]. Most of these AEs are similar to the signs and symptoms of a parasitic infection. However, to differentiate the true AEs associated with the MDA from the parasite infection symptoms, before the MDA, the study participants were interviewed to see if they had any pre-existing clinical symptoms (pre-MDA event) and the participants who reported similar symptoms at the baseline and at the post-MDA follow-up were excluded from the analysis.

The incidence of AEs was significantly higher among female participants compared to male ones (15.4% versus 11.3%). Similar sex difference in the incidence of AEs was reported in the previous studies [35,38,39]. Recent studies conducted on the safety of a MDA for the control and elimination of lymphatic filariasis in east Africa also reported a difference in the incidence of AEs across the sexes [41,42]. An adverse drug reaction (ADR) analysis of half a century data from the global ADR database based on sex differences also reported a higher proportion of ADR among females [43]. A similar finding was reported by the national Pharmacovigilance Centre in the Netherlands from the analysis of their database based on sex [44]. The higher incidence of AEs among females could be explained by their physiologic difference, which may lead to differences in the activity of enzymes for the drug metabolism, resulting in pharmacokinetics and pharmacodynamics deviations [45,46]. However, the sex-dependent pharmacokinetic and pharmacodynamic variations and its role in the occurrence of AEs associated with praziquantel and albendazole MDA remains to be investigated.

We observed a higher incidence of AEs among the older age groups (10–15 years), which is in line with the reported findings from previous studies and meta-analyses [22]. Perhaps this can be explained by the higher dose of praziquantel taken by this age group, as the drug was given based on height. A higher dose of praziquantel is associated with an increased risk of AEs in the previously reported studies [35].

To investigate whether the incidence or type of AEs is influenced by a parasite infection, one fourth of the study participants were pre-screened for *S. mansoni* and STH two weeks prior to receiving the MDA. Interestingly, we found a significantly higher incidence of MDA-associated AEs in children infected with *S. mansoni* and STH than non-infected children. Although a treatment-associated AE is significantly influenced by infections intensity among infected children [21], to our knowledge, ours is the first study to compare the type and incidence of MDA-associated AEs between infected and non-infected children who received a praziquantel and albendazole MDA for PC. Praziquantel-associated AEs in schistosomiasis-infected children may occur due to the drug effect or by the parasite itself. Thus, the reported high AEs among the infected children could be due to dying parasites resulting from the effect of the drugs on the parasites [47]. Further safety surveillance studies which evaluate and compare the difference in the occurrence of AEs among infected and non-infected groups is recommended for supporting the further risk benefit analysis of PC among non-infected individuals, particularly in low endemic areas.

5. Conclusions

Preventive chemotherapy with a praziquantel and albendazole combination is generally safe and tolerated by school children. Most of the observed AEs were of a mild to moderate grading and transient, resolving themselves within a week. Being female, older age group (10–15 years), or having a helminth infection are significant independent risk factors for the occurrence of AEs following a praziquantel and albendazole MDA. Though few, the finding of severe AEs and the significantly increased risk of AEs among helminth-infected children underscore the need for the integration of pharmacovigilance in MDA campaigns, especially in high endemic areas for the timely detection and management of AEs and to boost public confidence in the program.

Author Contributions: Conceptualization, T.D.G., E.M., T.T., H.G., B.T.T., P.G. and E.A.; data curation, T.D.G., H.G. (Habtamu Gashaw), W.D. and E.A.; formal analysis, T.D.G., E.M., T.T. and E.A.; Funding acquisition, H.G. (Heran Gerba), E.M. and E.A.; investigation, T.D.G., E.M., T.T. and H.G. (Habtamu Gashaw), W.D., H.G. (Heran Gerba), B.T.T., P.G. and E.A.; methodology, T.D.G., E.M., T.T., H.G. (Habtamu Gashaw), W.D., H.G. (Heran Gerba), B.T.T., P.G. and E.A.; project administration, T.D.G., E.M., H.G. (Heran Gerba) and E.A.; resources, T.T. and H.G. (Heran Gerba); supervision, E.M. and E.A.; validation, T.D.G.; writing—original draft, T.D.G.; writing—review and editing, T.D.G., T.T., B.T.T., P.G., E.M. and E.A. All authors have read and agreed to the published version of the manuscript.

Funding: This research was funded by the European and Developing Countries Clinical Trials Partnership (EDCTP) 2 program supported by the European Union (PROFORMA project, Grant number CSA2016S-1618), and the Swedish International Development Cooperation Agency (SIDA) as part of the Pharmacovigilance infrastructure and post-marketing surveillance system capacity building for regional medicine regulatory harmonization in East Africa project.

Institutional Review Board Statement: The study was conducted in accordance with the Declaration of Helsinki and approved by the Institutional Review Board of the Southern Nations, Nationalities and Peoples Region Health Bureau ethical clearance committee (Ref no 902-6-19/14966) and the Ethiopian national research ethics review committee (Ref no MoSHE//RD/141/9848/20).

Informed Consent Statement: Informed consent from was obtained from all parents/guardians and assent from participants (if applicable). For participants ≤ 12 years of age, verbal and written informed consent was obtained from their parent or guardian. Whereas for participants > 12 years of age, verbal and written informed consent was obtained from the parent or guardian and an assent was obtained from the study participant.

Data Availability Statement: All data presented in this study are contained within the manuscript.

Acknowledgments: We thank the national and regional neglected tropical diseases control program teams for their support during the conduct of the study. We are also grateful to officials from Hawela Tula and Wondo Gennet district health and education offices, schoolteachers, and administrators for giving permission to collect data in the study schools. We thank schoolteachers and health care professionals for participating in the data collection. We would also like to extend our gratitude to EFDA staff members both at the head office and south branch for their participation in the planning, awareness creation, and supervision during the data collection. We also appreciate the study participants, their parents/guardians, and teachers from the six schools for their participation.

Conflicts of Interest: The authors declare no conflict of interest. The funders had no role in the design of the study; in the collection, analyses, or interpretation of data; in the writing of the manuscript; or in the decision to publish the results.

References

1. Hotez, P.J.; Molyneux, D.H.; Fenwick, A.; Kumaresan, J.; Sachs, S.E.; Sachs, J.D.; Savioli, L. Control of neglected tropical diseases. *N. Engl. J. Med.* **2007**, *357*, 1018–1027. [CrossRef] [PubMed]
2. Ezeamama, A.E.; Bustinduy, A.L.; Nkwata, A.K.; Martinez, L.; Pabalan, N.; Boivin, M.J.; King, C.H. Cognitive deficits and educational loss in children with schistosome infection-A systematic review and meta-analysis. *PLoS Negl. Trop. Dis.* **2018**, *12*, e0005524. [CrossRef] [PubMed]
3. Hotez, P.J.; Bundy, D.A.P.; Beegle, K.; Brooker, S.; Drake, L.; de Silva, N.; Montresor, A.; Engels, D.; Jukes, M.; Chitsulo, L.; et al. Helminth Infections: Soil-transmitted Helminth Infections and Schistosomiasis. In *Disease Control Priorities in Developing Countries*; Jamison, D.T., Breman, J.G., Measham, A.R., Alleyne, G., Claeson, M., Evans, D.B., Jha, P., Mills, A., Musgrove, P., Eds.; World Bank: Washington, DC, USA, 2006; ISBN 978-0-8213-6179-5. Available online: http://www.ncbi.nlm.nih.gov/books/NBK11748/ (accessed on 10 August 2022).
4. King, C.H.; Dangerfield-Cha, M. The unacknowledged impact of chronic schistosomiasis. *Chronic Illn.* **2008**, *4*, 65–79. [CrossRef]
5. Stephenson, L. The impact of schistosomiasis on human nutrition. *Parasitology* **1993**, *107*, S107–S123. [CrossRef]
6. Webster, J.P.; Molyneux, D.H.; Hotez, P.J.; Fenwick, A. The contribution of mass drug administration to global health: Past, present and future. *Philos. Trans. R. Soc. B Biol. Sci.* **2014**, *369*, 20130434. [CrossRef] [PubMed]
7. WHO_Africa Second Edition of National Neglected Tropical Diseases Master Plan for Ethiopia, 2016. Available online: https://www.afro.who.int/publications/second-edition-national-neglected-tropical-diseases-master-plan-ethiopia-2016 (accessed on 7 October 2020).
8. Jember, T.H. Challenges of schistosomiasis prevention and control in Ethiopia: Literature review and current status. *JPVB* **2014**, *6*, 80–86. [CrossRef]
9. World Health Organization. *Sustaining the Drive to Overcome the Global Impact of Neglected Tropical Diseases: Second WHO Report on Neglected Tropical Diseases*; World Health Organization: Geneva, Switzerland, 2013; ISBN 978-92-4-156454-0.
10. *Helminth Control in School-Age Children: A Guide for Managers of Control Programmes*, 2nd ed.; Montresor, A.; World Health Organization (Eds.) World Health Organization: Geneva, Switzerland, 2011; ISBN 978-92-4-154826-7.
11. Gabrielli, A.-F.; Montresor, A.; Chitsulo, L.; Engels, D.; Savioli, L. Preventive chemotherapy in human helminthiasis: Theoretical and operational aspects. *Trans. R. Soc. Trop. Med. Hyg.* **2011**, *105*, 683–693. [CrossRef]
12. Bergquist, R.; Zhou, X.-N.; Rollinson, D.; Reinhard-Rupp, J.; Klohe, K. Elimination of schistosomiasis: The tools required. *Infect. Dis. Poverty* **2017**, *6*, 158. [CrossRef]
13. World Health Organization Summary of global update on implementation of preventive chemotherapy against NTDs in 2020. *Wkly. Epidemiol. Rec.* **2021**, *96*, 468–475.
14. Montresor, A.; Mupfasoni, D.; Mikhailov, A.; Mwinzi, P.; Lucianez, A.; Jamsheed, M.; Gasimov, E.; Warusavithana, S.; Yajima, A.; Bisoffi, Z.; et al. The global progress of soil-transmitted helminthiases control in 2020 and World Health Organization targets for 2030. *PLoS Negl. Trop. Dis.* **2020**, *14*, e0008505. [CrossRef]
15. Montresor, A.; Gabrielli, A.F.; Chitsulo, L.; Ichimori, K.; Mariotti, S.; Engels, D.; Savioli, L. Preventive chemotherapy and the fight against neglected tropical diseases. *Expert Rev. Anti-Infect. Ther.* **2012**, *10*, 237–242. [CrossRef] [PubMed]
16. Preventive Chemotherapy. Available online: https://www.who.int/data/preventive-chemotherapy (accessed on 5 June 2022).
17. WHO Guideline on Control and Elimination of Human Schistosomiasis. Available online: https://www.who.int/publications-detail-redirect/9789240041608 (accessed on 3 June 2022).
18. Souza, D.K.d.; Dorlo, T.P.C. Safe mass drug administration for neglected tropical diseases. *Lancet Glob. Health* **2018**, *6*, e1054–e1055. [CrossRef]
19. Lima, R.M.; Ferreira, M.A.D.; Carvalho, T.M.d.J.P.; Fernandes, B.J.D.; Takayanagui, O.M.; Garcia, H.H.; Coelho, E.B.; Lanchote, V.L. Albendazole-praziquantel interaction in healthy volunteers: Kinetic disposition, metabolism and enantioselectivity. *Br. J. Clin. Pharmacol.* **2011**, *71*, 528–535. [CrossRef] [PubMed]
20. Zwang, J.; Olliaro, P. Efficacy and safety of praziquantel 40 mg/kg in preschool-aged and school-aged children: A meta-analysis. *Parasites Vectors* **2017**, *10*, 47. [CrossRef]
21. Mnkugwe, R.H.; Minzi, O.S.; Kinung'hi, S.M.; Kamuhabwa, A.A.; Aklillu, E. Efficacy and Safety of Praziquantel for Treatment of Schistosoma mansoni Infection among School Children in Tanzania. *Pathogens* **2020**, *9*, 28. [CrossRef]
22. Erko, B.; Degarege, A.; Tadesse, K.; Mathiwos, A.; Legesse, M. Efficacy and side effects of praziquantel in the treatment of Schistosomiasis mansoni in schoolchildren in Shesha Kekele Elementary School, Wondo Genet, Southern Ethiopia. *Asian Pac. J. Trop. Biomed.* **2012**, *2*, 235–239. [CrossRef]
23. Lemos, M.; Pedro, J.M.; Fançony, C.; Moura, S.; Brito, M.; Nery, S.V.; Sousa, C.P.; Barros, H. Schistosomiasis and soil-transmitted helminthiasis preventive chemotherapy: Adverse events in children from 2 to 15 years in Bengo province, Angola. *PLoS ONE* **2020**, *15*, e0229247. [CrossRef]
24. Barry, A.; Olsson, S.; Khaemba, C.; Kabatende, J.; Dires, T.; Fimbo, A.; Minzi, O.; Bienvenu, E.; Makonnen, E.; Kamuhabwa, A.; et al. Comparative Assessment of the Pharmacovigilance Systems within the Neglected Tropical Diseases Programs in East Africa—Ethiopia, Kenya, Rwanda, and Tanzania. *Int. J. Environ. Res. Public Health* **2021**, *18*, 1941. [CrossRef]
25. Kiguba, R.; Olsson, S.; Waitt, C. Pharmacovigilance in low- and middle-income countries: A review with particular focus on Africa. *Br. J. Clin. Pharmacol.* **2021**. Available online: https://onlinelibrary.wiley.com/doi/abs/10.1111/bcp.15193 (accessed on 12 August 2022). [CrossRef]

26. Pal, S.N.; Duncombe, C.; Falzon, D.; Olsson, S. WHO Strategy for Collecting Safety Data in Public Health Programmes: Complementing Spontaneous Reporting Systems. *Drug Saf.* **2013**, *36*, 75–81. [CrossRef]
27. Weltgesundheitsorganisation, Collaborating Centre for International Drug Monitoring. *The Importance of Pharmacovigilance: Safety Monitoring of Medicinal Products*; WHO: Geneva, Switzerland, 2002; ISBN 978-92-4-159015-0.
28. World Health Organization. *A Practical Handbook on the Pharmacovigilance of Antiretroviral Medicines*; World Health Organization: Geneva, Switzerland, 2009; ISBN 978-92-4-154794-9.
29. World Health Organization. *Protocol Template to Be Used as Template for Observational Study Protocols: Cohort Event Monitoring (CEM) for Safety Signal Detection after Vaccination with COVID-19 Vaccines*; World Health Organization: Geneva, Switzerland, 2021; ISBN 978-92-4-002739-8.
30. WHO. WHO Anthro Survey Analyser and Other Tools. Available online: https://www.who.int/tools/child-growth-standards/software (accessed on 7 June 2022).
31. WHO. WHO | Basic Laboratory Methods in Medical Parasitology (Archived). Available online: https://www.who.int/malaria/publications/atoz/9241544104_part1/en/ (accessed on 9 October 2020).
32. Gebreyesus, T.D.; Tadele, T.; Mekete, K.; Barry, A.; Gashaw, H.; Degefe, W.; Tadesse, B.T.; Gerba, H.; Gurumurthy, P.; Makonnen, E.; et al. Prevalence, Intensity, and Correlates of Schistosomiasis and Soil-Transmitted Helminth Infections after Five Rounds of Preventive Chemotherapy among School Children in Southern Ethiopia. *Pathogens* **2020**, *9*, 920. [CrossRef] [PubMed]
33. Montresor, A.; Odermatt, P.; Muth, S.; Iwata, F.; Raja'a, Y.A.; Assis, A.M.; Zulkifli, A.; Kabatereine, N.B.; Fenwick, A.; Al-Awaidy, S.; et al. The WHO dose pole for the administration of praziquantel is also accurate in non-African populations. *Trans. R. Soc. Trop. Med. Hyg.* **2005**, *99*, 78–81. [CrossRef] [PubMed]
34. NIH, National Cancer Institute Common Terminology Criteria for Adverse Events (CTCAE) | Protocol Development | CTEP. Available online: https://ctep.cancer.gov/protocoldevelopment/electronic_applications/ctc.htm (accessed on 3 June 2022).
35. Kabatende, J.; Barry, A.; Mugisha, M.; Ntirenganya, L.; Bergman, U.; Bienvenu, E.; Aklillu, E. Safety of Praziquantel and Albendazole Coadministration for the Control and Elimination of Schistosomiasis and Soil-Transmitted Helminths Among Children in Rwanda: An Active Surveillance Study. *Drug Saf.* **2022**, *45*, 909–922. [CrossRef] [PubMed]
36. Kabatende, J.; Mugisha, M.; Ntirenganya, L.; Barry, A.; Ruberanziza, E.; Mbonigaba, J.B.; Bergman, U.; Bienvenu, E.; Aklillu, E. Prevalence, Intensity, and Correlates of Soil-Transmitted Helminth Infections among School Children after a Decade of Preventive Chemotherapy in Western Rwanda. *Pathogens* **2020**, *9*, 1076. [CrossRef]
37. Raso, G.; N'Goran, E.K.; Toty, A.; Luginbühl, A.; Adjoua, C.A.; Tian-Bi, N.T.; Bogoch, I.I.; Vounatsou, P.; Tanner, M.; Utzinger, J. Efficacy and side effects of praziquantel against Schistosoma mansoni in a community of western Côte d'Ivoire. *Trans. R. Soc. Trop. Med. Hyg.* **2004**, *98*, 18–27. [CrossRef]
38. Njenga, S.M.; Ng'ang'a, P.M.; Mwanje, M.T.; Bendera, F.S.; Bockarie, M.J. A School-Based Cross-Sectional Survey of Adverse Events following Co-Administration of Albendazole and Praziquantel for Preventive Chemotherapy against Urogenital Schistosomiasis and Soil-Transmitted Helminthiasis in Kwale County, Kenya. *PLoS ONE* **2014**, *9*, e88315. [CrossRef]
39. N'Goran, E.K.; Gnaka, H.N.; Tanner, M.; Utzinger, J. Efficacy and side-effects of two praziquantel treatments against Schistosoma haematobium infection, among schoolchildren from Côte d'Ivoire. *Ann. Trop. Med. Parasitol.* **2003**, *97*, 37–51. [CrossRef]
40. VigiLyze. Available online: https://vigilyze.who-umc.org/ (accessed on 14 June 2022).
41. Fimbo, A.M.; Minzi, O.M.; Mmbando, B.P.; Gurumurthy, P.; Kamuhabwa, A.A.R.; Aklillu, E. Safety and Tolerability of Ivermectin and Albendazole Mass Drug Administration in Lymphatic Filariasis Endemic Communities of Tanzania: A Cohort Event Monitoring Study. *Pharmaceuticals* **2022**, *15*, 594. [CrossRef]
42. Khaemba, C.; Barry, A.; Omondi, W.P.; Bota, K.; Matendechero, S.; Wandera, C.; Siyoi, F.; Kirui, E.; Oluka, M.; Nambwa, P.; et al. Safety and Tolerability of Mass Diethylcarbamazine and Albendazole Administration for the Elimination of Lymphatic Filariasis in Kenya: An Active Surveillance Study. *Pharmaceuticals* **2021**, *14*, 264. [CrossRef]
43. Watson, S.; Caster, O.; Rochon, P.A.; Ruijter, H. den Reported adverse drug reactions in women and men: Aggregated evidence from globally collected individual case reports during half a century. *Eclinicalmedicine* **2019**, *17*, 100188. [CrossRef]
44. de Vries, S.T.; Denig, P.; Ekhart, C.; Burgers, J.S.; Kleefstra, N.; Mol, P.G.M.; van Puijenbroek, E.P. Sex differences in adverse drug reactions reported to the National Pharmacovigilance Centre in the Netherlands: An explorative observational study. *Br. J. Clin. Pharmacol.* **2019**, *85*, 1507–1515. [CrossRef] [PubMed]
45. Zucker, I.; Prendergast, B.J. Sex differences in pharmacokinetics predict adverse drug reactions in women. *Biol. Sex Differ.* **2020**, *11*, 32. [CrossRef] [PubMed]
46. Rademaker, M. Do Women Have More Adverse Drug Reactions? *Am. J. Clin. Dermatol.* **2001**, *2*, 349–351. [CrossRef]
47. Katz, N.; Rocha, R.S.; Chaves, A. Preliminary trials with praziquantel in human infections due to Schistosoma mansoni. *Bull. World Health Organ.* **1979**, *57*, 781–785. [PubMed]

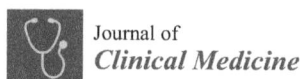 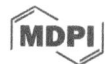

Journal of Clinical Medicine

Article

The Safety Profile of COVID-19 Vaccines in Patients Diagnosed with Multiple Sclerosis: A Retrospective Observational Study

Giorgia Teresa Maniscalco [1,2,†], Cristina Scavone [3,4,*,†], Annamaria Mascolo [3,4], Valentino Manzo [2], Elio Prestipino [1,2], Gaspare Guglielmi [5], Maria Luisa Aiezza [5], Santolo Cozzolino [6], Adele Bracco [6], Ornella Moreggia [1], Daniele Di Giulio Cesare [1], Antonio Rosario Ziello [1], Angela Falco [4], Marida Massa [5], Massimo Majolo [7], Eliana Raiola [7], Roberto Soprano [7], Giuseppe Russo [7], Giuseppe Longo [8], Vincenzo Andreone [1,2,‡] and Annalisa Capuano [3,4,‡]

1. Multiple Sclerosis Regional Center, "A. Cardarelli" Hospital, 80131 Naples, Italy
2. Neurological Clinic and Stroke Unit, "A. Cardarelli" Hospital, 80131 Naples, Italy
3. Department of Experimental Medicine, University of Campania "Luigi Vanvitelli", 80138 Naples, Italy
4. Regional Center of Pharmacovigilance and Pharmacoepidemiology of Campania Region, 80138 Naples, Italy
5. Pharmacy, "A. Cardarelli" Hospital, 80131 Naples, Italy
6. Biotechnology Center, "A. Cardarelli" Hospital, 80131 Naples, Italy
7. Healtcare Direction, "A. Cardarelli" Hospital, 80131 Naples, Italy
8. General Direction, "A. Cardarelli" Hospital, 80131 Naples, Italy
* Correspondence: cristina.scavone@unicampania.it; Tel.: +39-081-5665-805
† These authors contributed equally to this work.
‡ Co-lead authors.

Citation: Maniscalco, G.T.; Scavone, C.; Mascolo, A.; Manzo, V.; Prestipino, E.; Guglielmi, G.; Aiezza, M.L.; Cozzolino, S.; Bracco, A.; Moreggia, O.; et al. The Safety Profile of COVID-19 Vaccines in Patients Diagnosed with Multiple Sclerosis: A Retrospective Observational Study. *J. Clin. Med.* **2022**, *11*, 6855. https://doi.org/10.3390/jcm11226855

Academic Editor: Francisco J. De Abajo

Received: 21 October 2022
Accepted: 17 November 2022
Published: 21 November 2022

Publisher's Note: MDPI stays neutral with regard to jurisdictional claims in published maps and institutional affiliations.

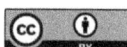

Copyright: © 2022 by the authors. Licensee MDPI, Basel, Switzerland. This article is an open access article distributed under the terms and conditions of the Creative Commons Attribution (CC BY) license (https://creativecommons.org/licenses/by/4.0/).

Abstract: In the current COVID-19 pandemic, patients diagnosed with multiple sclerosis (MS) are considered to be one of the highest priority categories, being recognized as extremely vulnerable people. For this reason, mRNA-based COVID-19 vaccines are strongly recommended for these patients. Despite encouraging results on the efficacy and safety profile of mRNA-based COVID-19 vaccines, to date, in frail populations, including patients diagnosed with MS, this information is rather limited. We carried out a retrospective observational study with the aim to evaluate the safety profile of mRNA-based COVID-19 vaccines by retrieving real-life data of MS patients who were treated and vaccinated at the Multiple Sclerosis Center of the Hospital A.O.R.N. A. Cardarelli. Three-hundred and ten medical records of MS patients who received the first dose of the mRNA-based COVID-19 vaccine were retrieved (63% female; mean age: 45.9 years). Of these patients, 288 also received the second dose. All patients received the Pfizer-BioNTech vaccine. Relapsing-Remitting Multiple Sclerosis (RRSM) was the most common form of MS. The Expanded Disability Status Scale (EDSS) values were <3.0 in 70% of patients. The majority of patients received a Disease Modifying Therapy (DMT) during the study period, mainly interferon beta 1-a, dimethyl fumarate, and natalizumab and fingolimod. Overall, 913 AEFIs were identified, of which 539 were after the first dose of the vaccine and 374 after the second dose. The majority of these AEFIs were classified as short-term since they occurred within the first 72 h. The most common identified adverse events were pain at injection site, flu-like symptoms, and headache. Fever was reported more frequently after the second dose than after the first dose. SARS-CoV-2 infection occurred in 3 patients after the first dose. Using historical data of previous years (2017–2020), the relapses' rate during 2021 was found to be lower. Lastly, the results of the multivariable analysis that assessed factors associated with the occurrence of AEFIs revealed a statistical significance for age, sex, and therapy with ocrelizumab ($p < 0.05$). In conclusion, our results indicated that Pfizer-BioNTech vaccine was safe for MS patients, being associated with AEFIs already detected in the general population. Larger observational studies with longer follow-up and epidemiological studies are strongly needed.

Keywords: COVID-19; mRNA-based vaccine; safety; multiple sclerosis; AEFI; observational study

1. Introduction

Since the beginning of the COVID-19 outbreak, a range of repurposed drugs against this new infection have been investigated with the aim to fight one of the largest international health emergencies [1–3]. Following the identification of the genetic sequence of SARS-CoV-2, the virus responsible for COVID-19, an intense research program on potential vaccines started worldwide. To date (November 2022), six vaccines have obtained marketing approval from the European Medicines Agency (EMA), including two RNA vaccines (Pfizer-BioNTech and Moderna), two adenovirus vaccines (AstraZeneca and Janssen), and one recombinant, adjuvanted vaccine (Novavax) and one inactivated, adjuvanted (COVID-19 Vaccine Valneva). The Pfizer-BioNTech vaccine is a modified mRNA-based vaccine that encodes a S protein of the virus. The RNA of this vaccine is produced by in vitro transcription from the corresponding DNA that encodes a S protein of SARS-CoV-2, which is responsible of the virus' attachment to the host's cells [4]. The Moderna vaccine has similar characteristics. Both vaccines are given as two injections, usually into the muscle of the upper arm, 3 and 4 weeks apart for the Pfizer and Moderna vaccine, respectively. The efficacy of both vaccines was evaluated in thousands of people aged 16 and above who had no sign of previous infection, resulting in an almost 95% reduction in the number of symptomatic COVID-19 cases in people who received the vaccination [5,6]. Preliminary data on their safety profile showed that adverse events following immunization (AEFIs) with mRNA-based COVID-19 vaccines are generally mild and consist of injection site reactions, headache, and asthenia [7].

According to the COVID-19 vaccination program of the Italian Ministry of Health, patients diagnosed with multiple sclerosis (MS) are considered to be one of the highest priority categories, being recognized as extremely vulnerable people. For this reason, mRNA-based COVID-19 vaccines are strongly recommended for these patients [8]. MS is an inflammatory-mediated demyelinating disease of the Central Nervous System caused by an immune dysregulation associated with genetic and environmental factors, including Epstein–Barr virus infection and cigarette smoking [9,10]. Worldwide, almost 2.5 million people are diagnosed with MS, mainly women aged 20–40 years [11]. Despite encouraging results on the efficacy and safety profile of mRNA-based COVID-19 vaccines, to date, in frail populations, including patients diagnosed with MS, this information is rather limited [12]. In addition, as both vaccines received conditional marketing authorization, the companies that market them must continue to provide results from the main clinical trials, which are still ongoing. These results, together with those provided by any other clinical study, will provide new data on the vaccine's long-term safety and benefit in the general population, including frail patients.

Based on these considerations, we carried out a retrospective observational study with the aim to evaluate the safety profile of COVID-19 vaccines by retrieving real-life data of MS patients who were treated and vaccinated at the Multiple Sclerosis Center of the Hospital A.O.R.N. A. Cardarelli. Specifically, we aimed to evaluate the safety profile of mRNA-based COVID-19 vaccines in MS patients, in terms of any AEFI occurring in the short- and long-term after each dose of these vaccines; identify any possible correlations between AEFIs and MS patients' demographic characteristics, clinical status, and their disease modifying therapies (DMTs); identify cases of relapses following mRNA-based COVID-19 vaccines and compare relapses' rate with those of previous years in the same population.

2. Methods

2.1. Study Design

This is a retrospective observational study carried out with data retrieved from medical records of SM patients treated and vaccinated at the MS Centre of the Cardarelli Hospital (Naples, South of Italy) for the period from March 2021 to September 2021 to assess the safety of mRNA-based COVID-19 vaccines in this population.

2.2. Demographic and Clinical Data Collection

The following data were retrieved: demographic data (MS diagnosis, age, gender); mRNA-based COVID-19 vaccine (date of vaccination, type of vaccine, vaccine batch); medical and clinical history, DMTs; all AEFIs that occurred after vaccination, in terms of number, time of occurrence and type (where available); patients' general clinical course.

2.3. AEFIs Data Collection

According to the European and Italian rules on the management of ICSRs [13,14], when an AEFI likely associated with the COVID-19 vaccine was identified from the medical records, the suspected reporting form established by the Italian Medicine Agency (AIFA) was filled in, if not previously performed. Then, the suspected reporting form was sent to the qualified person responsible for pharmacovigilance who recorded the ADR report into the Italian spontaneous reporting database (RNF).

We carried out a descriptive analysis of all identified AEFIs in terms of time of occurrence and Preferred term (PT), with a focus on MS relapses. Regarding the time of occurrence, AEFIs were classified as short-term when they occurred within 72 h the first and second dose of the vaccine and as long-term when they occurred within 20 days the first and second dose of the vaccine.

2.4. Statistical Analysis

Categorial variables were described as frequency and percentage, while continuous variables were reported by their median and mean. For the evaluation of the relapse rate following the vaccine, we retrieved historical data of previous years (from March to September during years 2017–2020) referred to the same population. This comparison was made in order to detect any differences with previous years' relapses considering the effects deriving both from the social distancing measures adopted across Italian territory and the immunization with the mRNA-based COVID-19 vaccine. We used a multivariable model (multiple logistic regression) to check for a difference of total AEFIs that occurred both after the first and the second doses, adjusted for age, sex, disease duration, Expanded Disability Status Scale (EDSS) and DMTs. Beta coefficients were calculated in order to compare the strength of the effect of each individual independent variable to the dependent variable. The EDSS is a method of quantifying disability in MS patients and monitoring changes in the level of disability over time.

2.5. Ethics

According to the Italian law, the retrospective study was notified to the Ethic Committee of A.O.R.N. A. Cardarelli/Santobono-Pausilipon. No written informed consent was necessary for the study conduction based on its retrospective nature.

3. Results

We retrieved 310 MS patients (63% female; mean age: 45.9 years) who received the first dose of the mRNA-based COVID-19 vaccine. Of these patients, 288 also received the second dose. All patients received the Pfizer-BioNTech vaccine. Relapsing-Remitting Multiple Sclerosis (RRSM) was the most common form of MS, which was identified in almost 87% of patients (n = 270), while almost 10% of patients were diagnosed with Secondary Progressive Multiple Sclerosis (SPSM) and 2.6% with Primary Progressive Multiple Sclerosis (PPSM). EDSS values were <3.0 in 70% of patients, equal to 3.5–5.5 in 22% of patients and ≥6.0 in 7% of patients. Approximately 10% of patients had a previous COVID-19 infection before the enrolment in our study (Table 1). The majority of retrieved patients (93.9%) were receiving a DMT during the study period. In particular, those prescribed in more than 10% of patients were interferon beta 1-a (19.7%), dimethyl fumarate (15.2%), and natalizumab (15.2%) and fingolimod (11.3%).

Table 1. Clinical and demographic variables of patients with multiple sclerosis who received COVID-19 vaccination.

Study Cohort	First Vaccine Dose	Second Vaccine Dose
Total patients	310	288
Gender, n (%)		
Female	195 (62.9)	179 (62.2)
Male	115 (37.1)	109 (37.8)
Mean age (years)	45.9	45.8
Disease duration, years (mean)	11.8	11.6
Median (years)	10.1	10.0
MS type, n (%)		
RRMS	270 (87.1)	251 (87.1)
SPMS	32 (10.3)	29 (10.1)
PPMS	8 (2.6)	8 (2.8)
Disability by EDSS, n (%)		
≤3.0	219 (70.6)	209 (72.6)
3.5–5.5	69 (22.3)	59 (20.5)
≥6.0	22 (7.1)	20 (6.9)
SARS-CoV-2 infection before vaccination, n (%)	34 (10.7)	19 (6.6)
DMTs, n (%)		
Interferon Beta 1-a	61 (19.7)	55 (19.2)
Glatiramer acetate	20 (6.5)	19 (6.7)
Teriflunomide	28 (9.0)	26 (9.0)
Dimethyl fumarate	47 (15.2)	45 (15.6)
Fingolimod	35 (11.3)	35 (12.1)
Natalizumab	47 (15.2)	43 (14.9)
Cladribine	17 (5.5)	12 (4.2)
Ocrelizumab	23 (7.4)	22 (7.7)
Interferon Beta 1-b	7 (2.3)	7 (2.4)
Azathioprine	1 (0.3)	1 (0.3)
Methotrexate	3 (0.9)	3 (1.0)
Rituximab	2 (0.6)	2 (0.7)
Untreated	19 (6.1)	18 (6.2)

RRMS: Relapsing Remitting Multiple Sclerosis; SPMS: Secondary Progressive Multiple Sclerosis; PPMS: Primary Progressive Multiple Sclerosis; EDSS: Expanded Disability Status Scale; DMTs: Disease Modifying Therapies.

Overall, 913 AEFIs were identified during the study period, of which 539 were after the first dose of the vaccine and 374 after the second dose. The majority of these AEFIs were classified as short-term since they occurred within the first 72 h (86.5% short-term vs. 13.5% long-term). This trend was confirmed after the first and second doses (Table 2).

Table 2. Distribution of Adverse Events Following Immunization (AEFIs) by time of occurrence (short- and long-term) and vaccine's dose.

	Total	First Vaccine Dose	Second Vaccine Dose
Study population	310	310	288
All AEFIs, n	913	539	374
Short-term AEFIs, n (%)	790 (86.5)	438 (81.3)	352 (94.1)
Long-term AEFIs, n (%)	123 (13.5)	101 (18.7)	22 (5.9)

The most common reported PTs were pain at injection site (n = 426; 46.7%), flu-like symptoms (n = 165; 18.1%), and headache (n = 123; 13.5%). No substantial differences were found in terms of PTs distribution by first and second dose (Figure 1). Fever was reported more frequently after the second dose than after the first dose. SARS-CoV-2 infection occurred in 3 patients after the first dose.

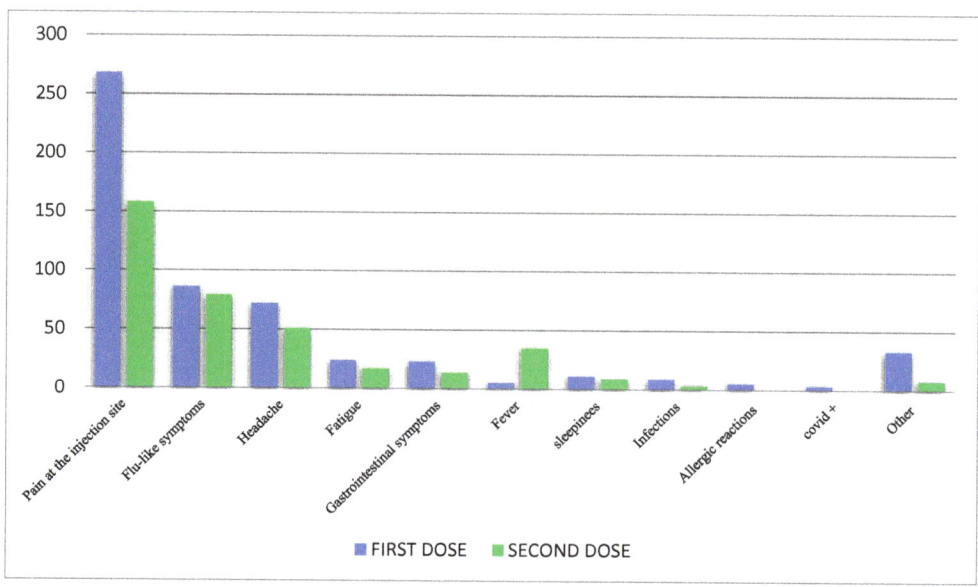

Figure 1. Distribution of Adverse Events Following Immunization (AEFIs) by Preferred Term (PT).

Regarding the relapse rate, a transient increase in MS symptoms following vaccination (pseudo-relapse) was reported in 6 patients out of 310 (1.9%), of which 2 were after the first dose (0.6% of vaccinated patients) and 4 after the second dose (1.4% of vaccinated patients). During the study period (March 2021–September 2021), relapses were identified in 5 patients, of which 3 were after first dose of the vaccine (0.9% of patients) and 2 after the second dose (0.7% of patients).

Using historical data from previous years (2017–2020), the relapse rates were found to be 6.1%, 6.1%, 7.4%, and 6.4%, respectively (Figure 2).

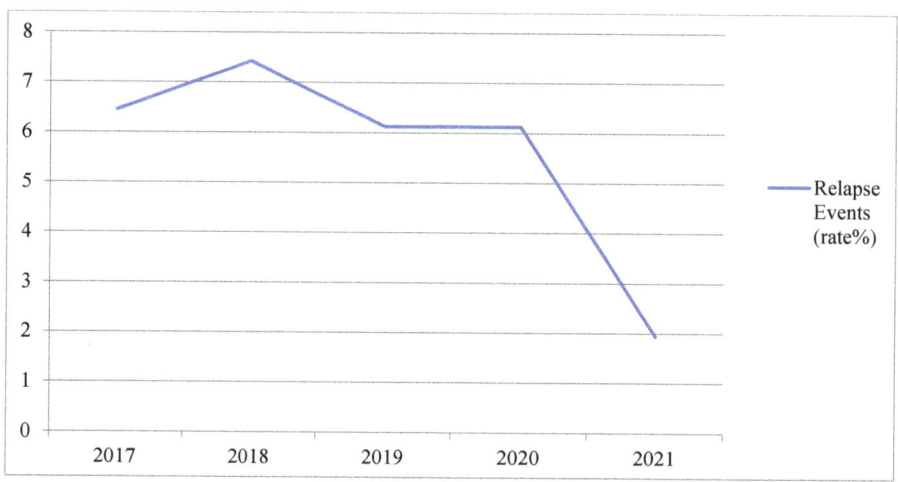

Figure 2. Trend of Relapses (%) during years 2017–2021 (periods considered: March–September).

Lastly, the results of the multivariable analysis that assessed factors associated with the occurrence of AEFIs revealed a statistical significance for age, sex, and therapy with ocrelizumab ($p < 0.05$) (Table 3), suggesting that AEFIs were less common in young patients (negative β coefficient = −0.02, $p = 0.03$), while they were more common in female patients (positive β coefficient = 0.361, $p = 0.03$) and in patients who were receiving ocrelizumab (positive β coefficient = 0.477, $p = 0.022$).

Table 3. Multivariable analysis assessing factors associated with Adverse Events Following Immunization (AEFIs).

Variable	Multivariable Analysis	
	Beta Coefficients (SE)	p Value
EDSS	−0.08 (0.08)	0.30
Disease duration	0.02 (0.01)	0.10
Age	−0.02 (0.01)	0.03
Sex (female vs. male)	0.361 (0.09)	<0.001
DMTs		
No therapy	Ref	Ref
Interferon Beta 1-a	0.263 (0.185)	0.156
Interferon Beta 1-b	−0.361 (0.367)	0.326
Glatiramer Acetate	0.071 (0.228)	0.756
Teriflunomide	0.118 (0.213)	0.579
Dimethyl fumarate	0.094 (0.193)	0.626
Natalizumab	0.068 (0.197)	0.730
Fingolimod	0.099 (0.202)	0.625
Ocrelizumab	0.477 (0.208)	0.022
Cladribine	0.101 (0.236)	0.669
Other treatment	−0.171 (0.357)	0.631

EDSS: Expanded Disability Status Scale; DMT: Disease Modifying Therapies; SE: Standard Error.

4. Discussion

We carried out a study with the aim to evaluate the safety profile of mRNA-based vaccine against COVID-19 in patients diagnosed with MS. Similar to any other medicine, vaccines can be associated with the occurrence of adverse events. An AEFI is defined as *"any untoward medical occurrence which follows immunization and which does not necessarily have a causal relationship with the usage of the vaccine"* [15]. AEFIs also include those events associated with vaccination, patient anxiety-related responses, and product quality defect [16–18]. Currently, AEFIs associated with mRNA COVID-19 vaccines in real-life settings are consistent with those already mentioned in the summary of product characteristics of these vaccines. For both vaccines, the most reported AEFIs are injection site pain, fever, asthenia, and muscle aches. Headache, paresthesia, dizziness, drowsiness, taste disturbances, nausea, and abdominal pain have also been observed with both vaccines. These AEFIs are generally not serious and resolve spontaneously. In line with our results, fever is reported more frequently after the second dose. Events occur mostly on the same day as vaccination or the day after [19].

We reported the results related to 310 MS patients who received the first dose of the Pfizer-BioNTech mRNA-based vaccine and 288 who received the second dose of the same vaccine. In our study, the mean age of patients was 45.9 years, and almost 63% were female. RRSM was the most common form of MS, while the most commonly prescribed DMTs were interferon, dimethyl fumarate, natalizumab, and fingolimod. These demographic characteristics were expected. Indeed, as we previously reported [20,21], MS shows the highest prevalence in the age group 35–64 years and with a well-known female predominance (the prevalence ratio of MS of women to men is 2.3–3.5:1) [22,23]. With regard to the most commonly prescribed DMTs, in our opinion the distribution in drugs' utilization could be related to the variegate population included in our study mainly in terms of age and MS type.

Other international research groups carried out clinical studies with the aim to evaluate the safety profile of COVID-19 vaccines in MS patients. For instance, Lotan I et al. carried out a survey among 425 MS patients with questions related to their general demographic and disease-related characteristics and the safety profile of COVID-19 vaccines. Out of the 425 patients, 262 completed the questionnaire, of which 239 had received the Pfizer-BioNTech vaccine. Almost 56% of patients (n = 136) experienced AEFIs, while 15% of them (n = 36) reported new or worsening neurological symptoms following the vaccination (mainly sensory disturbances). In line with our results, AEFIs commonly occurred within the first 24 h after vaccination and resolved within 3 days [24]. The safety profile of the Pfizer-BioNTech vaccine was evaluated in another observational study that enrolled 555 MS patients who received the first dose of the vaccine (of these, 435 received the second dose). This study was carried out in one clinical Centre in Israel where all patients received the Pfizer-BioNTech vaccine. In line with our findings, the PTs most commonly reported were pain at the injection site, fatigue, and headache, while the rate of patients with relapse was 2.1% and 1.6% following the first and second doses, respectively. The comparison of these rates with those from previous years highlighted no differences, although the short follow-up period could have resulted in lower relapse rates. As in our cohort, also in this study, three cases of COVID-19 infection were identified after the first dose [25].

Compared with previous years, we found a reduced relapse rate among MS patients who had received the vaccine during the study period [6 of 310 in 2021 (1.9%) vs. 19 of 310 in 2020 and 2019 (6.1%) vs. 23 of 310 in 2018 (7.4%) vs. 20 of 310 in 2017 (6.4%)]. In our opinion, this finding could be the result of the social distancing measures imposed by the Italian government to vulnerable patients, such as MS patients, which could have positively affected the risk of infection in general, leading to a reduction in relapses too. Indeed, the role of viral respiratory tract infections in increasing the risk of MS relapses [26–29] is widely recognized, especially considering that following a viral infection the activation of proinflammatory patterns, such as the host's T-cells, proinflammatory cytokines, and tumor necrosis factor (TNF)-α, increases the blood-brain barrier (BBB) permeability, allowing for transmigration of those molecules and promoting central nervous system inflammation [30]. In this respect, Landi et al. carried out a survey among MS patients followed at the MS center of Tor Vergata University hospital in Italy with the aim to explore adherence to social distancing habits. The results revealed that patients demonstrated good adherence to social distancing and use of protection equipment [31]. In addition, even though few cases of MS relapses following COVID-19 vaccines could be found in the literature [32–35], as recently reported by Di Filippo et al. [36], currently the evidence of a possible association between these vaccines and MS activity is still debated. Indeed, although mRNA-based COVID-19 vaccines might elicit a strong T and B cells response leading to the development of autoimmune processes [37,38], since systemic infections, such as COVID-19, can worsen MS, the vaccination can be able to reduce the risk of relapses by dropping the risk of infections [25]. Thus, no confirmed association between the Pfizer/BioNTech vaccine and the short-term risk of clinical reactivation in MS exists [36].

Finally, with regard to the results of the multivariable analysis, we found that AEFIs following the mRNA-based COVID-19 vaccine were less common in young patients, while they were more common in female patients and in patients who were receiving ocrelizumab. Contrary to our findings, Achiron et al. found a mild increase in the rate of AEFIs in younger patients and in those treated with immunomodulatory drugs [25]. With regard to the results of statistical analysis reporting a female predominance, many studies highlighted how differences in immunological, hormonal, and genetic mechanisms could explain disparities between men and women in vaccines' response (both in term of efficacy and safety) [18,39,40], leading to higher rate of AEFIs in female patients [39]. Indeed, compared with men, women typically develop higher antibody responses to vaccines, experiencing more local and systemic adverse reactions [40].

With regard to the association with ocrelizumab, to our knowledge, no other studies have evaluated the safety profile of mRNA vaccines in MS patients receiving this drug.

As we recently reported [41], it is known that some DMTs might induce immunomodulation through lymphocyte depletion, leading to different protective humoral and cellular responses to COVID-19 vaccines. For instance, rituximab, ocrelizumab, and fingolimod have been associated with changes in SARS-CoV-2 IgG antibody production in MS-treated subjects [25,42,43]. In this respect, as reported by Zabalza et al., 2021, less than 20% of MS patients treated with ocrelizumab generate an antibody response when naturally infected by COVID-19 [44]. Further studies evaluating humoral and cellular immune response to COVID-19 vaccines and their safety profiles among MS patients undergoing different DMTs are strongly needed.

5. Strengths and Limitations

Our study has several limitations, including its retrospective and monocentric nature and small sample size. Thus, our findings regarding the safety profile of the Pfizer-BioNTech vaccine in MS patients should be considered exploratory since we can't exclude the lack of important clinical data which might have led to different conclusions.

Nevertheless, to our knowledge, this is the first Italian study carried out in a real-life context among MS patients with the aim to evaluate the safety profile of mRNA-based COVID-19 vaccines. Even though the study was carried out in a single clinical center, it covers a population of approximately 800 MS patients. In addition, data collection and analysis have been performed by a multidisciplinary team of neurologists, pharmacologists, statisticians, and data managers. Lastly, using historical data from 2017 to 2020, we were able to make a comparison in term of relapses' rate and to provide possible explanations underlying the lower relapses' rate that we found during the period March–September 2021.

6. Conclusions

In conclusion, our results indicated that the Pfizer-BioNTech vaccine was safe for MS patients, being associated with AEFIs already detected in the general population. In addition, during the study period a reduced rate of MS relapse was found, which in our opinion could be related to the preventing measures introduced by the Italian government. The results of statistical analysis suggested that AEFIs might be more common in young and female MS patients and in those treated with ocrelizumab. While a higher rate of vaccine-induced AEFIs in young and female patients can be expected, no data are currently available regarding the association with ocrelizumab treatment. Larger observational studies with longer follow-up and epidemiological studies are strongly needed in order to collect more data on the safety profile of COVID-19 vaccines in the frail population [45–47].

Author Contributions: Conceptualization, G.T.M., C.S., V.A. and A.C.; Methodology, A.M., M.L.A., O.M. and D.D.G.C.; Software, D.D.G.C. and A.R.Z.; Validation, M.M. (Massimo Majolo), V.A. and A.C.; Formal analysis, A.M., O.M., D.D.G.C., A.R.Z. and M.M. (Marida Massa); Investigation, O.M.; Resources, G.G. and A.C.; Data curation, G.T.M., C.S., A.M., V.M., E.P., S.C., A.B., A.R.Z., A.F., M.M. (Marida Massa), M.M. (Massimo Majolo), E.R., R.S., G.R. and G.L.; Writing—original draft, G.T.M., C.S., V.A. and A.C.; Writing—review & editing, G.T.M., C.S., E.R., R.S., G.R., G.L., V.A. and A.C.; Visualization, V.M., E.P., G.G., M.L.A., S.C., A.B., A.F., M.M. (Marida Massa), M.M. (Massimo Majolo), E.R., R.S., G.R. and G.L. All authors have read and agreed to the published version of the manuscript.

Funding: The authors received no financial support for the research, authorship, and/or publication of this article.

Institutional Review Board Statement: The study was conducted according to the guidelines of the Declaration of Helsinki, and approved by the Ethics Committee of A. Cardarelli/Santobono-Pausilipon (with Resolution n. 2/2022).

Informed Consent Statement: This was a retrospective study, thus the informed consent was not obtained from patients.

Data Availability Statement: The data presented in this study are available on request from the corresponding author. The data are not publicly available due to privacy and ethical reasons.

Conflicts of Interest: The authors declare no conflict of interest. G.T.M. received personal compensation from Serono, Biogen, Novartis, Roche, and TEVA for public speaking and advisory boards. C.S., A.M., V.M., E.P., G.G., M.L.A., S.C., A.B., O.M., D.D.G.C., A.R.Z., A.F., M.M. (Marida Massa), M.M. (Massimo Majolo), E.R., R.S., G.R., G.L., V.A. and A.C. have no disclosures.

References

1. Scavone, C.; Brusco, S.; Bertini, M.; Sportiello, L.; Rafaniello, C.; Zoccoli, A.; Berrino, L.; Racagni, G.; Rossi, F.; Capuano, A. Current pharmacological treatments for COVID-19: What's next? *Br. J. Pharmacol.* **2020**, *177*, 4813–4824. [CrossRef] [PubMed]
2. Di Mauro, G.; Scavone, C.; Rafaniello, C.; Rossi, F.; Capuano, A. SARS-Cov-2 infection: Response of human immune system and possible implications for the rapid test and treatment. *Int. Immunopharmacol.* **2020**, *84*, 106519. [CrossRef] [PubMed]
3. Capuano, A.; Scavone, C.; Racagni, G.; Scaglione, F.; Italian Society of Pharmacology. NSAIDs in patients with viral infections, including COVID-19: Victims or perpetrators? *Pharmacol. Res.* **2020**, *157*, 104849. [CrossRef] [PubMed]
4. Scavone, C.; Mascolo, A.; Rafaniello, C.; Sportiello, L.; Trama, U.; Zoccoli, A.; Bernardi, F.F.; Racagni, G.; Berrino, L.; Castaldo, G.; et al. Therapeutic strategies to fight COVID-19: Which is the status artis? *Br. J. Pharmacol.* **2021**, *179*, 2128–2148. [CrossRef]
5. European Medicine Agency. Comirnaty (COVID-19 mRNA Vaccine [Nucleoside Modified]). An Overview of Comirnaty and Why It Is Authorised in the EU. Available online: https://www.ema.europa.eu/en/documents/overview/comirnaty-epar-medicine-overview_en.pdf (accessed on 16 September 2021).
6. European Medicine Agency. Spikevax1 (COVID-19 mRNA Vaccine [Nucleoside Modified]). An Overview of Spikevax and Why It Is Authorised in the EU. Available online: https://www.ema.europa.eu/en/documents/overview/spikevax-previously-covid-19-vaccine-moderna-epar-medicine-overview_en.pdf (accessed on 16 September 2021).
7. CDC. Possible Side Effects after Getting a COVID-19 Vaccine. Available online: https://www.cdc.gov/coronavirus/2019-ncov/vaccines/expect/after.html (accessed on 15 June 2021).
8. Raccomandazioni Aggiornate sul COVID-19 per le Persone con Sclerosi Multipla (SM)—12 Gennaio 2021 SIN ed AISM 12 Gennaio 2021 Ministero della Salute: Raccomandazioni ad Interim sui Gruppi Target della Vaccinazione Anti-SARS-CoV-2/COVID-19 8 Febbraio 2021. Available online: https://www.aism.it/sites/default/files/Raccomandazioni_COVID_SM_AISM_SIN.pdf (accessed on 16 November 2022).
9. Auricchio, F.; Scavone, C.; Cimmaruta, D.; Di Mauro, G.; Capuano, A.; Sportiello, L.; Rafaniello, C. Drugs approved for the treatment of multiple sclerosis: Review of their safety profile. *Expert Opin. Drug Saf.* **2017**, *16*, 1359–1371. [CrossRef]
10. Faissner, S.; Gold, R. Efficacy and Safety of the Newer Multiple Sclerosis Drugs Approved Since 2010. *CNS Drugs* **2018**, *32*, 269–287. [CrossRef]
11. Tullman, M.J. Overview of the epidemiology, diagnosis, and disease progression associated with multiple sclerosis. *Am. J. Manag. Care* **2013**, *19* (Suppl. S2), S15–S20.
12. Chilimuri, S.; Mantri, N.; Gongati, S.; Zahid, M.; Sun, H. COVID-19 vaccine failure in a patient with multiple sclerosis on ocrelizumab. *Vaccines* **2021**, *9*, 219. [CrossRef]
13. Mazzitello, C.; Esposito, S.; De Francesco, A.E.; Capuano, A.; Russo, E.; De Sarro, G. Pharmacovigilance in Italy: An overview. *J. Pharmacol. Pharmacother.* **2013**, *4* (Suppl. S1), S20–S28. [CrossRef]
14. ICH E2D Post-Approval Safety Data Management|European Medicines Agency. Available online: https://www.ema.europa.eu/en/documents/scientific-guideline/international-conference-harmonisation-technical-requirements-registration-pharmaceuticals-human-use_en-12.pdf (accessed on 16 September 2021).
15. World Health Organization. Adverse Events Following Immunization (AEFI). Available online: https://www.who.int/teams/regulation-prequalification/regulation-and-safety/pharmacovigilance/health-professionals-info/aefi (accessed on 15 September 2021).
16. WHO. *Casuality Assessment of an Adverse Event Following Immunizaiton (AEFI)*; WHO: Geneva, Switzerland, 2013; pp. 1–56.
17. Scavone, C.; Di Mauro, C.; Brusco, S.; Bertini, M.; di Mauro, G.; Rafaniello, C.; Sportiello, L.; Rossi, F.; Capuano, A. Surveillance of adverse events following immunization related to human papillomavirus vaccines: 12 years of vaccinovigilance in Southern Italy. *Expert Opin. Drug Saf.* **2019**, *18*, 427–433. [CrossRef]
18. Scavone, C.; Rafaniello, C.; Brusco, S.; Bertini, M.; Menditto, E.; Orlando, V.; Trama, U.; Sportiello, L.; Rossi, F.; Capuano, A. Did the New Italian Law on Mandatory Vaccines Affect Adverse Event Following Immunization's Reporting? A Pharmacovigilance Study in Southern Italy. *Front. Pharmacol.* **2018**, *9*, 1003. [CrossRef]
19. Agenzia Italiana del Farmaco. FAQ Vaccini a mRNA. Available online: https://www.aifa.gov.it/domande-e-risposte-su-vaccini-mrna (accessed on 21 December 2021).
20. Ziello, A.; Scavone, C.; Di Battista, M.E.; Salvatore, S.; Di Giulio Cesare, D.; Moreggia, O.; Allegorico, L.; Sagnelli, A.; Barbato, S.; Manzo, V.; et al. Influenza Vaccine Hesitancy in Patients with Multiple Sclerosis: A Monocentric Observational Study. *Brain Sci.* **2021**, *11*, 890. [CrossRef] [PubMed]
21. Maniscalco, G.T.; Brescia Morra, V.; Florio, C.; Lus, G.; Tedeschi, G.; Cianfrani, M.; Docimo, R.; Miniello, S.; Romano, F.; Sinisi, L.; et al. Preliminary Results of the FASM Study, an On-Going Italian Active Pharmacovigilance Project. *Pharmaceuticals* **2020**, *13*, 466. [CrossRef]

22. Koutsouraki, E.; Costa, V.; Baloyannis, S.J.; Koutsouraki, E. Epidemiology of multiple sclerosis in Europe: A Review. *Int. Rev. Psychiatry* **2010**, *22*, 2–13. [CrossRef]
23. Harbo, H.F.; Gold, R.; Tintoré, M. Sex and gender issues in multiple sclerosis. *Ther. Adv. Neurol. Disord.* **2013**, *6*, 237–248. [CrossRef] [PubMed]
24. Lotan, I.; Wilf-Yarkoni, A.; Friedman, Y.; Stiebel-Kalish, H.; Steiner, I.; Hellmann, M.A. Safety of the BNT162b2 COVID-19 vaccine in multiple sclerosis (MS): Early experience from a tertiary MS center in Israel. *Eur. J. Neurol.* **2021**, *28*, 3742–3748. [CrossRef] [PubMed]
25. Achiron, A.; Dolev, M.; Menascu, S.; Zohar, D.N.; Dreyer-Alster, S.; Miron, S.; Shirbint, E.; Magalashvili, D.; Flechter, S.; Givon, U.; et al. COVID-19 vaccination in patients with multiple sclerosis: What we have learnt by February 2021. *Mult. Scler.* **2021**, *27*, 864–870. [CrossRef] [PubMed]
26. Sibley, W.; Bamford, C.; Clark, K. Clinical viral infections and multiple sclerosis. *Lancet* **1985**, *325*, 1313–1315. [CrossRef]
27. Andersen, O.; Lygner, P.E.; Bergström, T.; Andersson, M.; Vablne, A. Viral infections trigger multiple sclerosis relapses: A prospective seroepidemiological study. *J. Neurol.* **1993**, *240*, 417–422. [CrossRef]
28. Tremlett, H.; Van Der Mei, I.A.; Pittas, F.; Blizzard, L.; Paley, G.; Mesaros, D.; Woodbaker, R.; Nunez, M.; Dwyer, T.; Taylor, B.V.; et al. Monthly ambient sunlight, infections and relapse rates in multiple sclerosis. *Neuroepidemiology* **2008**, *31*, 271–279. [CrossRef]
29. Correale, J.; Fiol, M.; Gilmore, W. The risk of relapses in multiple sclerosis during systemic infections. *Neurology* **2006**, *67*, 652–659. [CrossRef] [PubMed]
30. Marrodan, M.; Alessandro, L.; Farez, M.F.; Correale, J. The role of infections in multiple sclerosis. *Mult. Scler. J.* **2019**, *25*, 891–901. [CrossRef] [PubMed]
31. Landi, D.; Ponzano, M.; Nicoletti, C.G.; Cecchi, G.; Cola, G.; Mataluni, G.; Mercuri, N.B.; Sormani, M.P.; Marfia, G.A. Adherence to social distancing and use of personal protective equipment and the risk of SARS-CoV-2 infection in a cohort of patients with multiple sclerosis. *Mult. Scler. Relat. Disord.* **2020**, *45*, 102359. [CrossRef] [PubMed]
32. Maniscalco, G.T.; Manzo, V.; Di Battista, M.E.; Salvatore, S.; Moreggia, O.; Scavone, C.; Capuano, A. Severe Multiple Sclerosis Relapse After COVID-19 Vaccination: A Case Report. *Front. Neurol.* **2021**, *12*, 721502. [CrossRef]
33. Etemadifar, M.; Sigari, A.A.; Sedaghat, N.; Salari, M.; Nouri, H. Acute relapse and poor immunization following COVID-19 vaccination in a rituximab-treated multiple sclerosis patient. *Hum. Vaccin. Immunother.* **2021**, *20*, 1–3. [CrossRef]
34. Voysey, M.; Clemens, S.A.C.; Madhi, S.A.; Weckx, L.Y.; Folegatti, P.M.; Aley, P.K.; Angus, B.; Baillie, V.L.; Barnabas, S.L.; Bhorat, Q.E.; et al. Safety and efficacy of the ChAdOx1 nCoV-19 vaccine (AZD1222) against SARS-CoV-2: An interim analysis of four randomised controlled trials in Brazil, South Africa, and the UK. *Lancet* **2021**, *397*, 99–111. [CrossRef]
35. Nistri, R.; Barbuti, E.; Rinaldi, V.; Tufano, L.; Pozzilli, V.; Ianniello, A.; Marinelli, F.; De Luca, G.; Prosperini, L.; Tomassini, V.; et al. Case Report: Multiple Sclerosis Relapses After Vaccination Against SARS-CoV2: A Series of Clinical Cases. *Front. Neurol.* **2021**, *12*, 765954. [CrossRef]
36. Di Filippo, M.; Cordioli, C.; Malucchi, S.; Annovazzi, P.; Cavalla, P.; Clerici, V.T.; Ragonese, P.; Nociti, V.; Radaelli, M.; Laroni, A.; et al. mRNA COVID-19 vaccines do not increase the short-term risk of clinical relapses in multiple sclerosis. *J. Neurol. Neurosurg. Psychiatry* **2021**, *93*, 448–450. [CrossRef]
37. Sahin, U.; Muik, A.; Derhovanessian, E.; Vogler, I.; Kranz, L.M.; Vormehr, M.; Baum, A.; Pascal, K.; Quandt, J.; Maurus, D.; et al. COVID-19 vaccine BNT162b1 elicits human antibody and TH1 T cell responses. *Nature* **2020**, *586*, 594–599. [CrossRef]
38. Petersone, L.; Edner, N.M.; Ovcinnikovs, V.; Heuts, F.; Ross, E.M.; Ntavli, E.; Wang, C.J.; Walker, L.C.K. T Cell/B Cell Collaboration and Autoimmunity: An Intimate Relationship. *Front. Immunol.* **2018**, *9*, 1941. [CrossRef]
39. Harris, T.; Nair, J.; Fediurek, J.; Deeks, S.L. Assessment of sex-specific differences in adverse events following immunization reporting in Ontario, 2012–2015. *Vaccine* **2017**, *35*, 2600–2604. [CrossRef] [PubMed]
40. Fischinger, S.; Boudreau, C.M.; Butler, A.L.; Streeck, H.; Alter, G. Sex differences in vaccine-induced humoral immunity. *Semin. Immunopathol.* **2019**, *41*, 239–249. [CrossRef] [PubMed]
41. Maniscalco, G.T.; Manzo, V.; Ferrara, A.L.; Perrella, A.; Di Battista, M.; Salvatore, S.; Graziano, D.; Viola, A.; Amato, G.; Moreggia, O.; et al. Interferon Beta-1a treatment promotes SARS-CoV-2 mRNA vaccine response in multiple sclerosis subjects. *Mult. Scler. Relat. Disord.* **2021**, *58*, 103455. [CrossRef] [PubMed]
42. Sormani, M.P.; De Rossi, N.; Schiavetti, I.; Carmisciano, L.; Cordioli, C.; Moiola, L.; Radaelli, M.; Immovilli, P.; Capobianco, M.; Trojano, M.; et al. Disease-modifying therapies and coronavirus disease 2019 severity in multiple sclerosis. *Ann. Neurol.* **2021**, *89*, 780–789. [CrossRef]
43. Sormani, M.P.; Inglese, M.; Schiavetti, I.; Carmisciano, L.; Laroni, A.; Lapucci, C.; Da Rin, G.; Serrati, C.; Gandoglia, I.; Tassinari, T.; et al. Effect of SARS-CoV-2 mRNA vaccination in MS patients treated with disease modifying therapies. *EBioMedicine* **2021**, *72*, 103581. [CrossRef] [PubMed]
44. Zabalza, A.; Cárdenas-Robledo, S.; Tagliani, P.; Arrambide, G.; Otero-Romero, S.; Carbonell-Mirabent, P.; Rodriguez-Barranco, M.; Rodríguez-Acevedo, B.; Restrepo Vera, J.L.; Resina-Salles, M.; et al. COVID-19 in multiple sclerosis patients: Susceptibility, severity risk factors and serological response. *Eur. J. Neurol.* **2021**, *28*, 3384–3395. [CrossRef]
45. Moccia, M.; Erro, R.; Picillo, M.; Vassallo, E.; Vitale, C.; Longo, K.; Amboni, M.; Santangelo, G.; Palladino, R.; Nardone, A.; et al. Quitting smoking: An early non-motor feature of Parkinson's disease? *Parkinsonism Relat. Disord.* **2015**, *21*, 216–220. [CrossRef] [PubMed]

46. Singh, C.; Naik, B.; Pandey, S.; Biswas, B.; Pati, B.; Verma, M.; Singh, P. Effectiveness of COVID-19 vaccine in preventing infection and disease severity: A case-control study from an Eastern State of India. *Epidemiol. Infect.* **2021**, *149*, e224. [CrossRef]
47. Kampf, G. The epidemiological relevance of the COVID-19-vaccinated population is increasing. *Lancet Reg. Health Eur.* **2021**, *11*, 100272. [CrossRef]

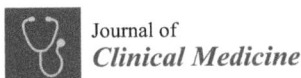

Article

Medication Adherence in Medicare-Enrolled Older Adults with Chronic Obstructive Pulmonary Disease before and during the COVID-19 Pandemic

Ligang Liu [1], Armando Silva Almodóvar [1] and Milap C. Nahata [1,2,*]

[1] Institute of Therapeutic Innovations and Outcomes (ITIO), College of Pharmacy, The Ohio State University, Columbus, OH 43210, USA
[2] College of Medicine, The Ohio State University, Columbus, OH 43210, USA
* Correspondence: nahata.1@osu.edu; Tel.: +1-614-292-2472

Abstract: Medication adherence to controller inhalers was unknown in older Medicare patients with chronic obstructive pulmonary disease (COPD) before and during the pandemic. This study evaluated changes in medication adherence to controller medications and factors associated with high adherence. This retrospective cohort study included older Medicare patients with COPD. The proportion of days covered (PDC) reflected changes in medication adherence from January to July in 2019 and in 2020. Paired *t*-test evaluated changes in adherence. Logistic regression determined the association of patient characteristics with high adherence (PDC $\geq$ 80%). Mean adherence decreased ($p < 0.001$) for long-acting beta-agonists, long-acting muscarinic antagonists, and inhaled corticosteroids in 2020. The percentage of patients with high adherence dropped from 74.4% to 58.1% ($p < 0.001$). The number of controllers, having $\geq$3 albuterol fills, and a 90-day supply were associated with high adherence in 2019 and 2020 ($p < 0.001$). The COVID-19 pandemic may negatively impact medication adherence. Patients with evidence of more severe diseases and a 90-day supply were more likely to adhere to therapy. Healthcare professionals should prioritize prescribing 90-day supplies of medications and monitor drug-related problems as components of pharmacovigilance to enhance adherence to therapies and the desired clinical outcomes among patients with COPD.

Keywords: COPD; Medicare; medication adherence; COVID-19 pandemic; geriatric

1. Introduction

Chronic obstructive pulmonary disease (COPD) and other chronic lower respiratory diseases were the sixth leading causes of death in 2020 [1]. These illnesses affected over 250 million people around the world, causing substantial burdens on healthcare systems [2]. Common comorbidities of COPD have included skeletal muscle dysfunction, cardiovascular disease, mental health disorders, and lung cancer [3–6].

Pharmacological therapies for patients with COPD include short-acting beta agonist(s) (SABA), short-acting muscarinic antagonist(s) (SAMA), long-acting muscarinic antagonist(s) (LAMA), long-acting β2-agonist(s) (LABA), and inhaled corticosteroid(s) (ICS) [7]. Adherence to guideline-directed medical therapy (GDMT) for COPD may improve clinical outcomes and reduce all-cause and respiratory-specific emergency department visits and hospitalizations [8,9].

Patient-specific factors, including mental health diagnoses (particularly depression), lower health literacy, medication-related problems, and lower sociodemographic status, have been associated with decreased medication adherence, increased readmission rates for acute COPD exacerbations, and poorer health outcomes [10,11]. Older adults are vulnerable to medication-related problems, and services such as comprehensive medication reviews need to be provided to improve adherence [12].

The COVID-19 pandemic limited access to healthcare for COPD patients [13]. Kahnert et al. found a deterioration of clinical status in the COPD population during the pandemic [14]. The GOLD Science Committee also emphasized that the COVID-19 pandemic had made COPD management challenges and urged actions to improve care for patients with COPD during the pandemic [15].

Conflicting data exist on medication adherence among patients with COPD. Several studies found increased medication adherence in older patients with asthma and/or COPD after the beginning of the pandemic [16,17]. However, Barrett et al. reported decreased prescription claims in COPD and asthma patients compared to the pre-pandemic time [18]. Zhang et al. observed similar adherence during the pandemic compared to the pre-pandemic period in the general COPD population [19]. Importantly, there are no data on medication adherence in Medicare-enrolled older adults with COPD alone from the COVID pandemic period.

The objectives of this study were to (1) examine medication adherence in older adults with COPD, (2) determine the impact of the COVID-19 pandemic on medication prescribing patterns and medication adherence in this population, and (3) evaluate the associations of specific sociodemographic and patient characteristics with medication adherence in older adults in the presence of the COVID-19 pandemic.

2. Materials and Methods

2.1. Study Design

This was a retrospective longitudinal cohort study of older Medicare patients with COPD. Eligible patients were individuals enrolled in medication therapy management (MTM) services, were diagnosed with COPD, and had at least two prescription claims for the same controller medication in 2019. Patients with cystic fibrosis or asthma or <65 years of age were excluded from this study. Medications included in this study were SABA, LABAs, LAMAs, and ICSs. Biologic medications were not included given they are largely covered under Medicare Part B; the MTM program did not have access to these data. The institutional review board at the Ohio State University approved this study (22 September 2020; study ID: 2020H0393).

2.2. Data Sources

Data were obtained from the MTM provider with permission from the insurance plan. These included the patient's age, sex, zip code, international classification of disease, tenth revision (ICD-10) codes, number of medications, number of prescribers, number of pharmacies, prescription claims data, medication-related problems identified by electronic review of prescription claims, and proportion of days covered (PDC) for inhalers for this study.

Medication refill histories based on pharmacy claim data were used to measure patient adherence to maintenance inhalers at a fixed time from 1 January to 31 July 2019, and 1 January to 31 July 2020. The proportion of days covered (PDC) was used to calculate a patient's adherence. The calculation for PDC equaled the number of covered days with a targeted medication divided by the number of days in a period. The tracking period started with the patient's first fill during the observation period. If a PDC could not be calculated, it was assumed that the patient had a PDC of 0%. Patients with a PDC below 80% were considered non-adherent, and greater or equal to 80% were considered highly adherent. Supplemental Table S1 shows a detailed list of medications assessed in this study.

2.3. Statistical Analysis

Microsoft Excel (Version 2209 Build 16.0.15629.20152) and IBM SPSS (version 28) were used to organize and analyze data. Nominal data were described by counts and percentages. Continuous data were presented by means and standard deviations (SDs). Age, prescribers, pharmacies, inhalers, and corticosteroids were transformed into ordinary variables.

Paired *t*-tests were used to assess differences in adherence to the same medication between 2019 and 2020. The percentage of patients adherent to medications in each period was reported and compared using McNemar's test.

Exploratory logistic regression was used to identify potential predictors of medication adherence in 2019 and 2020 separately. Variables used in this regression included age, sex, number of prescriptions, number of rescue inhalers, number of medication-related problems, the diagnosis of depression, number of pharmacies, number of prescribers, number of oral corticosteroids, and having a 90-day medication supply. The analysis in the regression for 2020 included a variable that reflected whether the patients were adherent to the inhalers in 2019. Bonferroni corrections were used to provide a conservative p value that would establish significance.

3. Results

A total of 1533 patients were included in this study. The mean patients' age was 76.14 ± 6.74 years, with 59% being female. They had 6.24 ± 3.38 prescribers, were prescribed 13.71 ± 4.70 medications, and went to 2.48 ± 1.46 pharmacies to fill their prescriptions in 2019. In this cohort, 32.2% of patients received oral corticosteroids, and 16.9% had depression. 77.9% of the patients needed more than one controller medication for COPD. Detailed information can be found in Table 1.

Table 1. Descriptive data and results from logistic regression evaluating the association between patient characteristics and adherence to controller inhalers in 2019 (N = 1533).

Characteristic	Overall Cohort	With High Adherence	With Nonadherence	p Value	B Value	Adjusted Odds Ratio (95% confidence interval)
	N = 1533	N = 1141	N = 392			
	N (%)	N (%)	N (%)			
Age, year				0.36		
65–74 (reference)	644 (42.0)	484 (42.4)	160 (40.8)			
75–84	656 (42.8)	496 (43.5)	160 (40.8)	0.81	0.03	1.04 (0.78–1.37)
≥85	233 (15.2)	161 (14.1)	72 (18.4)	0.23	−0.23	0.80 (0.55–1.15)
Sex						
Male (reference)	629 (41.0)	466 (40.8)	163 (41.6)			
Female	904 (59.0)	675 (59.2)	229 (58.4)	0.51	−0.09	0.509 (0.71–1.19)
Number of medications				0.31		
8–10 (reference)	456 (29.7)	315 (27.6)	141 (36.0)			
11–13	400 (26.1)	293 (25.7)	107 (27.3)	0.82	0.04	1.04 (0.75–1.44)
14–16	299 (19.5)	228 (20.0)	71 (18.1)	0.51	0.13	1.14 (0.78–1.65)
17–19	200 (13.0)	159 (13.9)	41 (10.5)	0.08	0.39	1.48 (0.95–2.31)
≥20	178 (11.6)	146 (12.8)	32 (8.2)	0.11	0.42	1.52 (0.91–2.53)
Number of medication-related problems				0.007		
0	179 (11.7)	144 (12.6)	35 (8.9)	0.01	−0.64	1.90 (1.16–3.10)
1	288 (18.8)	232 (20.3)	56 (14.3)	<0.001	−0.52	2.10 (1.38–3.18)
2	294 (19.2)	216 (18.9)	78 (19.9)	0.11	−0.49	1.37 (0.93–2.03)
3	220 (14.4)	161 (14.1)	59 (15.1)	0.47	−0.32	1.17 (0.77–1.77)
4	176 (11.5)	122 (10.7)	54 (13.8)	0.57	0.10	1.13 (0.74–1.75)
≥5 (reference)	376 (24.5)	266 (23.3)	110 (28.1)			
Number of prescribers				0.66		
1–5 (reference)	743 (48.5)	536 (47.0)	207 (52.8)			
6–10	635 (41.4)	479 (42.0)	156 (39.8)	0.55	0.09	1.089 (0.82–1.44)

Table 1. Cont.

Characteristic	Overall Cohort	With High Adherence	With Nonadherence	p Value	B Value	Adjusted Odds Ratio
11–15	131 (8.5)	106 (9.3)	25 (6.4)	0.29	0.29	1.329 (0.78–2.26)
≥16	24 (1.6)	20 (1.8)	4 (1.0)	0.44	0.47	1.592 (0.49–5.21)
Number of pharmacies				0.92		
1 (reference)	450 (29.4)	336 (29.4)	114 (29.1)			
2	449 (29.3)	336 (29.4)	113 (28.8)	0.95	−0.01	0.99 (0.71–1.37)
3	322 (21.0)	244 (21.4)	78 (19.9)	0.63	0.09	1.10 (0.76–1.58)
≥4	312 (20.4)	225 (19.7)	87 (22.2)	0.82	−0.04	0.96 (0.66–1.39)
Depression						
Yes	259 (16.9)	197 (17.3)	62 (15.8)	0.41	0.15	
No (reference)	1274 (83.1)	944 (82.7)	330 (84.2)			
Number of controlled medication classes				0.001		
1 (reference)	339 (22.1)	228 (20.0)	111 (28.3)			
2	598 (39.0)	380 (33.3)	218 (55.6)	0.15	−0.22	0.81 (0.60–1.09)
3	480 (31.3)	423 (37.1)	57 (14.5)	<0.001	1.06	2.89 (1.99–4.21)
≥4	116 (7.6)	110 (9.6)	6 (1.5)	<0.001	1.86	6.44 (2.68–15.46)
Number of oral corticosteroid fills				0.53		
0 (reference)	1040 (67.8)	767 (67.2)	273 (69.6)			
1	264 (17.2)	194 (17.0)	71 (18.1)	0.35	−0.16	0.85 (0.61–1.20)
2	98 (6.4)	72 (6.3)	26 (6.6)	0.35	−0.25	0.78 (0.46–1.31)
≥3	131 (8.5)	108 (9.5)	22 (5.6)	0.54	0.17	1.18 (0.69–2.03)
Number of albuterol inhalers						
≤2 (reference)	647 (42.2)	414 (36.3)	233 (59.4)			
≥3	886 (57.8)	727 (63.7)	159 (40.6)	<0.001	0.81	2.25 (1.74–2.91)
90-day supply of inhalers						
No (reference)	1088 (71.0)	759 (66.5)	329 (83.9)			
Yes	445 (29.0)	382 (33.5)	63 (16.1)	<0.001	0.95	2.57 (1.88–3.53)

Note. Bonferroni-adjusted p value = 0.0045.

About two-thirds of patients were highly adherent to their inhalers (LAMA [69.0%], LABA [66.8%], and ICS [65.9%]) in 2019. In the first several months of the pandemic, the average adherence rate to LABA [50.1%] and ICS [48.5%] decreased, and LAMA [69.1%] adherence did not change (Figure 1). Mean PDC for controller inhalers decreased significantly in 2020 compared with 2019 (LABA, 83.52 ± 20.09 vs. 58.36 ± 40.82; LAMA, 84.25 ± 19.88 vs. 59.76 ± 41.91; ICS 82.99 ± 20.47 vs. 56.60 ± 41.15 (all p values < 0.001) (Figure 2). The proportion of patients with an ICS-LABA, and a LABA-LAMA combination inhaler decreased; however, the proportion of patients having an ICS-LABA-LAMA combination inhaler decreased (Figure 3).

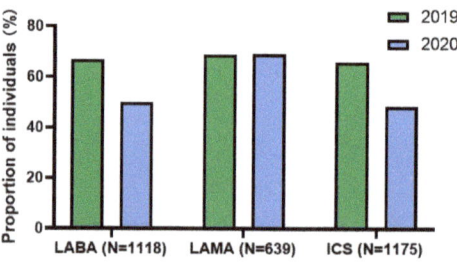

Figure 1. Proportion of individuals with high adherence to their controllers. Abbreviations: LABA, long-acting β2-agonists; LAMA, long-acting muscarinic antagonists; ICS, inhaled corticosteroid.

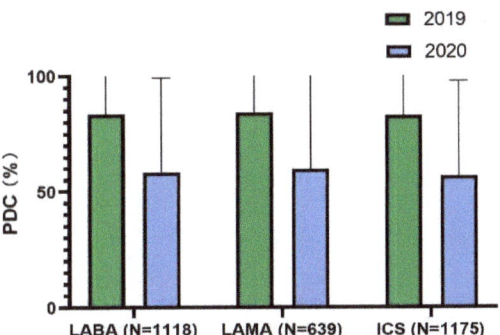

Figure 2. Mean proportion of days covered for controller inhalers. Abbreviations: LABA, long-acting β2-agonists; LAMA, long-acting muscarinic antagonists; ICS, inhaled corticosteroid.

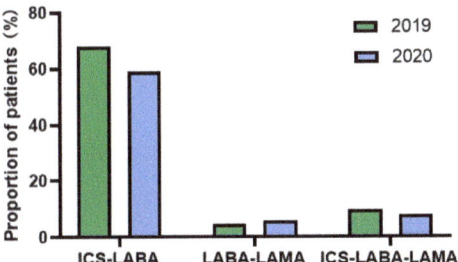

Figure 3. Proportion of patients with at least 1 combination inhaler. Abbreviations: LABA, long-acting β2-agonists; LAMA, long-acting muscarinic antagonists; ICS, inhaled corticosteroid.

The percentage of patients adhering to their treatment dropped from 74.4% in 2019 to 58.1% in 2020, with $p < 0.001$. The percentage of patients who received ICS and LABA decreased from 68% to 59%. However, the number of patients who used the combination of ICS, LABA, and LAMA increased from 71 to 91. The number of patients receiving oral corticosteroids decreased from 493 (32.2%) in 2019 to 414 (25.7%) in 2020.

In the regression model of 2019, the full model containing all predictors was statistically significant, X^2 (27, N = 1533) = 240.19, $p < 0.001$. The model as a whole explained between 14.5% (Cox and Snell R square) and 21.4% (Nagelkerke R squared) of the variance in sleep status, and correctly classified 77.3% of cases; variables that were associated with high adherence for controller inhalers were the number of maintenance inhalers ($p < 0.001$), having ≥3 albuterol inhalers (odds ratio [OR], 2.25; 95% confidence interval [CI], 1.74–2.91; $p < 0.001$), and a 90-day supply of controller medications (OR, 2.57; 95% CI, 1.88–3.53; $p < 0.001$). Patients with ≥3 controller medication classes had 2.89 to 6.44 times the odds of being adherent to COPD controller medications compared with patients with 1 controller ($p < 0.001$). A complete list of nonsignificant variables appears in Table 1.

In 2020, the full model containing all predictors was statistically significant, X^2 (28, N = 1533) = 182.45, $p < 0.001$. The model as a whole explained between 14.3% (Cox and Snell R square) and 21.3% (Nagelkerke R squared) of the variance in sleep status, and correctly classified 77.5% of cases. Variables related to high adherence to inhalers included the number of controller classes ($p < 0.001$), having ≥3 albuterol medication (OR, 2.44; 95% CI, 1.73–3.46; $p < 0.001$), a 90-day supply of controllers (OR, 3.06; 95% CI, 2.34–4.00; $p < 0.001$), and being adherent to controller medications in 2019 (OR, 2.24; 95% CI, 1.63–3.08; $p < 0.001$). A complete list of nonsignificant variables is provided in Table 2.

Table 2. Results from logistic regression evaluating the association between patient characteristics and adherence to controller medications in 2020 (N = 1533).

Characteristic	Overall Cohort	With High Adherence	With Non-Adherence	p Value	B Value	Adjusted Odds Ratio (95% confidence interval)
	N = 1533	N = 891 (58.1)	N = 642 (42.9)			
	N (%)	N (%)	N (%)			
Age, year				0.88		
65–74 (reference)	644 (42.0)	371 (41.6)	273 (42.5)			
75–84	656 (42.8)	401 (45.0)	255 (39.7)	0.77	0.05	1.05 (0.76–1.45)
≥85	233 (15.2)	119 (13.4)	114 (17.8)	0.79	−0.1	0.94 (0.61–1.46)
Sex						
Male (reference)	629 (41.0)	367 (41.2)	262 (40.8)			
Female	904 (59.0)	524 (58.8)	380 (59.2)	0.25	0.18	1.19 (0.88–1.62)
Number of medications				0.47		
8–10 (reference)	456 (29.7)	250 (28.1)	206 (32.1)			
11–13	400 (26.1)	235 (26.4)	165 (25.7)	0.56	0.12	1.12 (0.76–1.66)
14–16	299 (19.5)	181 (20.3)	118 (18.4)	0.83	−0.05	0.95 (0.62–1.47)
17–19	200 (13.0)	113 (12.7)	87 (13.6)	0.20	−0.32	0.72 (0.44–1.18)
≥20	178 (11.6)	112 (12.6)	66 (10.3)	0.62	0.14	1.15 (0.66–2.01)
Number of medication-related problems				0.03		
0	179 (11.7)	117 (13.1)	62 (9.7)	0.50	−0.20	1.22 (0.68–2.21)
1	288 (18.8)	181 (20.3)	107 (16.7)	0.35	0.21	0.80 (0.50–1.28)
2	294 (19.2)	154 (17.3)	140 (21.8)	0.08	−0.52	0.66 (0.41–1.05)
3	220 (14.4)	123 (13.8)	97 (15.1)	0.19	−0.62	0.73 (0.45–1.18)
4	176 (11.5)	104 (11.7)	72 (11.2)	0.14	−0.42	1.51 (0.87–2.63)
≥5 (reference)	376 (24.5)	212 (23.8)	164 (25.5)			
Number of prescribers				0.13		
1–5 (reference)	874 (57.0)	475 (53.3)	399 (62.1)			
6–10	544 (35.5)	335 (37.6)	209 (32.6)	0.80	−0.04	0.96 (0.70–1.32)
11–15	98 (6.4)	72 (8.1)	26 (4.0)	0.61	0.17	1.18 (0.63–2.22)
≥16	17 (1.1)	9 (1.0)	8 (1.2)	0.02	−1.35	0.26 (0.08–0.83)
Number of pharmacies				0.08		
1 (reference)	450 (29.4)	254 (28.5)	196 (30.5)			
2	449 (29.3)	271 (30.4)	178 (27.7)	0.05	0.38	1.46 (1.00–2.14)
3	322 (21.0)	180 (20.2)	142 (22.1)	0.87	0.03	1.03 (0.69–1.55)

Table 2. Cont.

Characteristic	Overall Cohort	With High Adherence	With Non-Adherence	p Value	B Value	Adjusted Odds Ratio
≥4	312 (20.4)	186 (20.9)	126 (19.6)	0.05	0.44	1.56 (1.01–2.41)
Depression						
Yes	259 (16.9)	152 (17.1)	107 (16.7)	0.38	0.19	1.21 (0.79–1.85)
No (reference)	1274 (83.1)	739 (82.9)	535 (83.3)			
Number of controlled medication classes				<0.001		
0–1 (reference)	595 (38.8)	175 (19.6)	420 (65.4)			
2	432 (28.2)	272 (30.5)	160 (24.9)	0.18	−0.25	0.78 (0.54–1.12)
3	397 (25.9)	340 (38.2)	57 (8.9)	<0.001	0.82	2.28 (1.50–3.47)
≥4	109 (7.1)	104 (11.7)	5 (0.8)	<0.001	1.88	6.55 (2.47–17.35)
Number of oral corticosteroids fills				0.57		
0 (reference)	1139 (74.3)	641 (71.9)	498 (77.6)			
1	187 (12.2)	115 (12.9)	72 (11.2)	0.21	−0.29	0.75 (0.48–1.18)
2	85 (5.5)	55 (6.2)	30 (4.7)	0.60	0.20	1.22 (0.59–2.51)
≥3	122 (8.0)	80 (9.0)	42 (6.5)	0.91	−0.03	0.97 (0.56–1.68)
Number of albuterol inhalers						
<3 (reference)	729 (47.6)	324 (36.4)	405 (63.1)			
≥3	804 (52.4)	567 (63.6)	237 (36.9)	0.01	0.39	1.48 (1.09–1.99)
90-day supply of inhalers						
No (reference)	1025 (66.9)	509 (57.1)	516 (80.4)			
Yes	508 (33.1)	382 (42.9)	126 (19.6)	<0.001	0.89	2.44 (1.73–3.46)
High adherence to any inhalers in 2019						
No (reference)	392 (25.6)	155 (17.4)	237 (36.9)			
Yes	1141 (74.4)	736 (82.6)	405 (63.1)	<0.001	0.81	2.24 (1.63–3.08)

Note. Bonferroni-adjusted p value = 0.0042.

4. Discussion

This was the first study to measure medication adherence and its changes during the COVID-19 pandemic compared to a pre-pandemic period using data from Medicare-enrolled, MTM-eligible older patients with COPD. We found a remarkable reduction in medication adherence to controller inhalers for COPD in the first several months of 2020. Significant indicators of adherence were patients receiving a 90-day supply of controller inhalers, ≥3 rescue inhalers, and the number of maintenance inhalers. Our findings suggested that access to medications and healthcare may have been disturbed in the pandemic's first few months given the observed decreases in medication claims.

Our data demonstrated that the percentage of patients adhering to maintenance controllers was suboptimal in 2019 and 2020. The proportion of patients who had high adherence, as measured by PDC, ranged from 65.9% to 69.0% in 2019 and 48.5% to 69.1% in 2020. Nishi et al. also used the PDC to measure the adherence to LABAs, LAMAs, and ICSs in Medicare-enrolled older patients with COPD from 2008 to 2013, and found that mean adherence to maintenance medication was about 55% [20]. Moreover, another study discovered that 69.8% of existing diagnosed and 84.4% of new COPD patients were non-adherent to maintenance therapy, which was defined as PDC < 80%, using Medicare real-world data from 2007 to 2014 [21]. In general, adherence to maintenance medication was still suboptimal in Medicare-enrolled MTM-eligible older adults with COPD before and during the COVID-19 pandemic. It is important to recognize barriers to adherence, and additional measures must be taken to improve medication adherence, especially during an event such as a pandemic.

This study importantly discovered that patients with a 90-day supply were more likely to be considered adherent. During the pandemic, access to medications may have been impeded in older people with chronic conditions [22]. Ismail et al. observed that about 20% of patients with chronic diseases had trouble obtaining medications during the pandemic [23]. It was assumed that patients who made regular visits to pharmacies to obtain refills were also at an increased risk of exposure to infections [24]. Vordenberg et al. reported that over one-half of older adults continued to go to the pharmacy for medicines despite the risk of infection [25]. A 90-day supply of medications would reduce the frequency of visits to the pharmacy and the risk of exposure to the virus. Several studies have reported that patients with a 90-day supply were more adherent to medications compared to patients with a non-90-day supply [26,27]. The Department of Health and Human Services also advocated for a 90-day supply of medications during the pandemic [28]. Therefore, a 90-day supply of medications should be prioritized to optimize the therapy during the pandemic in patients with chronic diseases, including COPD.

It is observed in this cohort that patients with a higher number of controller medications were more likely to be adherent to their medications. This finding supported the health belief model of behavior that patients' knowledge and perceptions of the disease and treatment were associated with good adherence [29]. Notably, patients adhering to medications in 2019 were more likely to adhere to medications in 2020, suggesting that evidence of previous medication adherence was an important predictor for adherence in the future [30].

It was found that 57.8% of patients in 2019 and 52.4% in 2020 had ≥3 rescue fills, possibly due to the patients being less active during the pandemic. This number may indicate the overutilization of rescue inhalers to control symptoms related to COPD, with implications of increased disease severity and high COPD burden [31,32]. Overuse of SABA may cause bronchodilator tolerance and decrease the response to rescue beta-agonist treatments [33]. Our study also discovered that oral corticosteroid fill claims decreased during the first few months of 2020. It is also reported that the number of patients with a moderate or severe exacerbation of COPD decreased during the pandemic [34], which may be explained by the use of face masks and other social distancing policies during the pandemic [35].

Older adults are more likely to experience medication-related problems due to polypharmacy and decreased liver and kidney functions [36], contributing to up to 30% of hospitalizations in the geriatric population [37]. In our study, we found patients with fewer medication-related problems were more likely to have high adherence, even though the association was weak. All patients included in this study were provided with MTM services, as a component of pharmacovigilance efforts made by pharmacists to identify and minimize medication nonadherence and maximize medication safety by detecting, assessing, and resolving drug-related problems to achieve desired clinical outcomes [38].

5. Limitations

This study only included Medicare-enrolled–MTM-eligible patients from one insurance company. Therefore, it may not represent the entire Medicare population. Further, this study only examined prescription claims in the first seven months of 2020 and did not capture the medication adherence changes during the entire pandemic period. Future research needs to be conducted to observe adherence trends amid the pandemic. Lastly, the status of the COVID-19 infection was not recorded in the system, and we were unable to assess the effects of a COVID-19 infection on adherence. The authors were unable to determine if providers discontinued medication therapies and could not assess the influence of cash claims that were not processed by the insurance. The authors were unable to assess historical trends of adherence prior to 2019 in this analysis.

6. Conclusions

The adherence to controller inhalers was suboptimal in Medicare–MTM-eligible older adults with COPD. Our study demonstrated that the COVID-19 pandemic might have had a negative impact on medication adherence during the initial months. Patients with signs of severe disease as evidenced by the receipt of a greater number of albuterol inhalers and more controller inhalers, and a 90-day supply, were more likely to adhere to the inhalers. Healthcare professionals should prioritize prescribing 90-day supplies of medications and monitor medication-related problems as components of pharmacovigilance efforts to achieve high adherence and desired clinical outcomes for the optimal care of COPD patients.

Supplementary Materials: The following supporting information can be downloaded at: https://www.mdpi.com/article/10.3390/jcm11236985/s1, Table S1: Medication included in each medication category.

Author Contributions: Conceptualization, M.C.N. and A.S.A.; methodology, M.C.N. and A.S.A.; software, L.L. and A.S.A.; validation, M.C.N.; formal analysis, L.L. and A.S.A.; data curation, A.S.A.; writing—original draft preparation, L.L.; writing—review and editing, A.S.A. and M.C.N.; supervision, M.C.N.; project administration, M.C.N. All authors have read and agreed to the published version of the manuscript.

Funding: This research received no external funding.

Institutional Review Board Statement: The study was conducted in accordance with the Declaration of Helsinki, and approved by the institutional review board at the Ohio State University (approved 22 September 2020; study ID: 2020H0393).

Informed Consent Statement: Not applicable.

Data Availability Statement: Not applicable.

Conflicts of Interest: The authors declare no conflict of interest.

References

1. Murphy, S.L.; Kochanek, K.D.; Xu, J.; Arias, E. Mortality in the United States, 2020. *NCHS Data Brief.* **2021**, *427*, 1–8.
2. Iheanacho, I.; Zhang, S.; King, D.; Rizzo, M.; Ismaila, A.S. Economic Burden of Chronic Obstructive Pulmonary Disease (COPD): A Systematic Literature Review. *Int. J. Chronic Obstr. Pulm. Dis.* **2020**, *ume 15*, 439–460. [CrossRef]
3. Chen, W.; Thomas, J.; Sadatsafavi, M.; FitzGerald, J.M. Risk of cardiovascular comorbidity in patients with chronic obstructive pulmonary disease: A systematic review and meta-analysis. *Lancet Respir. Med.* **2015**, *3*, 631–639. [CrossRef]
4. Fry, J.S.; Hamling, J.S.; Lee, P.N. Systematic review with meta-analysis of the epidemiological evidence relating FEV1decline to lung cancer risk. *BMC Cancer* **2012**, *12*, 498. [CrossRef] [PubMed]
5. Higham, A.; Mathioudakis, A.; Vestbo, J.; Singh, D. COVID-19 and COPD: A narrative review of the basic science and clinical outcomes. *Eur. Respir. Rev.* **2020**, *29*, 200199. [CrossRef] [PubMed]
6. Kühl, K.; Schürmann, W.; Rief, W. Mental disorders and quality of life in COPD patients and their spouses. *Int. J. Chronic Obstr. Pulm. Dis.* **2008**, *3*, 727–736. [CrossRef]
7. Global Initiative for Chronic Obstructive Lung Disease (GOLD). Global Strategy for the Diagnosis m, and Prevention of Chronic Obstructive Pulmonary Disease. 2022. Available online: https://goldcopd.org/2022-gold-reports-2/ (accessed on 20 July 2022).
8. Humenberger, M.; Horner, A.; Labek, A.; Kaiser, B.; Frechinger, R.; Brock, C.; Lichtenberger, P.; Lamprecht, B. Adherence to inhaled therapy and its impact on chronic obstructive pulmonary disease (COPD). *BMC Pulm. Med.* **2018**, *18*, 163. [CrossRef]
9. Mannino, D.M.; Yu, T.-C.; Zhou, H.; Higuchi, K. Effects of GOLD-Adherent Prescribing on COPD Symptom Burden, Exacerbations, and Health Care Utilization in a Real-World Setting. *Chronic Obstr. Pulm. Dis. J. COPD Found.* **2015**, *2*, 223–235. [CrossRef]
10. Albrecht, J.S.; Park, Y.; Hur, P.; Huang, T.-Y.; Harris, I.; Netzer, G.; Lehmann, S.W.; Langenberg, P.; Khokhar, B.; Wei, Y.-J.; et al. Adherence to Maintenance Medications among Older Adults with Chronic Obstructive Pulmonary Disease. The Role of Depression. *Ann. Am. Thorac. Soc.* **2016**, *13*, 1497–1504. [CrossRef]
11. Soones, T.N.; Lin, J.L.; Wolf, M.S.; O'Conor, R.; Martynenko, M.; Wisnivesky, J.P.; Federman, A.D. Pathways linking health literacy, health beliefs, and cognition to medication adherence in older adults with asthma. *J. Allergy Clin. Immunol.* **2016**, *139*, 804–809. [CrossRef] [PubMed]

12. Chan, D.-C.; Chen, J.-H.; Kuo, H.-K.; We, C.-J.; Lu, I.-S.; Chiu, L.-S.; Wu, S.-C. Drug-related problems (DRPs) identified from geriatric medication safety review clinics. *Arch. Gerontol. Geriatr.* **2012**, *54*, 168–174. [CrossRef]
13. Elbeddini, A.; Tayefehchamani, Y. Amid COVID-19 pandemic: Challenges with access to care for COPD patients. *Res. Soc. Adm. Pharm.* **2020**, *17*, 1934–1937. [CrossRef] [PubMed]
14. Kahnert, K.; Lutter, J.I.; Welte, T.; Alter, P.; Behr, J.; Herth, F.; Kauczor, H.-U.; Söhler, S.; Pfeifer, M.; Watz, H.; et al. Impact of the COVID-19 pandemic on the behaviour and health status of patients with COPD: Results from the German COPD cohort COSYCONET. *ERJ Open Res.* **2021**, *7*, 00242–2021. [CrossRef]
15. Halpin, D.M.G.; Criner, G.J.; Papi, A.; Singh, D.; Anzueto, A.; Martinez, F.J.; Agusti, A.A.; Vogelmeier, C.F. Global Initiative for the Diagnosis, Management, and Prevention of Chronic Obstructive Lung Disease. The 2020 GOLD Science Committee Report on COVID-19 and Chronic Obstructive Pulmonary Disease. *Am. J. Respir. Crit. Care Med.* **2021**, *203*, 24–36. [CrossRef] [PubMed]
16. Kaye, L.; Theye, B.; Smeenk, I.; Gondalia, R.; Barrett, M.A.; Stempel, D.A. Changes in medication adherence among patients with asthma and COPD during the COVID-19 pandemic. *J. Allergy Clin. Immunol. Pr.* **2020**, *8*, 2384–2385. [CrossRef] [PubMed]
17. Yıldız, M.; Aksu, F.; Yıldız, N.; Aksu, K. Clinician's perspective regarding medication adherence in patients with obstructive lung diseases and the impact of COVID-19. *Rev. Assoc. Med. Bras.* **2021**, *67*, 97–101. [CrossRef]
18. Barrett, R.; Barrett, R. Asthma and COPD medicines prescription-claims: A time-series analysis of England's national prescriptions during the COVID-19 pandemic (Jan 2019 to Oct 2020). *Expert Rev. Respir. Med.* **2021**, *15*, 1605–1612. [CrossRef]
19. Zhang, H.-Q.; Lin, J.-Y.; Guo, Y.; Pang, S.; Jiang, R.; Cheng, Q.-J. Medication adherence among patients with chronic obstructive pulmonary disease treated in a primary general hospital during the COVID-19 pandemic. *Ann. Transl. Med.* **2020**, *8*, 1179. [CrossRef]
20. Nishi, S.P.E.; Maslonka, M.; Zhang, W.; Kuo, Y.-F.; Sharma, G. Pattern and Adherence to Maintenance Medication Use in Medicare Beneficiaries with Chronic Obstructive Pulmonary Disease: 2008–2013. *Chronic Obstr. Pulm. Dis. J. COPD Found.* **2018**, *5*, 16–26. [CrossRef]
21. Le, T.T.; Bjarnadóttir, M.; Qato, D.M.; Magder, L.; Zafari, Z.; Simoni-Wastila, L. Prediction of treatment nonadherence among older adults with chronic obstructive pulmonary disease using Medicare real-world data. *J. Manag. Care Spec. Pharm.* **2022**, *28*, 631–644.
22. Bell, J.S.; Reynolds, L.; Freeman, C.; Jackson, J.K. Strategies to promote access to medications during the COVID-19 pandemic. *Aust. J. Gen. Pr.* **2020**, *49*, 530–532. [CrossRef]
23. Ismail, H.; Marshall, V.D.; Patel, M.; Tariq, M.; Mohammad, R.A. The impact of the COVID-19 pandemic on medical conditions and medication adherence in people with chronic diseases. *J. Am. Pharm. Assoc.* **2022**, *62*, 834–839.e1. [CrossRef] [PubMed]
24. Vordenberg, S.E.; Zikmund-Fisher, B.J. Older adults' strategies for obtaining medication refills in hypothetical scenarios in the face of COVID-19 risk. *J. Am. Pharm. Assoc.* **2020**, *60*, 915–922.e4. [CrossRef] [PubMed]
25. Khera, A.; Baum, S.; Gluckman, T.J.; Gulati, M.; Martin, S.S.; Michos, E.D.; Navar, A.M.; Taub, P.R.; Toth, P.P.; Virani, S.S.; et al. Continuity of care and outpatient management for patients with and at high risk for cardiovascular disease during the COVID-19 pandemic: A scientific statement from the American Society for Preventive Cardiology. *Am. J. Prev. Cardiol.* **2020**, *1*, 100009. [CrossRef] [PubMed]
26. Rymer, J.A.; Fonseca, E.; Bhandary, D.D.; Kumar, D.; Khan, N.D.; Wang, T.Y. Difference in Medication Adherence Between Patients Prescribed a 30-Day Versus 90-Day Supply After Acute Myocardial Infarction. *J. Am. Hear. Assoc.* **2021**, *10*, e016215. [CrossRef]
27. Ameli, N.; Jones, W.N. Evaluating Medication Day-Supply for Improving Adherence and Clinical Biomarkers of Hemoglobin A1c, Blood Pressure, and Low-Density Lipoprotein. *J. Pharm. Pract.* **2022**. [CrossRef]
28. Centers for Medicare & Medicaid Services. Information related to coronavirus disease 2019-COVID-19. 22 May 2020. Available online: https://www.cms.gov/files/document/covid-19-updated-guidance-ma-and-part-d-plan-sponsors-52220.pdf (accessed on 6 October 2022).
29. López-Pintor, E.; Grau, J.; González, I.; Bernal-Soriano, M.J.; Quesada, J.; Lumbreras, B. Impact of patients' perception of COPD and treatment on adherence and health-related quality of life in real-world: Study in 53 community pharmacies. *Respir. Med.* **2020**, *176*, 106280. [CrossRef]
30. Kumamaru, H.; Lee, M.P.; Choudhry, N.K.; Dong, Y.-H.; Krumme, A.A.; Khan, N.; Brill, G.; Kohsaka, S.; Miyata, H.; Schneeweiss, S.; et al. Using Previous Medication Adherence to Predict Future Adherence. *J. Manag. Care Spec. Pharm.* **2018**, *24*, 1146–1155. [CrossRef]
31. Fan, V.S.; Gylys-Colwell, I.; Locke, E.; Sumino, K.; Nguyen, H.Q.; Thomas, R.M.; Magzamen, S. Overuse of short-acting beta-agonist bronchodilators in COPD during periods of clinical stability. *Respir. Med.* **2016**, *116*, 100–106. [CrossRef]
32. Gondalia, R.; Bender, B.G.; Theye, B.; Stempel, D.A. Higher short-acting beta-agonist use is associated with greater COPD burden. *Respir. Med.* **2019**, *158*, 110–113. [CrossRef]
33. Haney, S.; Hancox, R.J. Recovery From Bronchoconstriction and Bronchodilator Tolerance. *Clin. Rev. Allergy Immunol.* **2006**, *31*, 181–196. [CrossRef] [PubMed]
34. Sarc, I.; Dolinar, A.L.; Morgan, T.; Sambt, J.; Ziherl, K.; Gavric, D.; Selb, J.; Rozman, A.; Bonca, P.D. Mortality, seasonal variation, and susceptibility to acute exacerbation of COPD in the pandemic year: A nationwide population study. *Ther. Adv. Respir. Dis.* **2022**, *16*. [CrossRef] [PubMed]
35. Faria, N.; Costa, M.I.; Gomes, J.; Sucena, M. Reduction of Severe Exacerbations of COPD during COVID-19 Pandemic in Portugal: A Protective Role of Face Masks? *COPD: J. Chronic Obstr. Pulm. Dis.* **2021**, *18*, 226–230. [CrossRef] [PubMed]

36. Plácido, A.I.; Herdeiro, M.T.; Morgado, M.; Figueiras, A.; Roque, F. Drug-related Problems in Home-dwelling Older Adults: A Systematic Review. *Clin. Ther.* **2020**, *42*, 559–572.e14. [CrossRef]
37. Somers, A.; Petrovic, M. Major drug related problems leading to hospital admission in the elderly. *J. Pharm. Belg.* **2014**, *2*, 34–38.
38. Liu, M.; Liu, J.; Geng, Z.; Bai, S. Evaluation of outcomes of medication therapy management (MTM) services for patients with chronic obstructive pulmonary disease (COPD). *Pak. J. Med Sci.* **2021**, *37*, 1832–1836. [CrossRef]

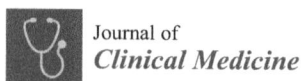

Article

Exposures and Suspected Intoxications to Pharmacological and Non-Pharmacological Agents in Children Aged 0–14 Years: Real-World Data from an Italian Reference Poison Control Centre [†]

Valentina Brilli [1,‡], Giada Crescioli [1,2,‡], Andrea Missanelli [3], Cecilia Lanzi [3], Massimo Trombini [3], Alessandra Ieri [3], Francesco Gambassi [3], Alfredo Vannacci [1,2,*], Guido Mannaioni [1,3,‡] and Niccolò Lombardi [1,2,‡]

[1] Department of Neurosciences, Psychology, Drug Research and Child Health, Section of Pharmacology and Toxicology, University of Florence, 50139 Florence, Italy
[2] Tuscan Regional Centre of Pharmacovigilance, 50122 Florence, Italy
[3] Toxicology Unit, Poison Control Center, Careggi University Hospital, 50134 Florence, Italy
* Correspondence: alfredo.vannacci@unifi.it; Tel.: +39-055-27-58-206
[†] Original Research Article for Special Issue "Medication Safety and Pharmacovigilance in Clinical: From the Researcher Bench to the Patient Bedside".
[‡] These authors contributed equally to this manuscript.

Abstract: This study describes the exposures and suspected intoxications in children (0–14 years) managed by an Italian reference poison control center (PCC). A seven-year observational retrospective study was performed on the medical records of the Toxicology Unit and PCC, Careggi University Hospital, Florence (Italy). During the study period (2015–2021), a total of 27,212 phone call consultations were managed by the PCC, of which 11,996 (44%) involved subjects aged 0–14 years. Most cases occurred in males (54%) aged 1–5 years (73.8%), mainly at home (97.4%), and with an oral route of intoxication (93%). Cases mainly occurred involuntarily. Consultations were generally requested by caregivers; however, in the age group 12–14 years, 70% were requested by healthcare professionals due to voluntary intoxications. Cleaners (19.44%) and household products (10.90%) were the most represented suspected agents. Pharmacological agents accounted for 28.80% of exposures. Covariates associated with a higher risk of emergency department visit or hospitalization were voluntary intoxication (OR 29.18 [11.76–72.38]), inhalation route (OR 1.87 [1.09–3.23]), and pharmacological agents (OR 1.34 [1.23–1.46]), particularly central nervous system medications. Overall, consultations do not burden national and regional healthcare facilities, revealing the activity of PCCs as having a strategic role in reducing public health spending, even during the COVID-19 pandemic.

Keywords: clinical toxicology; intoxication; poison control centre; clinical practice; children; emergency department; hospitalisation

Citation: Brilli, V.; Crescioli, G.; Missanelli, A.; Lanzi, C.; Trombini, M.; Ieri, A.; Gambassi, F.; Vannacci, A.; Mannaioni, G.; Lombardi, N. Exposures and Suspected Intoxications to Pharmacological and Non-Pharmacological Agents in Children Aged 0–14 Years: Real-World Data from an Italian Reference Poison Control Centre. *J. Clin. Med.* **2023**, *12*, 352. https://doi.org/10.3390/jcm12010352

Academic Editor: Ricardo Jorge Dinis-Oliveira

Received: 7 December 2022
Revised: 27 December 2022
Accepted: 29 December 2022
Published: 2 January 2023

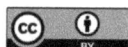

Copyright: © 2023 by the authors. Licensee MDPI, Basel, Switzerland. This article is an open access article distributed under the terms and conditions of the Creative Commons Attribution (CC BY) license (https://creativecommons.org/licenses/by/4.0/).

1. Introduction

Acute pediatric intoxication is a common and preventable cause of morbidity and mortality worldwide. Exposure to toxic substances can occur at all stages of the child's development and in different ways, depending on age, environmental factors, and the characteristics of various toxic substances [1].

A study conducted by the Pediatric Emergency Research Networks Poisoning Working Group, which included children younger than 18 years with acute poisonings presenting to 105 emergency departments (EDs) in 20 countries (8 different global regions), showed that 0.47% of pediatric ED admissions were due to intoxications, occurring at home for the most part (80.6%) and with a bimodal peak age distribution [2]. According to the 38th annual report of the American Association of Poison Control Centers' National Poison Data System, during 2020, more than two million human exposure cases were reported, of which 41.7% involved children ≤5 years [3]. In this age class, the top five most common exposures were cosmetics/personal care products (11.8%), household cleaning substances (11.3%), analgesics (7.57%), foreign bodies/toys/miscellaneous (6.71%), and dietary supplements/herbals/homeopathic (6.44%). Overall, the report showed that medical information requests had shown a 32.6 fold increase, reflecting COVID-19 pandemic calls to poison control centers (PCCs).

Data on large populations are relatively lacking in the literature, particularly in Europe; therefore, it is difficult to estimate the actual incidence of toxic exposure in children. Recently, three retrospective studies on pediatric poisoning were published in Italy. A six-year retrospective study by Berta et al. (2020) showed that 72.9% of cases of pediatric acute intoxication occurred in children <5 years, 85% of intoxications were unintentional, and non-pharmaceutical agents accounted for 59% of cases [4]. A three-year retrospective study by Marano et al. (2021) on Pediatric Poison Control Centre registry data showed that 74.1% of cases involved children aged 1–5 years, 98.2% of intoxications were accidental, and the causative agents were non-pharmaceutical products in 66.7% of cases [5].

In light of this, the aims of this study were to describe the demographics and clinical characteristics of exposures and suspected pediatric (0–14 years) intoxications through the analysis of data collected by an Italian reference PCC and to highlight the role of clinical toxicologists in the early evaluation/management of suspected intoxication in this subset.

2. Materials and Methods

This study was performed on data retrieved during phone call consultations by the Toxicology Unit and PCC of Careggi University Hospital, Florence (Italy), from 1 January 2015 to 31 December 2021. Data concerning exposures and probable or acute intoxications from any causative agent in subjects aged 0–14 years, from private individuals or health professionals, were included in the analysis.

For each phone call counselling (first contact), after obtaining the patient's parents or caregivers' informed consent to participate in the study, trained clinical toxicologists collected the following information: (1) patient's demographic characteristics (age, sex); (2) number and characteristics of suspected toxic agents; (3) the place of intoxication occurrence (home, public closed places, open environment/outdoors); (4) description of the event and its circumstances (accidental/involuntary exposure, voluntary intoxication, secondary effect); (5) intoxication route; and (6) symptomatology.

Toxic agents were categorized as follows: pharmacological agents (classified according to the anatomical therapeutic chemical (ATC) classification system); food toxins; animal poisons; mushrooms; plant poisons; CO and other gases; non-pharmacological agents (pesticides; cosmetics and personal hygiene products; substances of abuse; industrial products; other chemical compounds; household products). Household products were further classified into the following subgroups: detergents; hand-wash detergents; laundry detergents; other cleaners; bleaches; caustics; glues; fertilizers; thermometer liquids; toys; button batteries; silica gel; chlorine vapors; varnishes.

A toxicological evaluation was then performed, in order to calculate the poisoning severity score (PSS) [6] (PSS score 0–NONE: no signs or symptoms related to exposure; PSS score 1–MINOR: mild, transient symptoms with spontaneous resolution; PSS score 2–MODERATE: evident or prolonged symptoms; PSS score 3–SEVERE: severe or life-threatening symptoms; PSS score 4–FATAL: death), and to define the plausibility of the intoxication. Intoxications were defined as "absent" (no intoxication), "doubtful", "possible", and "confirmed". Toxicologists could also judge the patient's symptoms as "independent from the intoxication".

The phone call consultations were grouped according to the age of the patients (<1 years old; 1–5 years old; 6–10 years old; 11–14 years old), and divided in two cohorts, depending on whether the caller was a private individual or a healthcare professional.

The compilation, archiving of electronic folders, and data extrapolation were carried out using the "ARCHICAV" electronic registry version 1.0. Data were described as numbers and percentages and compared using a Chi-squared test. Multivariate logistic regression (crude and adjusted models) was performed to estimate the odds ratios (ORs) of ED visit or hospitalization according to subjects' demographic and clinical characteristics (sex, age, number of toxic agents, circumstances, toxic agents, route of exposure) and the most frequently reported pharmacological drug classes.

Statistical significance was considered with a p-value ≤ 0.05. Statistical analyses were carried out using Stata 17 (StataCorp).

3. Results

During the study period (2015–2021 years), a total of 27,212 phone call consultations were managed by our PCC, of which 11,996 (44.08%) involved subjects aged 0–14 years (Table 1). The majority of exposures and suspected intoxications occurred in males (53.98%) aged 1–5 years (N = 8854). Among all age groups, the most frequently reported route of exposure was the oral route, involving 92.87% of subjects aged 0–11 months, 93.51% of those aged 1–5 years, 87.04% of those aged 6–11 years, and 86.62% of those 12–14 years. The majority of consultations were requested by caregivers; however, in the age group 12–14 years, 70.28% of consultations were requested by healthcare professionals. More than 90% of all exposures and suspected intoxications took place in a domestic environment, through an involuntary means, with a mean time from exposure to consultation that ranged from 2.76 to 6.13 h. Of interest, the majority of voluntary intoxications occurred in the age group 12–14 years (23.14%). Overall, most subjects reported no symptoms at the moment of phone call consultation, followed by those reporting gastrointestinal and neurological symptoms. Among all consultations (N = 11,996), clinical toxicologists advised home observation in 68.58% of case (N = 8228), ED visit in 8.81% (N = 1057), ED observation in 15.04% (N = 1805), and hospitalization in 7.55% (N = 906). A total of 3358 (27.99%) pediatric subjects needed a pharmacological treatment, in particular a symptomatic therapy was prescribed in 22.09% (N = 2651), followed by decontamination in 5.06% (N = 607), and antidotal therapy in 0.83% (N = 100). Notably, none of the exposures and suspected intoxications resulted in the patient's death.

As reported in Table 2, the majority of subjects were exposed to only one suspected toxic agent (N = 11,833, 98.64%). Overall, the exposures and suspected intoxications managed by our PCC regarded non-pharmacological toxic agents in 68.40% (N = 8206) of cases. Among this subset, cleaners (19.44%) and other household products (10.90%), toys (9.26%), cosmetics (8.15%), and plant poisons (7.18%) were the most represented agents involved in the suspected intoxications. On the other hand, pharmacological agents accounted for 28.80% (N = 3785) of the total suspected intoxications, involving analgesics in 3.39% of cases, antibacterials for systemic use in 2.30%, NSAIDs and antirheumatic products in 2.30%, and psycholeptics in 2.02%, and thyroid therapy in 1.63%. Another class of suspected agents with therapeutic potential, i.e., products belonging to complementary and alternative medicine (CAM), accounted for 2.71% (N = 326) of exposures and suspected intoxications.

Table 1. Demographic and clinical characteristics (N = 11,996).

Demographic and Clinical Characteristics	0–11 Months N = 1220 (%)	1–5 Years N = 8854 (%)	6–11 Years N = 1451 (%)	>12 Years N = 471 (%)	p-Value
Sex					
Male	633 (51.89)	4779 (53.98)	855 (58.92)	222 (47.13)	<0.001
Female	587 (48.11)	4075 (46.02)	596 (41.08)	249 (52.87)	
Route of exposure					
Oral	1133 (92.87)	8279 (93.51)	1263 (87.04)	408 (86.62)	
Skin	15 (1.23)	220 (2.48)	64 (4.41)	24 (5.10)	
Ocular	16 (1.31)	215 (2.43)	33 (2.27)	10 (2.12)	<0.001
Inhalation	35 (2.87)	108 (1.22)	77 (5.31)	27 (5.73)	
Other route of exposure	21 (1.72)	32 (0.36)	14 (0.96)	2 (0.42)	
Qualification					
Caregiver	768 (62.95)	5050 (57.04)	745 (51.34)	140 (29.72)	<0.001
Healthcare professional	452 (37.05)	3804 (42.96)	706 (48.66)	331 (70.28)	
Location of exposure					
Home	1189 (97.46)	8656 (97.76)	1343 (92.56)	418 (88.75)	<0.001
Others	31 (2.54)	198 (2.24)	108 (7.44)	53 (11.25)	
Circumstances					
Involuntary intoxication	1220 (100)	8854 (100)	1445 (99.59)	362 (76.86)	
Domestic exposure	980	8333	1198	287	
Therapeutic error	231	511	242	74	
Adverse reactions	9	10	5	1	<0.001
Voluntary intoxications	-	-	6 (0.41)	109 (23.14)	
Suicide attempt	-	-	6	94	
Substance abuse	-	-	-	15	
Time from exposure					
Mean ± SD (hours)	5.75 ± 40.66	2.76 ± 17.68	5.20 ± 19.58	6.13 ± 30.09	0.997
<30 min	621 (50.90)	4388 (49.56)	563 (38.80)	134 (28.45)	
30–60 min	204 (16.72)	1776 (20.06)	247 (17.02)	79 (16.77)	<0.001
60 min–24 h	341 (27.95)	2447 (17.02)	555 (38.25)	232 (49.26)	
≥24 h	54 (4.43)	243 (2.74)	86 (5.93)	26 (5.52)	
Symptoms					
Absent	1067 (87.46)	7494 (84.64)	1054 (72.64)	271 (57.54)	
Gastrointestinal	77 (6.31)	755 (8.53)	190 (13.90)	78 (16.56)	
Neurologic	35 (2.87)	140 (1.58)	72 (4.96)	70 (14.86)	
Cutaneous	12 (0.98)	159 (1.80)	67 (4.62)	24 (5.10)	<0.001
Ocular	6 (0.49)	174 (1.97)	23 (1.59)	9 (1.91)	
Respiratory	10 (0.82)	92 (1.04)	31 (2.14)	13 (2.76)	
Cardiac	4 (0.33)	13 (0.15)	9 (0.62)	5 (1.06)	
Other	9 (0.74)	27 (0.30)	5 (0.34)	1 (0.21)	
Toxicologist advices					
Observation at home	908 (74.43)	6165 (69.63)	967 (66.64)	188 (39.92)	
ED visit for outpatients	89 (7.30)	795 (8.98)	118 (8.13)	55 (11.68)	<0.001
ED observation for inpatients	146 (11.97)	1318 (14.89)	224 (15.44)	117 (24.84)	
Hospitalisation	77 (6.31)	576 (6.51)	142 (9.79)	111 (23.57)	
Prescribed therapies					
No	989 (81.07)	6433 (72.66)	997 (68.71)	219 (46.50)	
Yes	231 (18.93)	2421 (27.34)	454 (31.29)	252 (53.50)	
Symptomatic therapies	190	1933	358	170	<0.001
Decontamination	31	444	69	63	
Antidotal therapies	10	44	27	19	

ED: emergency department; SD: standard deviation.

Table 2. Description of toxic agents according to age classes (N = 11,996).

	0–11 Months N = 1220 (%)	1–5 Years N = 8854 (%)	6–11 Years N = 1451 (%)	>12 Years N = 471 (%)
Number of toxic agents				
One	1211 (99.26)	8754 (98.87)	1434 (98.83)	434 (92.14)
More than one	9 (0.74)	100 (1.13)	17 (1.17)	37 (7.86)
Toxic agents				
Non-pharmacological agents	854 (70.00)	6144 (69.39)	952 (65.61)	256 (54.35)
Cleaners	160	1947	171	55
Other household products	126	951	190	41
Toys	105	844	145	18
Cosmetics	90	817	52	19
Plant poisons	164	589	95	14
Pesticides	120	449	66	8
Foods	32	193	85	23
Caustics	12	219	49	16
Animal poisons	12	80	59	24
Substances of abuse	16	44	9	28
Carbon monoxide or other gasses	17	33	34	12
Pharmacological agents [§]	366 (30.00)	2707 (30.57)	499 (34.39)	213 (45.22)
Analgesics (ATC N02)	63	269	43	32
Antibacterials for systemic use (ATC J01)	30	182	49	15
NSAIDs and antirheumatic products (ATC M01)	8	209	38	22
Psycholeptics (ATC N05)	11	118	51	63
Thyroid therapy (ATC H03)	7	170	16	3
Psychoanaleptics (ATC N06)	9	98	37	24
Drugs for obstructive airway diseases (ATC R03)	13	120	17	0
Sex hormones and modulators of the genital system (ATC G03)	0	116	11	1
Antihistamines for systemic use (ATC R06)	9	81	19	5
Agents acting on the renin–angiotensin system (ATC C09)	5	98	6	7
Antiepileptics (ATC N03)	4	59	29	23
Nasal preparations (ATC R01)	19	66	9	2
Mineral supplements (ATC A12)	27	52	9	0
Cough and cold preparations (ATC R05)	4	61	11	4
Beta blocking agents (ATC C07)	2	57	5	6
Complementary and alternative medicine	36 (2.95)	238 (2.68)	44 (3.03)	8 (1.69)
Dietary supplements	25	144	32	2
Phytotherapy	9	56	7	4
Homeopathy	2	38	5	2

ATC: anatomical, therapeutic, chemical classification system; NSAIDs: non-steroidal anti-inflammatory drugs. The distribution of variables was statistically different among age groups for the number of toxic agents and for toxic agents' description. [§] Only the first 15 most frequently reported pharmacological agents are depicted in the table.

The multivariate logistic regression analysis showed that the risk of ED visit or hospitalization was lower for females (adjusted OR 0.88 [95% CI: 0.81–0.95]), and this increased with age, ranging from 1.27 (1–5 years) to 2.52 (12–14 years) (Table 3). Furthermore, in the adjusted models, the analysis showed that the exposure to more than one suspected agent (OR 3.79 [95% CI: 2.65–5.42]), voluntary intoxication (OR 29.18 [95% CI: 11.76–72.38]), pharmacological agents (OR 1.34 [95% CI: 1.23–1.46]), concomitant exposure to pharmacological and non-pharmacological agents (OR 2.03 [95% CI: 0.20–20.13]), and inhalation as route of exposure (OR 1.87 [95% CI: 1.09–3.23]) were the covariates associated with a higher risk of ED visit or hospitalization.

Table 3. Risk of ED visit or hospitalization according to demographic and clinical characteristics.

	Crude Odds Ratio (95% Confidence Interval)	Adjusted Odds Ratio (95% Confidence Interval)
Sex		
Male	1	1
Female	0.92 (0.86–1.00)	0.88 (0.81–0.95)
Age		
0–11 months	1	1
1–5 years	1.27 (1.11–1.45)	1.27 (1.10–1.45)
6–11 years	1.46 (1.23–1.72)	1.35 (1.14–1.60)
>12 years	4.38 (3.50–5.48)	2.52 (1.97–3.22)
Number of toxic agents		
One	1	1
More than one	5.53 (3.93–7.78)	3.79 (2.65–5.42)
Circumstances		
Involuntary intoxication	1	1
Voluntary intoxications	51.31 (20.94–125.74)	29.18 (11.76–72.38)
Toxic agents		
Non-pharmacological agents	1	1
Pharmacological agents	1.40 (1.29–1.52)	1.34 (1.23–1.46)
Pharmacological and non-pharmacological agents	9.76 (1.09–87.39)	2.03 (0.20–20.13)
Route of exposure		
Other route of exposure	1	1
Oral	0.53 (0.33–0.86)	0.57 (0.35–0.93)
Skin	0.60 (0.35–1.01)	0.68 (0.40–1.16)
Ocular	0.91 (0.54–1.55)	1.07 (0.63–1.84)
Inhalation	1.74 (1.02–2.98)	1.87 (1.09–3.23)

Considering the suspected pharmacological agents (Table 4), the multivariate logistic regression analysis showed that beta blocking agents (OR 10.99 [95% CI: 5.38–22.44]), psycholeptics (OR 4.25 [95% CI: 3.13–5.78]), agents acting on the renin–angiotensin system (OR 4.13 [95% CI: 2.69–6.34]), psychoanaleptics (OR 3.68 [95% CI: 2.60–5.20]), and antiepileptics (OR 2.08 [95% CI: 1.40–3.07]) were the classes associated with a higher risk of ED visit or hospitalization observed in our cohort.

Table 4. Risk of ED visit or hospitalization according to the most frequently reported pharmacological drug classes.

	Crude Odds Ratio (95% Confidence Interval)	Adjusted Odds Ratio (95% Confidence Interval)
Analgesics (ATC N02)	1.07 (0.87–1.33)	1.05 (0.84–1.30)
NSAIDs and antirheumatics (ATC M01)	0.65 (0.49–0.86)	0.65 (0.49–0.86)
Antibacterials for systemic use (ATC J01)	0.41 (0.30–0.55)	0.37 (0.27–0.50)
Psycholeptics (ATC N05)	4.81 (3.56–6.50)	4.25 (3.13–5.78)
Thyroid therapy (ATC H03)	0.62 (0.45–0.86)	0.67 (0.48–0.93)
Psychoanaleptics (ATC N06)	3.88 (2.75–5.47)	3.68 (2.60–5.20)
Drugs for obstructive airway diseases (ATC R03)	0.44 (0.29–0.67)	0.46 (0.30–0.69)
Sex hormones (ATC G03)	0.42 (0.27–0.65)	0.45 (0.29–0.71)
Agents acting on the renin–angiotensin system (ATC C09)	3.85 (2.51–5.89)	4.13 (2.69–6.34)
Antiepileptics (ATC N03)	2.36 (1.61–3.47)	2.08 (1.40–3.07)
Antihistamines for systemic use (ATC R06)	1.92 (1.30–2.82)	1.92 (1.30–2.84)
Nasal preparations (ATC R01)	0.41 (0.24–0.69)	0.42 (0.25–0.71)
Mineral supplements (ATC A12)	0.82 (0.52–1.30)	0.89 (0.56–1.40)
Cough and cold preparations (ATC R05)	0.80 (0.50–1.30)	0.80 (0.49–1.29)
Beta blocking agents (ATC C07)	10.23 (5.02–20.84)	10.99 (5.38–22.44)

ATC: anatomical therapeutic chemical; NSAIDs: non-steroidal anti-inflammatory drugs.

During the seven-year study period, a consistent number of phone call consultations were observed, ranging from approximately 1600 to 1800 each year (Figure 1).

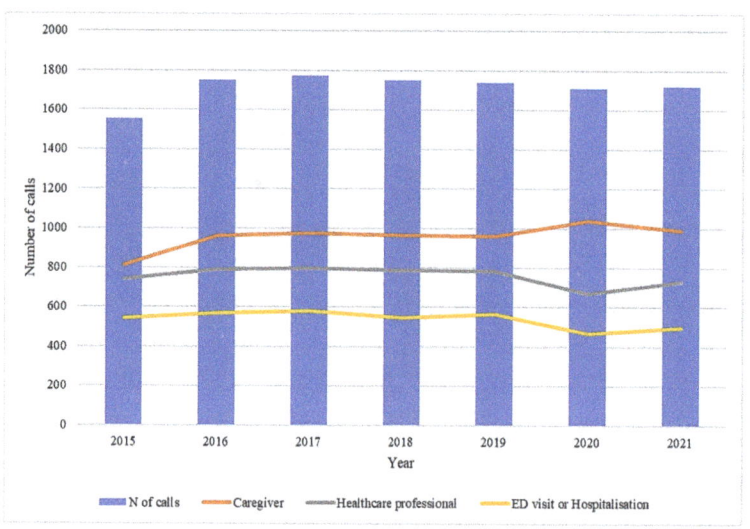

Figure 1. Distribution of calls, qualification and ED visits or hospitalizations during the study period (years 2015–2021).

Considering the pharmacological drug classes involved in the exposures and suspected intoxications in our cohort (Figure 2), a statistically significant risk of an ED visit or hospitalization was observed for the following ATC classes: beta blocking agents (OR 10.23 [95% CI: 5.02–20.84]), psycholeptics (OR 4.81 [95% CI: 3.56–6.50]), psychoanaleptics (OR 3.88 [95% CI: 2.75–5.47]), agents acting on the renin–angiotensin system (OR 3.85 [95% CI: 2.51–5.89]), antiepileptics (OR 2.36 [95% CI: 1.61–3.47]), and antihistamines for systemic use (OR 1.92 [95% CI: 1.30–2.82]).

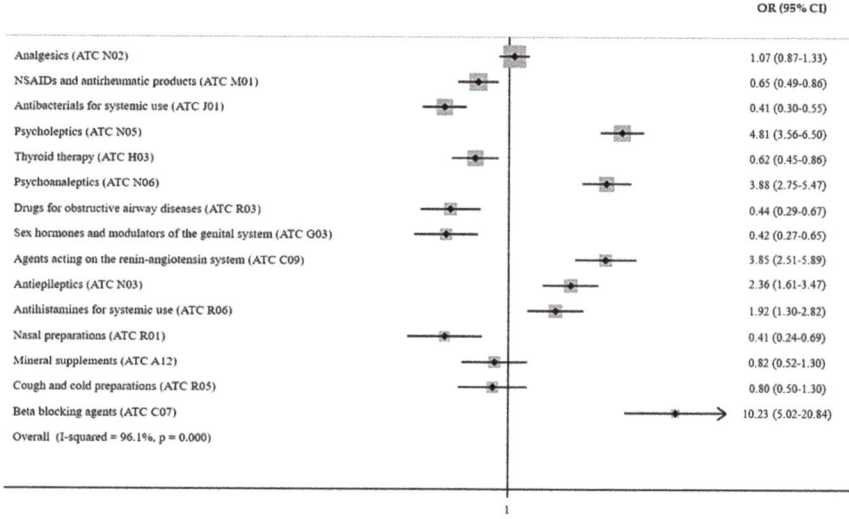

Figure 2. Risk of ED visit or hospitalization according to the most frequently reported pharmacological drug classes.

Although there was no statistically significant difference, exposures and suspected intoxications due to both pharmacological and non-pharmacological agents presented the shortest mean time to clinical toxicology consultation (Table S1). Additionally, caregivers consulted the PCC approximately one hour earlier than healthcare professionals.

Finally, the majority of phone call consultations requested by both caregivers (N = 6703) and healthcare professionals (N = 5293) were due to exposures and suspected intoxications associated with non-pharmacological agents (71.59% and 64.37%, respectively) (Table S2).

4. Discussion

Exposures and suspected intoxications in children are a frequent cause of ED visit and hospitalization worldwide; however, there is a lack of information on this preventable public health issue and on the associated potentially life-threatening clinical conditions, particularly in frail subsets. The present epidemiological analysis from a reference PCC in central Italy gives real-world insight into the main demographic, clinical, and pharmacotoxicological characteristics of intoxications in subjects aged 0–14 before and the during COVID-19 pandemic. To date, this retrospective analysis is the only one conducted in Italy on a representative sample of children over a study period of 7 years. It is relevant that all consultations described here were handled exclusively by clinical toxicology specialists. Furthermore, this study represents the extended epidemiological investigation that followed our preliminary study performed in the general population during the COVID-19 pandemic [7].

In the last two years, particularly in the context of COVID-19 pandemic, several observational studies evaluating the impact of suspected exposures and intoxications in children have been conducted.

Considering that real-world data about acute poisoning in Italian pediatric patients are lacking, different clinical research groups have recently reported new insights on this topic [4,5,8]. The majority of these observational investigations were conducted by pediatricians or other healthcare professionals (i.e., anesthesiologists) working in a pediatric ED, often equipped with a dedicated PCC. On the contrary, our analysis was performed only on the clinical activity of a medical toxicology unit and PCC, where specialists in clinical pharmacology and toxicology probably have the best expertise, in terms of the management of exposures and suspected intoxications in the general population, including children.

In 2020, Berta et al. performed a six-year retrospective evaluation of the Children's Emergency Department database at the Regina Margherita Hospital of Turin (Italy), where 1030 children under age 14 were accepted with a diagnosis of acute intoxication [4]. In their study, similarly to what was observed in our analysis, the majority of patients were male, with events occurring mostly in children aged 1–4 years, while 59% of patients were exposed to non-pharmaceutical agents. Among these, household cleaning products were the more frequently (49%) reported suspected agents. Regarding exposures to pharmaceuticals, the most frequently involved agents were analgesics (20.8%), psychotropics (18.2%), and cardiovascular (12.6%) drugs. Likewise, in our cohort, analgesics represented the main pharmacological class involved in exposures and suspected intoxications in children, thus indicating the need for additional monitoring of the appropriate use of these medications in clinical practice, especially in the domestic environment. Furthermore, Berta et al. found that 85% of intoxications occurred accidentally, 10.6% as therapeutic error, 2.3% as suicide attempts, and 1.5% for recreational purposes. Additionally, in our sample, the majority of cases were associated with an involuntary toxic exposure, underlining the need to both better store potentially dangerous products, which should always be kept out of reach of children, and to monitor them closely at home, especially with those aged 1–5.

Another study, published in 2021, aimed to describe the characteristics of a large pediatric cohort exposed to xenobiotics, through the analysis of a pediatric PCC registry [5]. This study, conducted in the Pediatric Hospital Bambino Gesù of Rome (Italy), a reference national pediatric hospital, collected data of children whose parents or caregivers contacted the pediatric PCC by phone or who presented to the ED, during a 3 year period (2014–2016). The authors collected data of a total of 2686 children, exposed to both pharmaceutical and non-pharmaceutical agents. Correspondingly to what we observed in our analysis, the authors found that pharmaceutical agent exposure increased with age and that the most common route of exposure was oral with gastrointestinal symptoms. Intentional exposure (substance abuse and suicide attempt), was associated with older age and was comparable to our results.

In 2022, Soave et al. identified risk factors associated with pediatric acute poisoning and proposed prevention strategies for children admitted to ED [8]. They performed a retrospective study in a tertiary care hospital, describing data of 436 children admitted for acute poisoning. In this analysis, the age group 1–5 and male sex were the most represented, with a higher frequency of unintentional poisoning and drug ingestion as the leading cause of intoxication.

International differences in the epidemiology of acute poisonings in children may help to improve prevention. In light of this, in 2019, the Pediatric Emergency Research Networks (PERN) Poisoning Working Group sought to evaluate the international epidemiological differences in acute poisonings in children presenting to EDs from different global regions, including eight different Italian pediatric hospitals [2]. Mintegi et al. conducted this international multicenter cross-sectional prospective study, including children younger than 18 years old with acute poisonings, presenting to a total of 105 EDs in 20 countries, and with a mean follow-up of 1 year. During the study period, 363,245 pediatric ED presentations were registered, of which 1727 were for poisoning, with a significant variation in incidence between the regions. Most poisonings (80.6%) occurred at home with either ingestion (89.0%) or inhalation (7.6%) as the route of exposure. Unintentional exposures accounted for 68.5% of poisonings, with pharmaceuticals (42.7%), household products (26.8%), and pesticides (5.1%) being the most common toxic agents. Furthermore, suicide attempts accounted for 13.8% of total exposures, with pharmaceuticals, mainly psychotropics and acetaminophen, being the most common suspected agents.

Overseas, Desai et al. characterized trends in clinically significant toxic exposures and their management, performing a retrospective review of patients 18 years or younger in the American College of Medical Toxicology's Toxicology Investigators Consortium (ToxIC) Registry, a self-reporting database completed by bedside consulting medical toxicologists [9]. From 2010 to 2015, the authors analyzed 11,616 cases reported in their registry. Unlike what has been observed in Europe, exposures were most commonly reported in females (57.8%) and adolescents (59.4%). Moreover, intentional ingestions (55.5%) comprised the majority of cases. The most frequent agents of exposure were analgesics (21.0%), and 0.9% of cases resulted in death.

Of interest, the 38th Annual Report of the American Association of Poison Control Centers' (AAPCC) National Poison Data System (NPDS) [3] reported that children younger than 3 years of age were involved in 30.3% of exposures and children ≤5 years accounted for 41.7% of human exposures in 2020. A prevalence of males was found among cases involving children ≤12 years, but this sex-based distribution was reversed in teenagers and adults. Overall, unintentional exposures outnumbered intentional ones, including children ≤5 years (57.14%). Moreover, the substance categories most frequently involved in pediatric (≤5 years) exposures were cosmetics/personal care products (11.82%), household products (11.30%), analgesics (7.57%), foreign bodies/toys (6.71%), and dietary supplements/herbals/homeopathic products (6.44%). Although children ≤5 years were involved in the majority of exposures, they comprised only 1.27% of fatalities.

From a pharmacological point of view, a result that should not be underestimated regards drugs with action on the central nervous system (CNS). In fact, our study highlighted that most of the ATC classes involved in exposures and suspected intoxications concerned drugs belonging to ATC class N (i.e., analgesics, psycholeptics, psychoanaleptics, and antiepileptics). This is a clinically relevant issue, since several studies have indicated a potential association between parental/caregiver CNS disorders and child mortality [10], particularly an increased risk of child poisoning, burns, and fractures before 5 years of age [11,12]. Our findings, combined with those described by other authors, emphasize the importance of specific interventions for parents/caregivers with CNS disorders. In this context, the clinical pharmacologist and toxicologist operating in a PCC could have a central role in communicating to parents/caregivers with CNS disorders the importance of the proper storage and management of medicines, with the aim of minimizing the risk of intoxication in children.

Considering the COVID-19 pandemic, for the three groups of substances that appear to be associated with COVID-19 cases, human exposure cases had two peaks [3]: one around 31 March to 3 April associated with increased exposures to cleaning/disinfectant agents (primarily bleaches), and one around July 15th, associated with a smaller peak in cleaning/disinfecting agents (primarily bleaches) and in hand sanitizer exposures. This trend was confirmed by a previous publication by our research group, where a higher frequency of suspected intoxications associated with both sanitizers/cleaners and bleaches was observed between the two study periods of January–April 2019 and January–April 2020 [7]. Considering the pediatric subjects analyzed in our study, from 2015 to 2019, the number of calls both from caregivers and healthcare professionals remained quite stable, as well as the ED visits or hospitalizations requested by clinical toxicologists. On the contrary, during the COVID-19 pandemic (first wave) experienced in 2020, an increase of calls from caregivers was observed. Accordingly, the number of calls received by healthcare professionals and the number of ED visits or hospitalizations requested by clinical toxicologists decreased, probably due to the social restrictions imposed by the pandemic emergency.

Limitations and Strengths

The present study has several limitations. First of all, it is necessary to remember that our analysis is a retrospective investigation, and for this reason, data collection might be inaccurate, since some patients' demographic and clinical variables were not always available. Moreover, we do not have a global overview of exposures and suspected intoxications in children, since they only come to healthcare professionals' attention if suspected agents are perceived as dangerous by parents/caregivers. Thus, an underestimation of total exposures and suspected intoxications could not be completely excluded. Additionally, it is difficult to compare the different series, because some papers, both at a national or international level, include patients up to 16 or 18 years of age. Although our data consider exposures and suspected intoxications that mainly occurred in children in central Italy, this study is not representative of Italy as a whole.

The major strength of our study relies on the fact that a large cohort of children aged 0–14 were evaluated over a relatively long follow-up period. In fact, this allowed us to evaluate changing trends in consultations for exposures and suspected intoxications in children before and during the COVID-19 pandemic in Italy. The utilization of a local validated electronic database (ArchiCav), which includes all demographic and clinical information of all the subjects who came into contact with our toxicology unit and PCC, allowed us to perform a detailed and extensive epidemiological analysis. This approach, as already demonstrated in our previously published analysis [7,13–16], could represent a useful source of new scientific insights for clinical toxicologists into the management of phone call consultations in the general population, particularly in children.

5. Conclusions

Despite exposures and suspected intoxications being a relevant problem in children aged 0–14, our results confirmed the clinical characteristics of these potential life threatening occurrences, being comparable with those reported both at the Italian and international level by other colleagues. Furthermore, our results highlighted the need for public health authorities to program preventive interventions, which should involve the daily clinical practice of all healthcare professionals, including general physicians and community pharmacists.

Of course, it is necessary to identify shared national best practices for prevention of acute poisonings in childhood. Understanding which pediatric exposures and suspected intoxications require a clinical toxicologist management, the agents most frequently involved, and the circumstances is paramount for providing education for parents/caregivers and providers.

In the context of a venerable subset, such as the pediatric population, our results showed the utility of the PCC counselling in avoiding unnecessary visits to the ED, which is a relevant achievement, particularly in the time of COVID-19 pandemic, as well as the value of specialized clinical toxicologists in managing serious exposures.

Supplementary Materials: The following supporting information can be downloaded at: https://www.mdpi.com/article/10.3390/jcm12010352/s1, Table S1: Time elapsed between the exposure and the calling to the poison control center; Table S2: Classification of toxic agents according to the qualification of the caller.

Author Contributions: Conceptualization, V.B., G.C. and N.L.; methodology, G.C. and N.L.; formal analysis, G.C.; data curation, V.B. and G.C.; writing—original draft preparation, V.B., G.C. and N.L.; writing—review and editing, A.M., C.L., M.T. and A.I.; supervision, F.G., A.V. and G.M. All authors have read and agreed to the published version of the manuscript.

Funding: This research received no external funding.

Institutional Review Board Statement: The study was approved by the Regional Ethics Committee for Clinical Trials of the Tuscany Region (Italy)-Section: Pediatric Ethics Committee (approval: 30 March 2022). The study was performed following all the guidelines for observational studies with human subjects required by the institution with which the authors are affiliated.

Informed Consent Statement: Informed consent was obtained from all subjects involved in the study.

Data Availability Statement: Data that support the findings of this study are available upon reasonable request from the corresponding author, A.V.

Acknowledgments: We would like to thank all the healthcare professionals of the Medical Toxicology Unit and Poison Control Centre, Careggi University Hospital (Florence, Italy), who directly collaborated in the collection of clinical data used for this study.

Conflicts of Interest: The authors declare no conflict of interest.

References

1. Toce, M.S.; Burns, M.M. The Poisoned Pediatric Patient. *Pediatr. Rev.* **2017**, *38*, 207–220. [CrossRef] [PubMed]
2. Mintegi, S.; Azkunaga, B.; Prego, J.; Qureshi, N.; Dalziel, S.R.; Arana-Arri, E.; Acedo, Y.; Martinez-Indart, L.; Urkaregi, A.; Salmon, N.; et al. International Epidemiological Differences in Acute Poisonings in Pediatric Emergency Departments. *Pediatr. Emerg. Care* **2019**, *35*, 50–57. [CrossRef] [PubMed]
3. Gummin, D.D.; Mowry, J.B.; Beuhler, M.C.; Spyker, D.A.; Bronstein, A.C.; Rivers, L.J.; Pham, N.P.T.; Weber, J. 2020 Annual Report of the American Association of Poison Control Centers' National Poison Data System (NPDS): 38th Annual Report. *Clin. Toxicol. (Phila.)* **2021**, *59*, 1282–1501. [CrossRef] [PubMed]
4. Berta, G.N.; Di Scipio, F.; Bosetti, F.M.; Mognetti, B.; Romano, F.; Carere, M.E.; Del Giudice, A.C.; Castagno, E.; Bondone, C.; Urbino, A.F. Childhood acute poisoning in the Italian North-West area: A six-year retrospective study. *Ital. J. Pediatr.* **2020**, *46*, 83. [CrossRef] [PubMed]
5. Marano, M.; Rossi, F.; Ravà, L.; Ramla, M.K.; Pisani, M.; Bottari, G.; Genuini, L.; Zampini, G.; Nunziata, J.; Reale, A.; et al. Acute toxic exposures in children: Analysis of a three year registry managed by a Pediatric poison control Center in Italy. *Ital. J. Pediatr.* **2021**, *47*, 125. [CrossRef] [PubMed]
6. Persson, H.E.; Sjöberg, G.K.; Haines, J.A.; Pronczuk de Garbino, J. Poisoning severity score. Grading of acute poisoning. *J. Toxicol. Clin. Toxicol.* **1998**, *36*, 205–213. [CrossRef] [PubMed]
7. Crescioli, G.; Lanzi, C.; Gambassi, F.; Ieri, A.; Ercolini, A.; Borgioli, G.; Bettiol, A.; Vannacci, A.; Mannaioni, G.; Lombardi, N. Exposures and suspected intoxications during SARS-CoV-2 pandemic: Preliminary results from an Italian poison control centre. *Intern. Emerg. Med.* **2021**, *17*, 535–540. [CrossRef] [PubMed]
8. Soave, P.M.; Curatola, A.; Ferretti, S.; Raitano, V.; Conti, G.; Gatto, A.; Chiaretti, A. Acute poisoning in children admitted to pediatric emergency department: A five-years retrospective analysis. *Acta Biomed.* **2022**, *93*, 2022004. [CrossRef]
9. Desai, N.M.; Mistry, R.D.; Brou, L.; Boehnke, M.E.; Lee, J.S.; Wang, G.S. Pediatric Exposures Reported to the Toxicology Investigators Consortium, 2010-2015. *Pediatr. Emerg. Care* **2021**, *37*, e1039–e1043. [CrossRef] [PubMed]

10. Yang, S.-W.; Kernic, M.A.; Mueller, B.A.; Simon, G.E.; Chan, K.C.G.; Stoep, A.V. Association of Parental Mental Illness With Child Injury Occurrence, Hospitalization, and Death During Early Childhood. *JAMA Pediatr.* **2020**, *174*, e201749. [CrossRef] [PubMed]
11. Baker, R.; Kendrick, D.; Tata, L.J.; Orton, E. Association between maternal depression and anxiety episodes and rates of childhood injuries: A cohort study from England. *Inj. Prev.* **2017**, *23*, 396–402. [CrossRef] [PubMed]
12. Orton, E.; Kendrick, D.; West, J.; Tata, L.J. Independent Risk Factors for Injury in Pre-School Children: Three Population-Based Nested Case-Control Studies Using Routine Primary Care Data. *PLoS ONE* **2012**, *7*, e35193. [CrossRef] [PubMed]
13. Crescioli, G.; Lanzi, C.; Mannaioni, G.; Vannacci, A.; Lombardi, N. Adverse drug reactions in SARS-CoV-2 hospitalised patients: A case-series with a focus on drug-drug interactions-reply. *Intern. Emerg. Med.* **2021**, *16*, 799–800. [CrossRef] [PubMed]
14. Missanelli, A.; Lombardi, N.; Bettiol, A.; Lanzi, C.; Rossi, F.; Pacileo, I.; Donvito, L.; Garofalo, V.; Ravaldi, C.; Vannacci, A.; et al. Birth outcomes in women exposed to diagnostic radiology procedures during first trimester of pregnancy: A prospective cohort study. *Clin. Toxicol.* **2022**, *60*, 175–183. [CrossRef] [PubMed]
15. Sartori, S.; Crescioli, G.; Brilli, V.; Traversoni, S.; Lanzi, C.; Vannacci, A.; Mannaioni, G.; Lombardi, N. Phenobarbital use in benzodiazepine and z-drug detoxification: A single-centre 15-year observational retrospective study in clinical practice. *Intern. Emerg. Med.* **2022**, *17*, 1631–1640. [CrossRef] [PubMed]
16. Crescioli, G.; Bonaiuti, R.; Corradetti, R.; Mannaioni, G.; Vannacci, A.; Lombardi, N. Clinical Medicine Pharmacovigilance and Pharmacoepidemiology as a Guarantee of Patient Safety: The Role of the Clinical Pharmacologist. *J. Clin. Med.* **2022**, *11*, 3552. [CrossRef] [PubMed]

Disclaimer/Publisher's Note: The statements, opinions and data contained in all publications are solely those of the individual author(s) and contributor(s) and not of MDPI and/or the editor(s). MDPI and/or the editor(s) disclaim responsibility for any injury to people or property resulting from any ideas, methods, instructions or products referred to in the content.

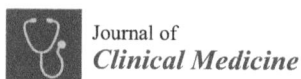

Article

The Interplay of Perceived Risks and Benefits in Deciding to Become Vaccinated against COVID-19 While Pregnant or Breastfeeding: A Cross-Sectional Study in Italy

Teresa Gavaruzzi [1,2,*,†], Marta Caserotti [2,†], Roberto Bonaiuti [3], Paolo Bonanni [4], Giada Crescioli [3], Mariarosaria Di Tommaso [4], Niccolò Lombardi [3], Lorella Lotto [2], Claudia Ravaldi [3], Enrico Rubaltelli [2], Alessandra Tasso [5], Alfredo Vannacci [3,†] and Paolo Girardi [6,†]

1. Department of Medical and Surgical Sciences, University of Bologna, 40126 Bologna, Italy
2. Department of Developmental Psychology and Socialization, University of Padova, 35122 Padova, Italy
3. PeaRL Perinatal Research Laboratory, CiaoLapo Foundation for Perinatal Health, Department of Neurosciences, Psychology, Drug Research and Child Health, University of Firenze, 50139 Firenze, Italy
4. Department of Health Science, University of Firenze, 50121 Firenze, Italy
5. Department of Humanities, University of Ferrara, 44121 Ferrara, Italy
6. Department of Environmental Sciences, Informatics and Statistics, Ca' Foscari University of Venezia, 30123 Venezia, Italy
* Correspondence: teresa.gavaruzzi@unibo.it
† These authors contributed equally to this work.

Abstract: The present study examined the role of the perception of risks and benefits for the mother and her babies in deciding about the COVID-19 vaccination. In this cross-sectional study, five hypotheses were tested using data from a convenience sample of Italian pregnant and/or breastfeeding women (N = 1104, July–September 2021). A logistic regression model estimated the influence of the predictors on the reported behavior, and a beta regression model was used to evaluate which factors influenced the willingness to become vaccinated among unvaccinated women. The COVID-19 vaccination overall risks/benefits tradeoff was highly predictive of both behavior and intention. Ceteris paribus, an increase in the perception of risks for the baby weighed more against vaccination than a similar increase in the perception of risks for the mother. Additionally, pregnant women resulted in being less likely (or willing) to be vaccinated in their status than breastfeeding women, but they were equally accepting of vaccination if they were not pregnant. COVID-19 risk perception predicted intention to become vaccinated, but not behavior. In conclusion, the overall risks/benefits tradeoff is key in predicting vaccination behavior and intention, but the concerns for the baby weigh more than those for the mother in the decision, shedding light on this previously neglected aspect.

Keywords: decision making; risk perception; risk/benefit tradeoff; COVID-19 vaccination; pregnancy; breastfeeding; maternal vaccination

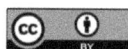

1. Introduction

While an individual's vaccination involves a trade-off between risks and benefits for the single individual, pregnant women have to consider the benefits and risks not only for themselves, but also for the baby they are carrying. Additionally, breastfeeding women have to consider the benefits and risks for themselves and their nursling. Comparing the two groups may help reveal the similarities or differences of the decision process; indeed, the risks for a nursling are usually smaller than those for the fetus, and, also, the potential risks for the mother do not directly affect the baby [1].

The psychological literature suggests that risk perception plays an important role in preventive behaviors, including immunization [2], and events or stimuli are often judged based on the positive–negative feelings they evoke (affect heuristic [3]). Indeed, many studies preceding the COVID-19 pandemic showed that being concerned about the risks for the baby is the most common barrier to vaccination during pregnancy [4–6], but, also, vice versa, the desire to protect the baby is the most common facilitator [4,7,8]. When compared directly, the concern for the safety of the vaccine for the baby is cited as a primary concern more frequently (95%) than the safety for the mother (82%) [9]. A systematic review of 120 articles and a meta-analysis of 49 of them [10] showed that both the benefits for the baby and those for the mother were similarly predictive of vaccine uptake, whereas the concern for the risks for the baby (referred to as "risk of vaccine harm during pregnancy") had a stronger negative effect on vaccine uptake than the concern for the risks of side effects for the mother [10]. However, it remains unclear how the interplay between perceived benefits and risks for the mother and baby contributes to the decision to receive a vaccination during pregnancy or lactation.

Several studies have examined the acceptability of COVID-19 vaccines in pregnant and (to a lesser extent) in breastfeeding women, showing a high heterogeneity in vaccine acceptance and hesitancy in several countries and at different timing of the pandemic [11–13]. At the same time, most studies showed that the main reasons for vaccine hesitancy in pregnant and breastfeeding women were similar to those expressed by the general population. Specifically, they included concerns over safety and fear of adverse events and lack of information or lack of recommendation from healthcare professionals [11–14]. These reasons were amplified by the lack of safety data for pregnant women and also by concerns about the possibility of harm to the fetus [15,16] and long-term adverse events in children, including children of breastfeeding women [17]. Conversely, factors favoring the acceptance of the COVID-19 vaccination were: trust in the importance (i.e., knowing the risks of the illness) and effectiveness of the COVID-19 vaccine and other vaccines and, more generally, trust in health institutions [13]. However, no study has examined in details the role of the perceived risks and benefits for the mother and for the baby.

The aim of the present study was to examine the role of the perception of risks and benefits for the mother and her babies in deciding about the COVID-19 vaccination in pregnant and breastfeeding women. Based on the literature, it was expected that:

H1: *The mother's status is predictive of COVID-19 vaccination self-reported behavior and intention: pregnant women are less likely than breastfeeding women to have been vaccinated and to intend to be vaccinated while in the current status.*

Indeed, in earlier studies, vaccine hesitancy was higher in pregnant women than in breastfeeding women [18,19], although later studies showed more mixed results and a high heterogeneity [12]. Earlier on, pregnant women were less likely to accept a vaccine (52% vs. 73%), they were more often concerned about possible harmful side effects for their baby (66% vs. 28%), and they were more interested in safety and effectiveness data specific for them (49% vs. 33%) than were mothers considering vaccinating their children [19]. Similarly, in a large study in six European countries, pregnant women were less likely to accept a vaccine than breastfeeding women (62% vs. 69%) [18].

H2: *Similarly to the general population, COVID-19 risk perception is predictive of COVID-19 vaccination self-reported behavior and intention: women who (a) are more worried about COVID-19 (b) perceive themselves as more likely to become infected, (c) perceived it as a severe disease, and (d) are more concerned about variants, and they are more likely to be vaccinated or intending to become vaccinated.*

Indeed, COVID-19 risk perception has been repeatedly found to be a predictor of vaccine acceptance in the general population [20–22] and also in pregnant women some evidence suggests this link [13] although this seems more linked to an emotional level than a cognitive level of risk perception as only a very weak positive correlation was found between C19 knowledge and C19 vaccine acceptance [12].

H3: *The trade-off between the perceived risks and the perceived benefits of vaccination is predictive of COVID-19 vaccination self-reported behavior and intention, regardless of the specific consideration for mother and baby. When the benefits of vaccination clearly outweigh the risks, women are more likely to be vaccinated or intend to be vaccinated than when the risks outweigh the benefits or they are similar.*

H4: *The concerns for the baby are more important than those for the mother in predicting vaccination behavior and intention. For the same value of trade-off between risks and benefits of vaccination, as the risks for the baby increase, the likelihood that women have been vaccinated or intend to be vaccinated decreases.*

Both these predictions are based on the literature reviewed above about the role of perceived benefits and risks, especially on the review and meta-analysis by Kilich and colleagues [10].

H5: *During pregnancy, the concerns for the baby weigh more than during breastfeeding in the decision to become vaccinated.*

This prediction stems from H1 and from considerations about the actual potential for risks of adverse events for the fetus and the nursling.

2. Materials and Methods

2.1. Participants

Participants were recruited through social media posts, with a link to an online questionnaire, and informed consent was obtained from all women involved in the study. Data were collected nation-wide between late July and early September 2021. Inclusion criteria were being pregnant, breastfeeding, or both. The study information sheet was read by 1720 potential participants, and 1484 consented to participate. Of those, 52 (3.5%) participants did not meet the inclusion criteria, 270 (18.2%) participants dropped out during the survey, 50 (3.4%) were excluded because they were vaccinated before being pregnant or before knowing they were pregnant, and eight (0.5%) were excluded because they provided incoherent answers, leaving 1104 (77%) participants for the analyses. The final sample consisted of 572 (52%) breastfeeding women and 532 (48%) pregnant women (of whom 34 were both pregnant and breastfeeding). The study was approved by the ethical committee for psychological studies of the first authors' university (protocol: 4220, approved 7 July 2021).

2.2. Procedure

Participants who consented to participate indicated whether they were pregnant and whether they were breastfeeding. They were then asked personal information, including: age, level of education (middle school, high school, university degree, higher degrees), employment (employee, unemployed, freelancer), and whether they had other children (no, one, two, or more). Pregnant women were asked to report their current pregnancy week. Breastfeeding women were asked the age of the breastfed baby. The *C19 Vaccine Status* was assessed by asking all women if they had received at least one dose of a COVID-19 vaccine (Yes, No) during pregnancy and/or during breastfeeding. Women who had not yet been vaccinated were asked to indicate their *willingness to become vaccinated (WTV)*, i.e., how likely they were to become vaccinated against COVID-19 (from 0 = *Not at all likely* to 100 = *Extremely likely*), with a vaccine recommended for their case. This question was asked twice, once referring to their status at the time of the questionnaire and once referring to their intention if they were not pregnant nor breastfeeding. Four questions assessed the perception of benefits and risks for the mother and for the baby associated with the mother's COVID-19 vaccination (all measured on a scale from 1 = *Completely disagree* to 5 = *Completely agree*). These four questions were combined in two indexes (see also Figure S1):

$$C19\ Vaccination\ risks/benefits\ overall\ ratio = \frac{(risk\ for\ baby + risk\ for\ mother)}{(benefit\ for\ baby + benefit\ for\ mother)} \quad (1)$$

The index *C19 Vaccination risks/benefits overall ratio* (1) can range from a minimum of 0.2 (when risks are both judged to be equal to the minimum value of 1 and benefits are both judged to be equal to the maximum value of 5) to a maximum of 5 (when risks are both equal to 5 and benefits are both equal to 1). The index is equal to 1 when risks and benefits are judged to be equal overall; values smaller than 1 indicate lower risks than the benefits, whereas values bigger than 1 indicate that the risks are judged higher than the benefits.

$$C19\ Vaccination\ baby/mother\ risk/benefit\ ratio = \frac{\frac{risk\ for\ baby}{benefit\ for\ baby}}{\frac{risk\ for\ mother}{benefit\ for\ mother}} \quad (2)$$

The index *C19 Vaccination baby/mother risk/benefit ratio* (2) can range from a minimum of 0.04 (when the risk/benefit ratio for the baby is equal to the minimum of 0.2 and the risk/benefit ratio for mother is equal to the maximum of 5), to a maximum of 25 (when risk/benefit ratio for the baby has the highest possible value of 5 and that for the mother the lowest possible value of 0.2). The index is equal to 1 when the two risks-benefits ratios are judged to be equal; values lower than 1 indicate a lower risks-benefits ratio for the baby than for the mother (e.g., when the benefits are perceived as equal, the risks for the mother are higher than those for the baby), and values higher than 1 indicate the opposite (risks–benefits ratio higher for the baby than for the mother).

Similarly to previous studies [20,23], COVID-19 risk perception was assessed by asking participants to report their perceived severity of the disease, the perceived likelihood of being infected, how scared they felt about the disease, and the concern for possible variants (all measured on a scale from 0 = *Not at all* to 100 = *Extremely*). Participants were then asked to complete the Pandemic Fatigue scale, assessing a general distress and sense of fatigue related to the pandemic, indicating their degree of agreement (1 = *Not at all*; 7 = *Very much*) with six items, such as "I feel challenged by following all of the rules and behavioral rules regarding C19." [24]. Further, participants completed a previously used ad hoc scale, investigating the sense of conspiracy related to the COVID-19 context, indicating their degree of agreement (1 = *Not at all*; 7 = *Very much*) with seven items, such as "The C19 virus was created in a laboratory" and "Vaccines against C19 can alter people's DNA" [25]. Finally, participants were asked to answer an eight-item scale to assess the perception of vaccines in general, indicating their agreement (1 = *Not at all*; to 5 = *Very much*) on items such as "Vaccines are important to human health" and "Vaccines are produced and recommended only for the economic interest of pharmaceutical companies" [26].

2.3. Statistical Analyses

2.3.1. Descriptive Analysis

The variables in the study were summarized by frequency, for categorical variables, as well as median (and Inter Quartile Range, IQR) for continuous variables (see Table 1). Wilcoxon rank sum tests were computed to compare variables on an ordinal Likert scale or on continuous scores across mother status (pregnancy or breastfeeding), while, for categorical variables, the Pearson chi-squared test was used. Statistical significance was assumed at the 5% level. Tables S1–S4 provide additional descriptive analyses not reported in the main article.

Table 1. Main characteristics of the mothers by COVID-19 vaccine status.

Variable	Overall, N = 1104 [1]	C19 Vaccine Status Not Vaccinated, N = 592 [1]	C19 Vaccine Status Vaccinated, N = 512 [1]	p-Value [2]
Age (years)	34.0 (31.0, 37.0)	34.0 (31.0, 37.0)	35.0 (32.0, 37.0)	**0.012**
Education				**<0.001**
Middle school	25 (2.3%)	15 (2.5%)	10 (2.0%)	
High school	318 (29%)	212 (36%)	106 (21%)	
University degree	581 (53%)	289 (49%)	292 (57%)	
Higher level degree	180 (16%)	76 (13%)	104 (20%)	
Employment				0.516
Private or public employee	735 (67%)	392 (66%)	343 (67%)	
Unemployed or Other	182 (16%)	104 (18%)	78 (15%)	
Self-employed	187 (17%)	96 (16%)	91 (18%)	
Other Children				0.238
No	476 (43%)	266 (45%)	210 (41%)	
1	481 (44%)	244 (41%)	237 (46%)	
2+	147 (13%)	82 (14%)	65 (13%)	
Mother Status				**<0.001**
Breastfeeding	572 (52%)	188 (32%)	384 (75%)	
Pregnancy	532 (48%)	404 (68%)	128 (25%)	
C19 Risk Perception	0.19 (−0.58, 0.70)	−0.19 (−1.09, 0.58)	0.41 (−0.02, 0.77)	**<0.001**
Pandemic Fatigue	0.04 (−0.62, 0.64)	0.21 (−0.50 0.79)	−0.18 (−0.68, 0.39)	**<0.001**
Pro-vax Attitude	0.17 (−0.57, 0.74)	−0.25 (−0.96, 0.47)	0.48 (0.01, 0.99)	**<0.001**
C19 Conspiracy score	−0.30 (−0.79, 0.66)	0.51 (−0.36, 1.26)	−0.70 (−0.96, −0.32)	**<0.001**

[1] Median (IQR) or frequency (%). [2] Wilcoxon rank sum test; Pearson's chi-squared test. Abbreviation: C19 for COVID-19, vax for vaccination. Bold: statistically significant results.

2.3.2. Dimensionality Reduction—Factor Analyses

Four different factor analyses were performed for the Pandemic Fatigue scale [24], as well as for the group of variables related to COVID-19 risk perception [20,23], COVID-19 conspiracy [25], and to vaccine perception in general [26]. For all the factor analyses, the amount of variance explained by the one factor solution was acceptable (see Table S5).

2.3.3. Logistic and Beta Regressions

To estimate the influence of the perceived risks/benefits ratios (overall and baby/mother) from COVID-19 vaccination on the probability to have received the vaccine against COVID-19, a logistic regression model was employed, in which the dependent variable was the COVID-19 Vaccine Status (0 = not yet received; 1 = received). Covariates (mother status, vaccine perception, COVID-19 risk perception, COVID-19 conspiracy, and pandemic fatigue) were included, minimizing the AIC index with a forward selection criteria. The presence of interactions between covariates and risks/benefits ratio indices was tested employing a Chi-squared test, fixing a significance level equal to 5%. The model included the mother's age (in continuous form), the educational level, the employment, and the presence of other kids to adjust for non-probability sampling. The results are presented by means of Odds Ratios (ORs) by exponentiating the estimated coefficients from the logistic regression, calculating the relative 95% Confidence Interval (95%CI).

To evaluate which factors influenced the WTV among mothers who had not yet received the vaccine, a beta regression model, which is commonly used to model variables that assume values in the standard unit interval (0,1), was used. The WTV was divided by 100, applying to the new scale correction [27] to have values strictly between 0 and 1, extremes excluded. Two separate models were estimated, one for the WTV in the current status and one for the WTV assuming not to be pregnant and/or in breastfeeding. For these models, the same selection variables scheme adopted for the logistic regression was considered. The results are presented using ORs by exponentiating the estimated coefficients reporting the relative 95%CI.

Regression analyses were performed by R 4.2 statistical software using the package betareg for the beta regression model.

3. Results

3.1. Demographic

The main characteristics of the sample are reported in Table 1.

Mothers reported an average age of 34.2 years (min–max: 20–48 years), with a predominant high educational level (53% and 16% obtained a degree or a higher education, respectively). The majority was employed as a private or public employee (67%) and had no other child (44%) or one other child (43%). With respect to their mother status, pregnant women were between six and forty-three weeks of gestation (average: 28.4, Standard Deviation (SD): 9.21), while, for breastfeeding women, 25% of the lactated children were below three months, 25% were between four and eight months, 25% were between nine and fifteen months, and 5.3% were older than three years.

The distribution of the scores for the perceived risks and benefits for the baby and the mother is depicted in Figure 1. All scores differed between vaccinated and unvaccinated women (Table 2). Both overall and baby/mother risks/benefits ratios differed between vaccinated and unvaccinated women and between pregnant and breastfeeding women (Table 3).

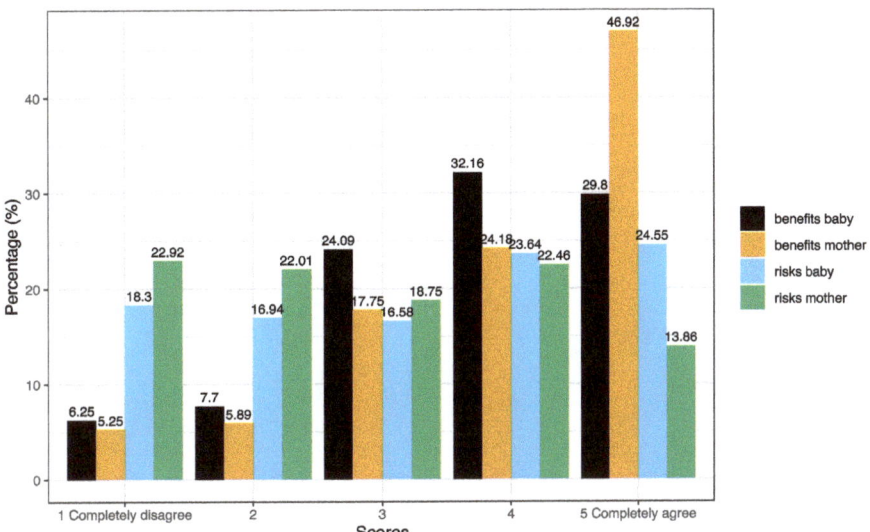

Figure 1. Distribution of the scores of the perception of COVID-19 vaccination risks and benefits for the baby and the mother, each assessed on a scale from 1 (=completely disagree) to 5 (=completely agree).

Table 2. COVID-19 vaccine perception of risks and benefits for the baby and the mother by COVID-19 vaccine status.

| C19 Vaccine Perception of | Overall, N = 1104 [1] | C19 Vaccine Status | | p-Value [2] |
		Not Vaccinated, N = 592	Vaccinated, N = 512 [1]	
Risks for baby	3 (2, 4)	4 (4, 5)	2 (1, 3)	**<0.001**
Risks for mother	3 (2, 4)	4 (2, 4)	2 (1, 3)	**<0.001**
Benefits for baby	4 (3, 5)	3 (3, 4)	5 (4, 5)	**<0.001**
Benefits for mother	4 (3, 5)	4 (3, 4)	5 (5, 5)	**<0.001**

[1] Median (IQR) or frequency (%). [2] Wilcoxon rank sum test. Abbreviation: C19 for COVID-19. Bold: statistically significant results.

Table 3. C19 Vaccination risks/benefits ratio and COVID-19 vaccination baby/mother ratio by mother status and COVID-19 vaccine status.

C19 Vax	Mother Status				C19 Vaccine Status		
	Overall, N = 1104 [1]	Breastfeeding, N = 572 [1]	Pregnancy, N = 532 [1]	p-Value [2]	Not Vaccinated, N = 592 [1]	Vaccinated, N = 512 [1]	p-Value [2]
Risks/benefits ratio	0.75 (0.44, 1.17)	0.62 (0.40, 1.00)	0.89 (0.56, 1.33)	**<0.001**	1.14 (0.80, 1.60)	0.44 (0.30, 0.67)	**<0.001**
Baby/mother ratio	1.00 (1.00, 2.00)	1.00 (0.83, 1.67)	1.25 (1.00, 2.00)	**<0.001**	1.25 (1.00, 2.02)	1.00 (0.83, 1.33)	**<0.001**

[1] Median (IQR) or frequency (%). [2] Wilcoxon rank sum test. Abbreviation: C19 for COVID-19; vax for vaccination. Bold: statistically significant results.

3.2. Logistic Regression Model

The factors associated with a reduction in the probability to be vaccinated (Table 4) were: the current status, with pregnant women reporting a heavy reduction (−73%) in the probability to be vaccinated relative to those breastfeeding (OR: 0.27, 95%CI: 0.10–0.76), perceiving that, overall, the vaccination risks exceed the benefits (+1 point increase in the risks/benefits overall index: OR: 0.19, 95%CI: 0.04–0.74), and having a higher COVID-19 conspiracy score (+1 point increase: OR: 0.36, 95%CI: 0.24–0.54). Whereas higher values on the pandemic fatigue scale were associated with an increased probability to become vaccinated (+1 point increase: OR: 1.44, 95%CI: 1.13–1.83).

Table 4. Odds ratios (ORs) estimated by a logistic regression model for the probability to be vaccinated by the COVID-19 vaccine with respect to the reference category [1].

Predictors	OR	95%CI	p-Values
COVID-19 vax risks/benefits overall ratio	0.19	0.04–0.74	**0.021**
COVID-19 vax baby/mother risks/benefits ratio	1.52	0.81–2.90	0.193
Mother Status [Pregnancy]	0.27	0.10–0.76	**0.012**
Age (+1 years)	1.04	0.98–1.09	0.175
Education [High school]	0.89	0.23–3.15	0.858
Education [University Degree]	1.04	0.27–3.63	0.955
Education [High level degree]	1.10	0.27–4.21	0.891
Employment [Unemployed or Other]	1.14	0.64–2.03	0.666
Employment [Self-employed]	1.21	0.69–2.14	0.512
Other Children [1]	1.03	0.66–1.59	0.905
Other Children [2+]	0.81	0.42–1.55	0.513
COVID-19 Conspiracy score [2]	0.36	0.24–0.54	**<0.001**
Pandemic Fatigue [2]	1.44	1.13–1.83	**0.003**
COVID-19 vax risks/benefits ratio × Mother Status [Pregnancy]	0.20	0.05–0.82	**0.029**
COVID-19 vax risks/benefits ratio × COVID-19 vax baby/mother ratio	0.23	0.08–0.60	**0.003**
Observations		1104	
R^2 Tjur		0.636	

[1] Mother Status [Breastfeeding], Education [Middle School], Employment [Private or public employee], Other Children [No]. [2] 1-point increase. Abbreviation: C19 for COVID-19; vax for vaccination. Bold: statistically significant results.

Although no marginal effect was found for the COVID-19 vaccination baby/mother risks/benefits ratio, results showed a significant interaction between this index and COVID-19 vaccination risks/benefits overall ratio, leading mothers who perceived a higher risks/benefits ratio for their baby than for themselves to be more hesitant (OR: 0.23, 95%CI: 0.08–0.60; Figure 2, left panel). Further, COVID-19 vaccination risks/benefits overall ratio also interacted with the mother status, accentuating the reduction in the likelihood of being vaccinated among pregnant women (OR: 0.20, 95%CI: 0.05–0.82; Figure 2, right panel).

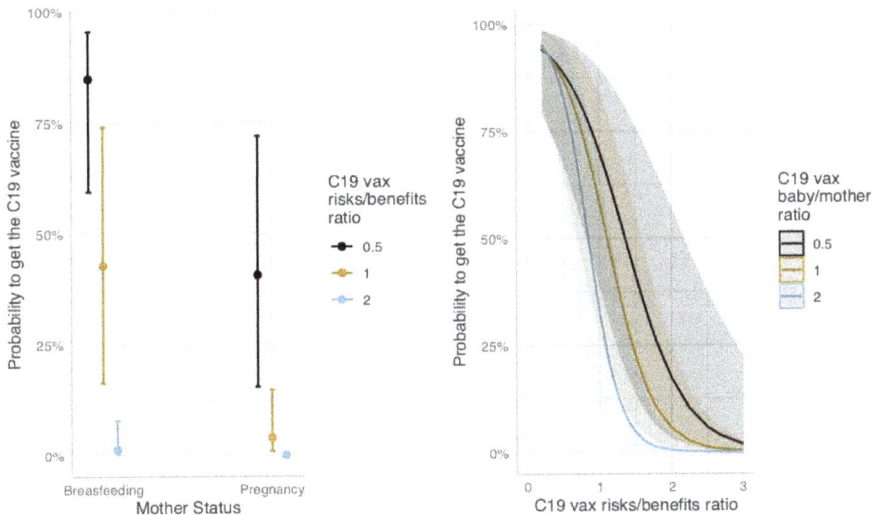

Figure 2. Predicted probability and 95%CI to be vaccinated, considering the interaction between mother status and COVID-19 vaccination risks/benefits ratio (**left**) and COVID-19 vaccination risks/benefits ratio and COVID-19 vax baby/mother ratio (**right**).

3.3. Beta Regression Models

As shown in Table 5, the higher the risks/benefits overall ratio, the lower the WTV of unvaccinated women, both at the time of the survey (+1 point increase: OR: 0.83, 95%CI: 0.73–0.94) and if they were not pregnant or breastfeeding (+1 point increase: OR: 0.79, 95%CI: 0.69–0.90). The risks/benefits baby/mother ratio decreased the WTV in the current status (+1 point increase: OR: 0.87, 95%CI: 0.83–0.92), while it slightly increased if women were neither pregnant nor breastfeeding (+1 point increase: OR: 1.05, 95%CI: 1.00–1.11). Being pregnant decreased the WTV in the current status (+1 point increase: OR: 0.61, 95%CI: 0.49–0.76), whereas having a general attitude towards vaccination increased the WTV if not pregnant or breastfeeding (+1 point increase: OR: 1.18, 95%CI: 1.02–1.36). C19 Risk perception increased WTV in both models, respectively (+1 point increase: OR: 1.24, 95%CI: 1.20–1.39 for current status and OR: 1.43, 95%CI: 1.27–1.61 if not pregnant or breastfeeding); to the contrary, COVID-19 conspiracy decreased the WTV in both models, respectively (OR: 0.57, 95%CI: 0.49–0.67 for current status and OR: 0.59, 95%CI: 0.49–0.71 if not pregnant or breastfeeding).

Table 5. Odds Ratio, estimated by a beta regression model for the willingness to become vaccinated in the current status and if not pregnant/breastfeeding, with respect to the reference category [1].

Predictors	WTV in Current Status			WTV if Not Preg./Breast.		
	OR	95%CI	p-Values	OR	95%CI	p-Values
COVID-19 vax risks/benefits ratio	0.83	0.73–0.94	**0.003**	0.79	0.69–0.90	**<0.001**
COVID-19 vax baby/mother ratio	0.87	0.83–0.92	**<0.001**	1.05	1.00–1.11	**0.045**
Mother Status [Pregnancy]	0.61	0.49–0.76	**<0.001**	NS	-	-
Age (+1 years)	0.99	0.96–1.01	0.234	0.98	0.95–1.00	0.075
Education [High school]	0.68	0.36–1.30	0.246	0.97	0.51–1.84	0.924
Education [University Degree]	0.74	0.39–1.41	0.362	0.86	0.45–1.64	0.643
Education [High level degree]	0.78	0.39–1.57	0.487	0.96	0.48–1.91	0.898
Employment [Unemployed or Other]	0.98	0.74–1.29	0.882	0.90	0.69–1.18	0.460
Employment [Self-employed]	0.84	0.63–1.11	0.223	0.89	0.67–1.17	0.401
Other Children [1]	1.03	0.82–1.29	0.804	0.94	0.75–1.16	0.548
Other Children [2+]	1.11	0.81–1.53	0.517	0.83	0.61–1.14	0.247

Table 5. Cont.

Predictors	WTV in Current Status			WTV if Not Preg./Breast.		
	OR	95%CI	p-Values	OR	95%CI	p-Values
COVID-19 Risk Perception [2]	1.24	1.10–1.39	**<0.001**	1.43	1.27–1.61	**<0.001**
COVID-19 Conspiracy score [2]	0.57	0.49–0.67	**<0.001**	0.59	0.49–0.71	**<0.001**
Pro-vax Attitude [2]	NS	-	-	1.18	1.02–1.36	**0.026**
Observations		592			592	
R²		0.406			0.611	

[1] Mother Status [Breastfeeding], Education [Middle School], Employment [Private or public employee], Other Children [No]. [2] 1-point increase. Abbreviation: C19 for COVID-19; vax for vaccination. Bold: statistically significant results.

4. Discussion

In a convenience sample of over a thousand women, this study examined the interplay of perceived risks and benefits for the mother and the baby in deciding to become vaccinated against C19 while pregnant or breastfeeding, confirming most of the hypotheses based on the literature and highlighting some important relationships.

In the present sample, only about a quarter of pregnant women had received the vaccine while pregnant, whereas about two thirds of breastfeeding women received it while breastfeeding. In other words, pregnant women were less likely to be vaccinated or to be willing to become vaccinated than breastfeeding women (supporting H1, in line with [18,19]), but they were equally likely to intend to be vaccinated if they were not pregnant, suggesting that their attitude is attributable to their current status. This result is further supported by the finding that a general positive attitude towards immunization was a positive predictor only when modeling the intention to become vaccinated if not pregnant or breastfeeding. These findings suggest that the hesitancy shown by pregnant women in our sample was highly context-specific and temporary. It remains to be ascertained whether this type of hesitancy could still affect attitudes towards other vaccines and childhood vaccines, which are often formed during pregnancy [28].

In line with the literature [2,20–22], findings also confirmed that COVID-19 risk perception plays a role in women's WTV, with higher risk perception yielding a higher intention to become vaccinated, both in the current status and if not pregnant or breastfeeding. However, COVID-19 risk perception was not a predictor of actually being vaccinated at the time of the survey, only partially supporting H2. A possible explanation is that, after being vaccinated, women's COVID-19 risk perception decreased, showing no predictive value. In other words, if COVID-19 risk perception was measured before these women were vaccinated, it is expected that it would predict the decision to become vaccinated. This interpretation is supported by evidence showing that COVID-19 risk perception decreases after being vaccinated [29].

The predictive power of the trade-off between perceived risks and benefits was confirmed in all three models, fully supporting H3. The higher the risks–benefits trade-off, the lower the probability that women have been vaccinated against C19 while pregnant or breastfeeding and, if not yet vaccinated, the lower their willingness to be vaccinated, both at the time of the survey and if they were not pregnant or breastfeeding. This is in line with the psychological literature on the affect heuristic [3], whereby people often heavily rely on their feelings to make judgments and decisions, in this case on the perceived risks and benefits of the vaccination.

The distinctive role of the risks–benefit ratio for the baby and for the mother also emerged in the analyses, supporting H4. This finding is corroborated by the interaction found in the logistic model: the higher the baby–mother ratio, the steeper the drop in the probability of being vaccinated when the risks–benefits ratio increases (Figure 2, right panel). For example, for women whose general risks–benefits trade-off is equal to 1, the probability of being vaccinated against C19 is around 55–60% when the baby–mother ratio is also equal to 1. It lowers to around 35% when the baby–mother ratio is equal to 2 (i.e., when the risks–benefits trade-off for the baby is twice the risks–benefits trade-off for the mother). Whereas it reaches about 70% when the baby–mother ratio is equal to 0.5 (i.e., when the risks–benefits trade-off for the mother is twice the risks–benefits trade-off for the baby). This finding suggests that, all other things being equal, an increase in the perception of risks for the baby weighed more against the decision to vaccinate than a similar increase in the perception of risks for the mother, shedding light on this previously neglected aspect [10].

Among unvaccinated women, the risks–benefits ratio for the baby and for the mother had a direct effect on the intention to become vaccinated at the time of the survey: the higher the baby–mother ratio, the lower the intention to become vaccinated while being pregnant or breastfeeding (in line with H4). However, the opposite was found when modeling the intention to become vaccinated if women were not pregnant or breastfeeding. Considering that most unvaccinated women were pregnant, this result suggests that the relevance of the risks for the baby in the decision decreases once a woman is no longer pregnant, providing support for H5. Additionally, an interaction between the mother's current status and the risks–benefits trade-off was found: the level of risks–benefits ratio being equal, breastfeeding women are more likely to be vaccinated than pregnant women, and the effect of the risks–benefits ratio is stronger in breastfeeding women (Figure 2, left panel). For example, when the benefits of the vaccination are judged to be two times greater than the risks, on average, lactating women are around 85% likely to have been vaccinated, whereas pregnant women are around 40% likely to have been vaccinated. When the benefits are judged to be equal to the risks, the probability of breastfeeding women to be vaccinated is around 40–45%, but, for pregnant women, it is around 5%. While not directly expected, this is in line with H5, as, for a pregnant woman, the benefits have to outweigh the risks more than for a breastfeeding woman to have decided to vaccinate.

Moreover, COVID-19 conspiracy was a consistent predictor in all models: the higher the conspiracy score, the lower the probability that women were vaccinated and their WTV now or if not pregnant/breastfeeding. This is not surprising, as conspiracy mentality has been repeatedly associated with vaccine hesitancy in general [30,31] in the COVID-19 context [32,33] and also during pregnancy [34].

Finally, the level of pandemic fatigue (i.e., being tired of information about COVID-19 and of behavioral measures to counter it [24]) was positively associated with having been vaccinated during pregnancy or breastfeeding, but not with WTV among unvaccinated women. This seems to contrast with previous findings, showing that pandemic fatigue is a strong predictor of non-adherence to health protective measures [24]. However, it is possible that high pandemic fatigue leads to avoidance of information and to a reluctance to adhere to behavioral measures, such as wearing masks, keeping distance, and washing hands, but vaccination could be seen as a solution to the pandemic [35]; this would explain why a positive association between pandemic fatigue and vaccine uptake was found.

This study has limitations that should be considered. While the sample recruited was not representative of the population of pregnant and lactating women, the sample reached was ample and varied, and the use of social media through which participants were recruited has become even more widespread than in the past. Nonetheless, also due to the drop-out of about 25% of participants during the questionnaire, the generalizability of the findings should be taken cautiously and compared with other findings. However, in the regression analyses, all the confounders (age, educational level, employment, and presence of other children) were included to adjust the effect estimate. Finally, as the pandemic is constantly evolving, and the recommendations for immunization against C19 during pregnancy have changed since the study was conducted (when it was still recommended to discuss with healthcare professionals the benefits and risks of C19 vaccination for each pregnant or breastfeeding woman), it is important to consider the context when data were collected when interpreting the findings.

5. Conclusions

To summarize and conclude, the study focused on pregnant and breastfeeding women's decision making about COVID-19 vaccination, especially about the role of the perception of risks and benefits for themselves and for their babies. The COVID-19 vaccination risks/benefits tradeoff was highly predictive of behavior and intention. Ceteris paribus, an increase in the perception of risks for the baby weighed more against the decision to vaccinate than a similar increase in the perception of risks for the mother, shedding light on this previously neglected aspect. When counseling pregnant and breastfeeding women about vaccinations, it is important to be aware that their decision is likely based on the risks and benefits tradeoff in general, but also that they are particularly worried about the baby and may not fully appreciate the indirect benefits to the baby conveyed by the mother's vaccination. Indeed, it is also possible that women underappreciate the benefits for their babies in vaccinating themselves, as being less likely to experience severe COVID-19 illness also reduces the risks of negative events for the fetus (for pregnant women) and makes them more available to care for their babies (for breastfeeding women). While pregnant women's hesitancy seems transient, it is important to foster decision-making, improving women's understanding and awareness of the risks and benefits for them and for their babies and helping women to weighing them.

Supplementary Materials: The following supporting information can be downloaded at: https://www.mdpi.com/article/10.3390/jcm12103469/s1, Table S1. Selection Criteria. Questionnaire completion of at least 85%, vaccination before pregnancy, and completeness of the analyzed variables; Table S2. Main characteristics by Mother Status; Table S3. Main characteristics of not vaccinated mothers by Mother Status; Table S4. C19 vaccine perception of Risks and Benefits for baby and mother by Mother Status; Table S5. Dimensionality reduction—factor analyses; Figure S1. Joint and marginal distribution of the scores for C19 vax risks/benefits ratio and C19 vax baby/mother ratio. With the dotted lines the ratios equal to the unity.

Author Contributions: Conceptualization, T.G., M.C., R.B., P.B., G.C., M.D.T., N.L., L.L., C.R., E.R., A.T., A.V. and P.G.; methodology, T.G., M.C., R.B., P.B., G.C., M.D.T., N.L., L.L., C.R., E.R., A.T., A.V. and P.G.; formal analysis, T.G., M.C. and P.G.; investigation, T.G. and M.C.; data curation, T.G., M.C. and P.G.; writing—original draft preparation, T.G., M.C. and P.G.; writing—review and editing, R.B., P.B., G.C., M.D.T., N.L., L.L., E.R., A.T. and A.V.; visualization, T.G., M.C. and P.G.; supervision, A.V.; project administration, T.G., M.C. and A.V. All authors have read and agreed to the published version of the manuscript.

Funding: This research received no external funding.

Institutional Review Board Statement: The study was conducted in accordance with the Declaration of Helsinki and approved by the Ethics Committee for psychological studies of the University of Padova (protocol: 4220, approved 7 July 2021).

Informed Consent Statement: Informed consent was obtained from all subjects involved in the study.

Data Availability Statement: Data are available upon request to the authors.

Acknowledgments: Participants who volunteered their time to fill the questionnaire, the CiaoLapo Foundation for disseminating the research link, and the student Laura Salvi for contributing to the data collection.

Conflicts of Interest: The authors declare no conflict of interest.

References

1. Luxi, N.; Giovanazzi, A.; Capuano, A.; Crisafulli, S.; Cutroneo, P.M.; Fantini, M.P.; Trifirò, G. COVID-19 vaccination in pregnancy, paediatrics, immunocompromised patients, and persons with history of allergy or prior SARS-CoV-2 infection: Overview of current recommendations and pre-and post-marketing evidence for vaccine efficacy and safety. *Drug Saf.* **2021**, *44*, 1247–1269. [CrossRef] [PubMed]
2. Brewer, N.T.; Chapman, G.B.; Gibbons, F.X.; Gerrard, M.; McCaul, K.D.; Weinstein, N.D. Meta-analysis of the relationship between risk perception and health behavior: The example of vaccination. *Health Psychol.* **2007**, *26*, 136. [CrossRef] [PubMed]

3. Slovic, P.; Finucane, M.L.; Peters, E.; MacGregor, D.G. The affect heuristic. *Eur. J. Oper. Res.* **2007**, *177*, 1333–1352. [CrossRef]
4. Meharry, P.M.; Colson, E.R.; Grizas, A.P.; Stiller, R.; Vázquez, M. Reasons why women accept or reject the trivalent inactivated influenza vaccine (TIV) during pregnancy. *Matern. Child Health J.* **2013**, *17*, 156–164. [CrossRef]
5. Song, Y.; Zhang, T.; Chen, L.; Yi, B.; Hao, X.; Zhou, S.; Greene, C. Increasing seasonal influenza vaccination among high risk groups in China: Do community healthcare workers have a role to play? *Vaccine* **2017**, *35*, 4060–4063. [CrossRef] [PubMed]
6. Yun, X.; Xu, J. Survey of attitude toward immunization of H1N1 influenza A vaccine of pregnant women in Guangzhou. *J. Trop. Med.* **2010**, *10*, 1136–1140.
7. McCarthy, E.A.; Pollock, W.E.; Tapper, L.; Sommerville, M.; McDonald, S. Increasing uptake of influenza vaccine by pregnant women post H1N1 pandemic: A longitudinal study in Melbourne, Australia, 2010 to 2014. *BMC Pregnancy Childbirth* **2015**, *15*, 1–7. [CrossRef]
8. Goldfarb, I.; Panda, B.; Wylie, B.; Riley, L. Uptake of influenza vaccine in pregnant women during the 2009 H1N1 influenza pandemic. *Am. J. Obstet. Gynecol.* **2011**, *204*, S112–S115. [CrossRef]
9. Campbell, H.; Van Hoek, A.J.; Bedford, H.; Craig, L.; Yeowell, A.L.; Green, D.; Amirthalingam, G. Attitudes to immunisation in pregnancy among women in the UK targeted by such programmes. *Br. J. Midwifery* **2015**, *23*, 566–573. [CrossRef]
10. Kilich, E.; Dada, S.; Francis, M.R.; Tazare, J.; Chico, R.M.; Paterson, P.; Larson, H.J. Factors that influence vaccination decision-making among pregnant women: A systematic review and meta-analysis. *PLoS ONE* **2020**, *15*, e0234827. [CrossRef]
11. Bhattacharya, O.; Siddiquea, B.N.; Shetty, A.; Afroz, A.; Billah, B. COVID-19 vaccine hesitancy among pregnant women: A systematic review and meta-analysis. *BMJ Open* **2022**, *12*, e061477. [CrossRef]
12. Bianchi, F.P.; Stefanizzi, P.; Di Gioia, M.C.; Brescia, N.; Lattanzio, S.; Tafuri, S. COVID-19 vaccination hesitancy in pregnant and breastfeeding women and strategies to increase vaccination compliance: A systematic review and meta-analysis. *Expert Rev. Vaccines* **2022**, *21*, 1443–1454. [CrossRef]
13. Januszek, S.M.; Faryniak-Zuzak, A.; Barnaś, E.; Łoziński, T.; Góra, T.; Siwiec, N.; Kluz, T. The approach of pregnant women to vaccination based on a COVID-19 systematic review. *Medicina* **2021**, *57*, 977. [CrossRef]
14. Maltezou, H.C.; Effraimidou, E.; Cassimos, D.C.; Medic, S.; Topalidou, M.; Konstantinidis, T.; Rodolakis, A. Vaccination programs for pregnant women in Europe, 2021. *Vaccine* **2021**, *39*, 6137–6143. [CrossRef]
15. Goncu Ayhan, S.; Oluklu, D.; Atalay, A.; Menekse Beser, D.; Tanacan, A.; Moraloglu Tekin, O.; Sahin, D. COVID-19 vaccine acceptance in pregnant women. *Int. J. Gynecol. Obstet.* **2021**, *154*, 291–296. [CrossRef] [PubMed]
16. Mohan, S.; Reagu, S.; Lindow, S.; Alabdulla, M. COVID-19 vaccine hesitancy in perinatal women: A cross sectional survey. *J. Perinat. Med.* **2021**, *49*, 678–685. [CrossRef] [PubMed]
17. Jayagobi, P.A.; Ong, C.; Thai, Y.K.; Lim, C.C.; Jiun, S.M.; Koon, K.L.; Chien, C.M. Perceptions and acceptance of COVID-19 vaccine among pregnant and lactating women in Singapore: A cross-sectional study. *MedRxiv* **2021**, *2021*, 6. [CrossRef] [PubMed]
18. Ceulemans, M.; Foulon, V.; Panchaud, A.; Winterfeld, U.; Pomar, L.; Lambelet, V.; Nordeng, H. Vaccine willingness and impact of the COVID-19 pandemic on women's perinatal experiences and practices—A multinational, cross-sectional study covering the first wave of the pandemic. *Int. J. Environ. Res. Public Health* **2021**, *18*, 3367. [CrossRef]
19. Skjefte, M.; Ngirbabul, M.; Akeju, O.; Escudero, D.; Hernandez-Diaz, S.; Wyszynski, D.F.; Wu, J.W. COVID-19 vaccine acceptance among pregnant women and mothers of young children: Results of a survey in 16 countries. *Eur. J. Epidemiol.* **2021**, *36*, 197–211. [CrossRef]
20. Caserotti, M.; Girardi, P.; Rubaltelli, E.; Tasso, A.; Lotto, L.; Gavaruzzi, T. Associations of COVID-19 risk perception with vaccine hesitancy over time for Italian residents. *Soc. Sci. Med.* **2021**, *272*, 113688. [CrossRef]
21. Murphy, J.; Vallières, F.; Bentall, R.P.; Shevlin, M.; McBride, O.; Hartman, T.K.; Hyland, P. Psychological characteristics associated with COVID-19 vaccine hesitancy and resistance in Ireland and the United Kingdom. *Nat. Commun.* **2021**, *12*, 29. [CrossRef] [PubMed]
22. Khubchandani, J.; Sharma, S.; Price, J.H.; Wiblishauser, M.J.; Sharma, M.; Webb, F.J. COVID-19 vaccination hesitancy in the United States: A rapid national assessment. *J. Community Health* **2021**, *46*, 270–277. [CrossRef] [PubMed]
23. Caserotti, M.; Girardi, P.; Tasso, A.; Rubaltelli, E.; Lotto, L.; Gavaruzzi, T. Joint analysis of the intention to vaccinate and to use contact tracing app during the COVID-19 pandemic. *Sci. Rep.* **2022**, *12*, 793. [CrossRef] [PubMed]
24. Lilleholt, L.; Zettler, I.; Betsch, C.; Böhm, R. Pandemic fatigue: Measurement, correlates, and consequences. *PsyArXiv* **2020**, preprint. [CrossRef]
25. Caserotti, M.; Gavaruzzi, T.; Girardi, P.; Sellaro, R.; Rubaltelli, E.; Tasso, A.; Lotto, L. People's perspectives about COVID-19 vaccination certificate: Findings from a representative Italian sample. *Vaccine* **2022**, *40*, 7406–7414. [CrossRef] [PubMed]
26. Boccalini, S.; Vannacci, A.; Crescioli, G.; Lombardi, N.; Del Riccio, M.; Albora, G.; Bechini, A. Knowledge of university students in health care settings on vaccines and vaccinations strategies: Impact evaluation of a specific educational training course during the COVID-19 pandemic period in Italy. *Vaccines* **2022**, *10*, 1085. [CrossRef]
27. Smithson, M.; Verkuilen, J. A better lemon squeezer? Maximum-likelihood regression with beta-distributed dependent variables. *Psychol. Methods* **2006**, *11*, 54. [CrossRef]
28. Danchin, M.H.; Costa-Pinto, J.; Attwell, K.; Willaby, H.; Wiley, K.; Hoq, M.; Marshall, H. Vaccine decision-making begins in pregnancy: Correlation between vaccine concerns, intentions and maternal vaccination with subsequent childhood vaccine uptake. *Vaccine* **2018**, *36*, 6473–6479. [CrossRef]

29. Thorpe, A.; Fagerlin, A.; Drews, F.A.; Shoemaker, H.; Scherer, L.D. Self-reported health behaviors and risk perceptions following the COVID-19 vaccination rollout in the US: An online survey study. *Public Health* **2022**, *208*, 68–71. [CrossRef]
30. Attwell, K.; Leask, J.; Meyer, S.B.; Rokkas, P.; Ward, P. Vaccine rejecting parents' engagement with expert systems that inform vaccination programs. *J. Bioethical Inq.* **2017**, *14*, 65–76. [CrossRef]
31. Geiger, M.; Rees, F.; Lilleholt, L.; Santana, A.P.; Zettler, I.; Wilhelm, O.; Betsch, C.; Böhm, R. Measuring the 7Cs of vaccination readiness. *Eur. J. Psychol. Assess.* **2022**, *38*, 261–269. [CrossRef]
32. Allington, D.; McAndrew, S.; Moxham-Hall, V.; Duffy, B. Coronavirus conspiracy suspicions, general vaccine attitudes, trust and coronavirus information source as predictors of vaccine hesitancy among UK residents during the COVID-19 pandemic. *Psychol. Med.* **2021**, *53*, 236–247. [CrossRef] [PubMed]
33. Zarbo, C.; Candini, V.; Ferrari, C.; d'Addazio, M.; Calamandrei, G.; Starace, F.; De Girolamo, G. COVID-19 Vaccine Hesitancy in Italy: Predictors of Acceptance, Fence Sitting and Refusal of the COVID-19 Vaccination. *Front. Public Health* **2022**, *10*, 873098. [CrossRef] [PubMed]
34. Smith, S.E.; Sivertsen, N.; Lines, L.; De Bellis, A. Decision making in vaccine hesitant parents and pregnant women–An integrative review. *Int. J. Nurs. Stud. Adv.* **2022**, *4*, 100062. [CrossRef]
35. Caserotti, M.; Gavaruzzi, T.; Girardi, P.; Tasso, A.; Buizza, C.; Candini, V.; Lotto, L. Who is likely to vacillate in their COVID-19 vaccination decision? Free-riding intention and post-positive reluctance. *Prev. Med.* **2022**, *154*, 106885. [CrossRef]

Disclaimer/Publisher's Note: The statements, opinions and data contained in all publications are solely those of the individual author(s) and contributor(s) and not of MDPI and/or the editor(s). MDPI and/or the editor(s) disclaim responsibility for any injury to people or property resulting from any ideas, methods, instructions or products referred to in the content.

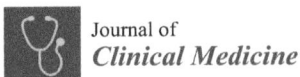
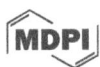

Article

Three Doses of COVID-19 Vaccines: A Retrospective Study Evaluating the Safety and the Immune Response in Patients with Multiple Sclerosis

Giorgia Teresa Maniscalco [1,2], Daniele Di Giulio Cesare [1], Valerio Liguori [3,4], Valentino Manzo [1,2], Elio Prestipino [1,2], Simona Salvatore [1,2], Maria Elena Di Battista [1,2], Ornella Moreggia [1], Antonio Rosario Ziello [1], Vincenzo Andreone [2], Cristina Scavone [3,4,*,†] and Annalisa Capuano [3,4,†]

1. Multiple Sclerosis Regional Center, "A. Cardarelli" Hospital, 80131 Naples, Italy; gtmaniscalco@libero.it (G.T.M.); d.cesaresm@gmail.com (D.D.G.C.); valentino.manzo@aocardarelli.it (V.M.); elio.prestipino@aocardarelli.it (E.P.); simona.salvatore@aocardarelli.it (S.S.); elena.dibattista@aocardarelli.it (M.E.D.B.); ornellamoreggia@gmail.com (O.M.); antonioziello@libero.it (A.R.Z.)
2. Neurological Clinic and Stroke Unit, "A. Cardarelli" Hospital, 80131 Naples, Italy; vincenzo.andreone@aocardarelli.it
3. Department of Experimental Medicine, University of Campania "Luigi Vanvitelli", 80138 Naples, Italy; valerio.liguori@unicampania.it (V.L.); annalisa.capuano@unicampania.it (A.C.)
4. Regional Center of Pharmacovigilance and Pharmacoepidemiology of Campania Region, 80138 Naples, Italy
* Correspondence: cristina.scavone@unicampania.it; Tel.: +39-0815665805
† These authors contributed equally to this work.

Abstract: Since the beginning of the mass immunization of patients with multiple sclerosis (MS), many data on the efficacy and safety of COVID-19 vaccines have been produced. Considering that MS is an autoimmune disease and that some disease-modifying therapies (DMTs) could decrease the antibody response against COVID-19 vaccines, we carried out this retrospective study with the aim to evaluate the safety of these vaccines in terms of AEFI occurrence and the antibody response after MS patients had received the third dose. Two hundred and ten patients (64.8% female; mean age: 46 years) received the third dose of the mRNA-based COVID-19 vaccine and were included in the study. Third doses were administered from October 2021 to January 2022. The majority of patients (n = 193) were diagnosed with RRMS and EDSS values were ≤3.0 in 72.4% of them. DMTs most commonly used by included patients were interferon Beta 1-a, dimethyl fumarate, natalizumab and fingolimod. Overall, 160 patients (68.8% female) experienced 294 AEFIs, of which about 90% were classified as short-term, while 9.2% were classified as long-term. The most commonly reported following the booster dose were pain at the injection site, flu-like symptoms, headache, fever and fatigue. Regarding the immune response, consistently with literature data, we found that patients receiving ocrelizumab and fingolimod had lower IgG titer than patients receiving other DMTs.

Keywords: COVID-19; mRNA-based vaccine; safety; multiple sclerosis; AEFI; observational study; three doses

1. Introduction

During the COVID-19 pandemic, recommendations from the Italian Ministry of Health highlighted the need to take care with much more attention of the frail population, including those suffering from chronic diseases, such as multiple sclerosis (MS), who were recognized as extremely vulnerable people and consequently being part of the highest-priority categories [1].

Thus, since the approval of COVID-19 vaccines and the beginning of the mass immunization of MS patients, many data on the efficacy and safety of these vaccines in a real-life context have been produced. In this context, our research group (composed of neurologists,

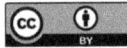

pharmacologists, psychologists, data managers and statisticians) has been actively engaged in the monitoring of MS patients who received flu and COVID-19 vaccines, documenting the main features of patients receiving vaccines in the COVID-19 era and the efficacy and safety profile of these vaccines [2–4]. In particular, in November 2022 we published the results of the first retrospective study in which we analyzed the safety profile of the mRNA COVID-19 vaccines in patients with MS vaccinated with the Pfizer-BioNTech vaccine at the MS Center of the Hospital A.O.R.N. A. Cardarelli [5]. In this study, 310 MS patients received the first dose and 288 the second dose. Patients were mainly diagnosed with Relapsing-Remitting Multiple Sclerosis (RRSM) and the majority of them were receiving a disease-modifying therapy (DMT) during the study period, mainly interferon beta 1-a, dimethyl fumarate, natalizumab and fingolimod. More than nine hundred Adverse Events Following Immunization (AEFIs) were identified, of which 539 were after the first dose of the vaccine and 374 after the second dose. The majority of these AEFIs were classified as short-term and were mainly represented by pain at injection site, flu-like symptoms and headache.

After the publication of this study, many of the patients included received the third dose of the vaccine, and for some of them the immunologic response was monitored in terms of Anti-SARS-CoV-2 IgG value. Considering that MS is an autoimmune disease whose pathology can be explained by an altered immune system [6], and that some DMTs, especially CD20 depleting agents such as ocrelizumab and sphingosine-1-phosphate receptor modulator (S1PRM) such as fingolimod, seem to be able to decrease the antibody response against COVID-19 vaccines [7], and given the collection of new data among our MS patients, we carried out this retrospective study with the aim to evaluate the safety in terms of AEFI occurrence and the antibody response after the third dose of COVID-19 vaccines in people with MS.

2. Methods

2.1. Study Design

This was a retrospective observational study carried out with the aim to assess the safety profile of mRNA-based COVID-19 vaccines and the antibody response among MS patients at the MS Centre of the Cardarelli Hospital (Naples). Third doses were administered from October 2021 to January 2022.

2.2. Demographic and Clinical Data Collection

The following data were retrieved: demographic data (MS diagnosis, age, gender); mRNA-based COVID-19 vaccine (date of vaccination, type of vaccine, vaccine batch); medical and clinical history, DMTs, all AEFIs that occurred after vaccination, patients' general clinical course, values of Anti-SARS-CoV-2 IgG (BAU/mL). The blood samples were collected during the routine clinical practice at least two weeks after the third vaccine dose.

We carried out a descriptive analysis of all identified AEFIs in terms of time occurrence and preferred term (PT). Regarding the time of occurrence, AEFIs were classified as short-term when they occurred within 72 h of the first, second and booster dose of the vaccine and as long-term when they occurred within 20 days of the first, second and booster dose of the vaccine.

2.3. Statistical Analysis

Categorial variables were described as frequency and percentage, while continuous variables were reported by their mean and standard deviation. Shapiro–Wilk test was used to assess the normality of data distribution. In the case of not normal distribution, no parametric test was applied.

For difference between DMTs in terms of SARS-humoral response, we used one-way ANOVA with Gamess-Howell (no parametric post hoc test) for differences between groups. p value less than 0.05 was considered significant.

2.4. Ethics

The retrospective study was reported to the Ethic Committee of A.O.R.N. A. Cardarelli/Santobono-Pausilipon. No written informed consent was necessary for the study conduction based on its retrospective nature.

3. Results

3.1. Overall Safety Results

Clinical and demographic characteristics of enrolled patients are reported in Table 1. We enrolled 210 MS patients (64.8% female; mean age: 46 years) who received the third dose (booster dose) of the mRNA-based COVID-19 vaccine. As for previous doses [5], all patients received the Pfizer-BioNTech vaccine. In addition, 91.9% of patients (n = 193) were diagnosed with RRMS, 5.7% of patients (n = 12) with Secondary Progressive Multiple Sclerosis (SPMS) and 1.9% (n = 4) with Primary Progressive Multiple Sclerosis (PPMS). The mean disease duration was 11.5 years (data not shown). EDSS values were ≤3.0 in 72.4% of patients, followed by equal 3.5–5.5 in 16.2% of patients, and ≥6.0 in 11.4% of patients. With regard to DMTs, many patients (n = 36; 17.1%) were receiving interferon Beta 1-a, followed by dimethyl fumarate (n = 34; 16.2%), natalizumab (n = 33; 15.7%) and fingolimod (n = 22; 10.5%) (Table 1).

Table 1. Clinical and demographic variables of patients with multiple sclerosis who received booster dose COVID-19 vaccination.

Study Cohort	Patients Who Received the Third Dose	Patients with Blood Test Collected
Total patients	210	60
Female, n (%)	136 (64.8)	27 (45)
Male, n (%)	74 (35.2)	33 (55)
Mean age (years) ± sd	46.3 ± 13.4	39.6 ± 10.5
MS type, n (%)		
RRMS	193 (91.9)	59 (98.3)
SPMS	12 (5.7)	1 (1.7)
PPMS	4 (1.9)	-
PRMS	1 (0.5)	-
Disability by EDSS, n (%)		
≤3.0	152 (72.4)	55 (91.7)
3.5–5.5	34 (16.2)	3 (5.0)
≥6.0	24 (11.4)	2 (3.3)
DMTs, n (%)		
ocrelizumab	20 (9.5)	8 (13.4)
fingolimod	22 (10.5)	7 (11.7)
interferon beta 1-a	36 (17.1)	9 (15)
natalizumab	33 (15.7)	11 (18.3)
dimethyl fumarate	34 (16.2)	11 (18.3)
cladribine	12 (5.7)	6 (10)
glatiramer acetate	15 (7.1)	3 (5)
teriflunomide	23 (11)	5 (8.3)
interferon beta 1-b	6 (2.9)	-

Table 1. *Cont.*

Study Cohort	Patients Who Received the Third Dose	Patients with Blood Test Collected
methotrexate	1 (0.5)	-
rituximab	3 (1.4)	-
alemtuzumab	1 (0.5)	-
Untreated	4 (1.9)	-

RRMS: Relapsing Remitting Multiple Sclerosis; SPMS: Secondary Progressive Multiple Sclerosis; PPMS: Primary Progressive Multiple Sclerosis; PRMS: Primary Relapsing Multiple Sclerosis; EDSS: Expanded Disability Status Scale; DMTS: Disease-Modifying Therapies.

During the study period, 160 patients (68.8% female) experienced at least one AEFI (data not shown). In particular, 294 AEFIs occurred, of which about 90.8% were classified as short-term, while 9.2% were classified as long-term (Table 2). Looking at the type of AEFIs, the most commonly reported following the booster dose were pain at the injection site (n = 112; 38.0%), flu-like symptoms (n = 62; 21.0%), headache (n = 39; 13.3%), fever (n = 32; 10.9%) and fatigue (n = 24; 8.2%) (Figure 1). More in detail, the most common short-term AEFIs after booster dose were pain at the injection site (n = 111; 41.6%), flu-like symptoms (n = 56; 20.9%) and headache (n = 34; 12.7%). Fever (n = 32; 12%) was more frequent after the second dose of the vaccine and the booster dose than after the first vaccine dose. However, compared to the second booster dose, fatigue symptoms were similar following the administration of the booster dose and following the administration of the first dose of the vaccine (Table 3).

Table 2. Distribution of Adverse Events Following Immunization (AEFIs) by time of occurrence (short- and long-term) and vaccine's dose.

	Total	First Dose	Second Dose	Booster Dose
Study population	310	310	288	210
All AEFIs, n	1207	539	374	294
Short-term AEFIs, n (%)	1057 (87.6)	438 (81.3)	352 (94.1)	267 (90.8)
Long-term AEFIs, n (%)	150 (12.4)	101 (18.7)	22 (5.9)	27 (9.2)

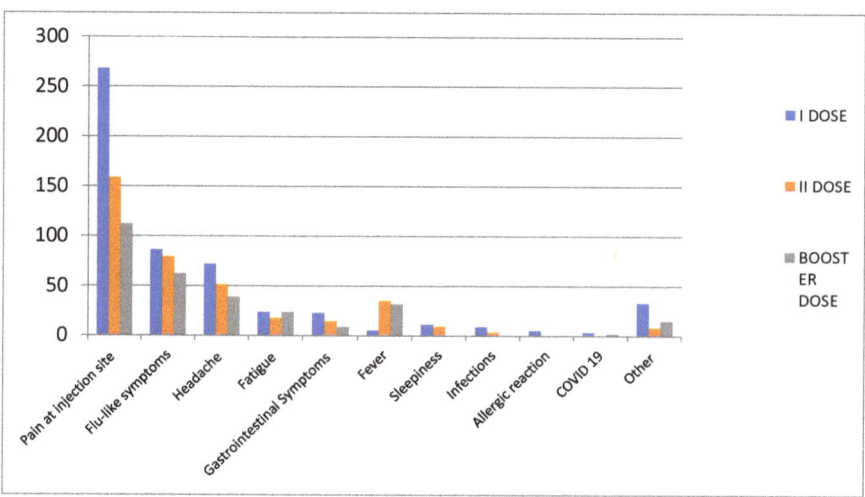

Figure 1. Distribution of Adverse Events Following Immunization (AEFIs) by Preferred Term (PT).

Table 3. Distribution of Adverse Events Following Immunization (AEFIs) by time of occurrence and Preferred term (PT) among MS patients.

	Short-Term AEFIs	Long-Term AEFIs
Any adverse events, n (%)	267	27
Pain at injection site	111 (41.6)	1 (3.7)
Flu-like symptoms	56 (20.9)	6 (22.2)
Headache	34 (12.7)	5 (18.5)
Fever	32 (12)	-
Fatigue	17 (6.4)	7 (25.9)
Gastrointestinal symptoms	8 (3)	1 (3.7)
Other symptoms	9 (3.4)	5 (18.5)
Infection with SARS-CoV-2 after vaccination	-	2 (7.5)

3.2. Immune Response Results

After having received the third dose of the vaccine, 60 patients (28.6% of the cohort, 55% females) underwent laboratory tests, including the detection of SARS-CoV-2 IgG level (Table 1). The IgG test was performed after a mean of 33.1 days (± 9.3), ranging from 15 to 60 days. The mean of Anti-SARS-CoV-2 IgG level following the booster dose was 8152 (± 4750).

A difference in IgG level by DMTs was found. In particular, significant differences were found between: interferon Beta 1-a vs. ocrelizumab (10,315; $p < 0.001$) and fingolimod (9573; $p < 0.001$). Natalizumab showed higher levels of Anti-SARS-CoV IgG than ocrelizumab (6262; $p = 0.019$) and fingolimod (5521; $p = 0.045$). Lastly, patients treated with dimethyl fumarate had higher IgG titer of Anti-SARS-CoV-2 than ocrelizumab (9651; $p < 0.001$) and fingolimod (8910; $p < 0.001$) (Figure 2).

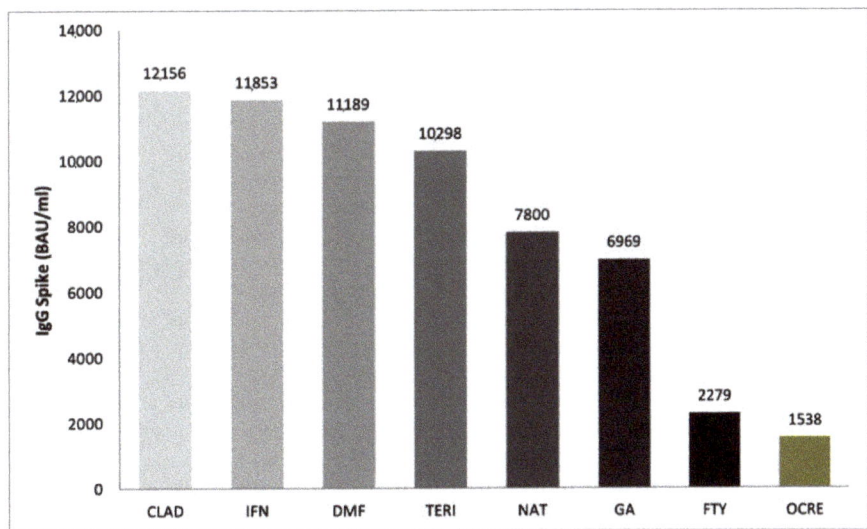

Figure 2. IgG Spike (BAU/mL) post booster dose in different DMTs. CLAD: Cladribine; IFN: Interferon B 1-a; DMF: Dimethyl Fumarate; TERI: Teriflunomide; NAT: Natalizumab; GA: Glatiramer Acetate; FTY: Fingolimod; OCRE: Ocrelizumab.

Among patients for whom IgG level were available, 42 (70%) experienced short-term AEFIs. Of these patients, 25 were female (59.5% of total) and 17 were male (40.5%); mean EDSS was higher in patients who reported short-term AEFIs (2 vs. 1.1), with lower mean age (39 vs. 42).

4. Discussion

Since the beginning of the COVID-19 vaccination campaign among MS patients, a huge amount of clinical and laboratory data has been collected, representing a valuable source of information for a frail population such as MS patients. Since then, many research groups started to collect and analyze these data, providing new evidence on the efficacy and safety of COVID-19 vaccines among MS patients. For instance, a group of Italian researchers [8] compared the COVID-19 course and outcomes in MS patients on ocrelizumab and fingolimod after receiving the third dose of mRNA vaccine vs. patients on natalizumab. They enrolled 290 patients, of whom 79 were treated with natalizumab, 126 with ocrelizumab and 85 with fingolimod. Their results showed that patients who had COVID-19 on ocrelizumab and fingolimod were more symptomatic with higher hospitalization rates compared to patients on natalizumab. Overall, the results supported the effectiveness of the third booster dose of mRNA-Vax against severe forms of COVID-19 in patients treated with ocrelizumab and fingolimod.

We carried out a retrospective study to examine the safety profile and the antibody response in 210 MS patients who received the third dose of a mRNA COVID-19 vaccine. More in detail, we carried out a descriptive analysis of the AEFIs by time of occurrence and PT.

Overall, our analysis showed that the mean age of 210 patients was 46.3 years, and almost 60% were females. These results are consistent with those of previous studies; indeed, as reported also by Harbo HF et al., women are more likely than men to get MS (the prevalence ratio of MS in women to men is 2.3–3.5:1) [9].

In our cohort, a total of 160 patients (76.2%) had at least one AEFI. Of these patients, almost 70% were female. In line with this finding, Peter Yamoah et al. reported that COVID-19 vaccine-induced AEFIs were more frequently observed in women than men and in patients of the age group 18–64 years [10]. Other studies reported similar difference in AEFIs distribution by gender [11,12].

RRMS was the most prevalent MS subtype among patients included in our study with interferon Beta 1-a, dimethyl fumarate and natalizumab the DMTs most frequently prescribed. These results are in line with previous findings [2–5] but also with another study that investigated the antibody response after the third dose of COVID-19 vaccine in MS patients affected by various MS subtypes [13]. According to our opinion, the distribution of drug use among MS patients may be related to the diverse population included in our study, especially in terms of age and MS type.

In our study, the most commonly reported AEFIs following the booster dose were pain at the injection site, flu-like symptoms, headache, fever and fatigue. Comparing our descriptive analysis of AEFIs with previous results [5], flu-like symptoms and fever were more frequent after the second dose of the vaccine, and in this analysis, following the booster dose than after the first dose. In most cases, these AEFIs are not serious and resolve on their own. Events occur mostly on the vaccination day or the day after. In line with our results, Sapir Dreyer-Alster et al. conducted a study on 211 MS patients (62% female, 74.8% treated with different DMTs) who received the third dose of the BNT162b2 vaccine. Following vaccination, no anaphylactic or life-threatening reactions occurred. The most commonly reported AEFIs were muscle or joint discomfort, fatigue, localized pain at the injection site and fever. Headaches and dizziness occurred in 7.6% and 1.9% of patients, respectively [14]. Regarding the occurrence of headache, Castaldo M et al. carried out a systematic review and meta-analysis of 84 articles (accounting for 1.57 million participants) to assess the pooled incidence of post-vaccine headache (after first and second dose) by vaccine type. In line with our results, headache was the third most common AE and a two-fold risk of developing headache within 7 days from injection was found. As reported by study's authors, patients developing a new-onset headache should be carefully monitored for the risk of developing cerebral venous thrombosis, especially those with risk factors, such as thrombocytopenia, anti-platelet factor 4 antibodies, and multiple organ thrombosis [15]. Even though the mechanism underlying the occurrence of post-vaccination headache is currently unknown, this symptom could be a consequence of a homoeostasis disorder deriving from humoral and cellular immunity induced by the vaccine, which are characterized by an increase in inflammatory cytokines (i.e., interferon gamma, interleukin-6, CXC ligand 10) leading to a plethora of symptoms that also include headache [16,17].

We aimed also to investigate the antibody response among 60 MS patients who underwent—during routine clinical practice—laboratory tests, including SARS-CoV-2 IgG. According to this analysis, we found a difference in IgG level for different DMTs (ANOVA test, $p < 0.001$). Significant differences were found for the comparison interferon Beta 1-a vs. ocrelizumab (10,315; $p < 0.001$) and interferon Beta 1-a vs. fingolimod (9573; $p < 0.001$). As reported by Pitzalis M et al. [18], who evaluated the SARS-CoV-2 response after the second dose of the COVID-19 vaccine among 912 Sardinian MS patients and 63 healthy controls, humoral response to BNT162b2 was significantly influenced by these specific DMTs. In addition, Garjani et al. showed that fingolimod and ocrelizumab are to blame for the reduced immune response following COVID-19 vaccinations [19]. Similarly, findings were reported by Baba et al. [13]. Wu X et al. [7] carried out a meta-analysis of 48 studies published until March 2022 to evaluate the risk of impaired response to vaccination among 6860 patients with MS receiving DMTs. An attenuated serologic response was observed in patients treated with anti-CD20 (OR = 0.02, 95% CI: 0.01–0.03) and S1PRM (OR = 0.03, 95% CI: 0.01–0.06) after full vaccination compared with patients not receiving any DMT. No other significant associations between other DMTs and humoral response to SARS-CoV-2 vaccines were found by the authors' study. Another study [20] found out that the effects of fingolimod on cellular immunity persisted for more than 2 years after a change to ocrelizumab; thus, clinicians should consider the possible failure to provide protection against SARS-CoV-2 when switching from fingolimod to ocrelizumab. König et al. evaluated the safety and immunogenicity profiles of the third dose of mRNA COVID-19 vaccine among MS patients already receiving fingolimod or anti-CD20 therapy. The results highlighted a better antibody response among patients who received anti-CD20 therapy than those who received fingolimod and that a higher absolute lymphocyte count was linked to both a better antibody response and more side effects [21]. In the same way, Achiron et al. compared the efficacy profile of the third dose of the COVID-19 vaccine respect to MS non-responder-patients treated with fingolimod. Specifically, a total of 20 patients were randomized into two groups, 10 patients in the fingolimod-continuation and 10 patients in the fingolimod-discontinuation. One month after receiving the third dose positive SARS-CoV-IgG antibodies were detected in two patients in the fingolimod-continuation group vs. eight patients in the fingolimod-discontinuation group, suggesting that fingolimod discontinuation is associated with beneficial humoral immune protection [22]. Lastly, Madelon et al. carried out a study where 20 patients that received ocrelizumab had a robust T-cell response recognizing spike proteins from the Delta and Omicron variants after vaccination. Following the third dose of the vaccine, there was an increase in the number of both CD4 and CD8 T cells that responded, showing that it was possible to improve individuals who had an undetectable memory response after the initial vaccination series [23].

5. Strengths and Limitations

The main limitations of our study include its retrospective and monocentric nature and the small sample size. In addition, the assessment of IgG response was used as a measure of assumed humoral immunity even though we are aware that antibody levels are not fully predictive of protection against infection and that the protective immune response to SARS-CoV-2 could also depend on T-cell responses. As we previously reported [5], considering that we cannot exclude the lack of important clinical data, our findings should be considered exploratory and interpreted with caution.

Nevertheless, we have provided new evidence collecting and analyzing clinical and laboratory data on the safety of the third dose COVID-19 vaccines in a frail population such as MS patients. As for previous studies, data collection and analysis have been performed by a multidisciplinary team of neurologists, pharmacologists, statisticians, and data managers with a long-standing experience in the management of studies focusing on the monitoring of the safety profile of medicines and vaccines [24–26].

6. Conclusions

In conclusion, our results indicated that the booster dose of the Pfizer-BioNTech vaccine was safe for MS patients, being associated with AEFIs already detected in the general population and with previous vaccine doses and shown in our previous publications. Specifically, in this study the booster dose was associated with 294 AEFIs which occurred in 160 patients (mainly women) and the most common AEFIs (mainly classified as short-term) were injection-site reactions, flu-like symptoms, headache, fever and fatigue. After having received the third dose of the vaccine, 60 patients underwent laboratory tests, including the detection of SARS-CoV-2 IgG levels. Consistently with literature data, we found that patients receiving ocrelizumab and fingolimod had lower IgG titer than patients receiving other DMTs.

Author Contributions: Conceptualization, G.T.M., C.S. and A.C.; methodology, O.M. and D.D.G.C.; software, O.M. and D.D.G.C.; formal analysis, V.L., D.D.G.C. and C.S.; investigation, V.M., E.P., S.S., M.E.D.B., O.M., A.R.Z. and V.A.; resources, V.M., E.P, S.S., M.E.D.B., O.M., A.R.Z. and V.A.; writing—original draft preparation, G.T.M., C.S. and A.C.; writing—review and editing, G.T.M., D.D.G.C., V.L., V.M., E.P., S.S., M.E.D.B., O.M., A.R.Z., V.A., C.S. and A.C.; supervision, G.T.M. and A.C.; project administration, G.T.M. All authors have read and agreed to the published version of the manuscript.

Funding: This research received no external funding.

Institutional Review Board Statement: The study was conducted in accordance with the Declaration of Helsinki, and approved by the Ethics Committee of A.O.R.N. A. Cardarelli/Santobono-Pausilipon (with Resolution n. 2/2022).

Informed Consent Statement: This was a retrospective study, thus the informed consent was not obtained from patients.

Data Availability Statement: The data presented in this study are available on request from the corresponding author. The data are not publicly available due to privacy and ethical reasons.

Conflicts of Interest: The authors declare no conflict of interest. G.T.M. received personal compensation from Serono, Biogen, Novartis, Roche, and TEVA for public speaking and advisory boards.

References

1. Raccomandazioni Aggiornate sul COVID-19 per le Persone con Sclerosi Multipla (SM)—12 Gennaio 2021 SIN ed AISM 12 Gennaio 2021 Ministero della Salute: Raccomandazioni ad Interim sui Gruppi Target della Vaccinazione Anti-SARS-CoV-2/COVID-19 8 Febbraio 2021. Available online: https://www.aism.it/sites/default/files/Raccomandazioni_COVID_SM_AISM_SIN.pdf (accessed on 16 November 2022).
2. Maniscalco, G.T.; Scavone, C.; Moreggia, O.; Cesare, D.D.G.; Aiezza, M.L.; Guglielmi, G.; Longo, G.; Maiolo, M.; Raiola, E.; Russo, G.; et al. Flu vaccination in multiple sclerosis patients: A monocentric prospective vaccine-vigilance study. *Expert Opin. Drug Saf.* **2022**, *21*, 979–984. [CrossRef] [PubMed]
3. Maniscalco, G.T.; Manzo, V.; Di Battista, M.E.; Salvatore, S.; Moreggia, O.; Scavone, C.; Capuano, A. Severe Multiple Sclerosis Relapse After COVID-19 Vaccination: A Case Report. *Front. Neurol.* **2021**, *12*, 721502. [CrossRef] [PubMed]
4. Ziello, A.; Scavone, C.; Di Battista, M.E.; Salvatore, S.; Cesare, D.D.G.; Moreggia, O.; Allegorico, L.; Sagnelli, A.; Barbato, S.; Manzo, V.; et al. Influenza Vaccine Hesitancy in Patients with Multiple Sclerosis: A Monocentric Observational Study. *Brain Sci.* **2021**, *11*, 890. [CrossRef]

5. Maniscalco, G.T.; Scavone, C.; Mascolo, A.; Manzo, V.; Prestipino, E.; Guglielmi, G.; Aiezza, M.L.; Cozzolino, S.; Bracco, A.; Moreggia, O.; et al. The Safety Profile of COVID-19 Vaccines in Patients Diagnosed with Multiple Sclerosis: A Retrospective Observational Study. *J. Clin. Med.* **2022**, *11*, 6855. [CrossRef]
6. Titus, H.E.; Chen, Y.; Podojil, J.R.; Robinson, A.P.; Balabanov, R.; Popko, B.; Miller, S.D. Pre-clinical and clinical implications of "inside-out" vs. "outside-in" paradigms in multiple sclerosis etiopathogenesis. *Front. Cell. Neurosci.* **2020**, *14*, 599717. [CrossRef] [PubMed]
7. Wu, X.; Wang, L.; Shen, L.; Tang, K. Response of COVID-19 vaccination in multiple sclerosis patients following disease-modifying therapies: A meta-analysis. *EBioMedicine* **2022**, *81*, 104102. [CrossRef]
8. Capuano, R.; Prosperini, L.; Altieri, M.; Lorefice, L.; Fantozzi, R.; Cavalla, P.; Guaschino, C.; Radaelli, M.; Cordioli, C.; Nociti, V.; et al. Symptomatic COVID-19 course and outcomes after three mRNA vaccine doses in multiple sclerosis patients treated with high-efficacy DMTs. *Mult. Scler. J.* **2023**, *29*, 856–865. [CrossRef]
9. Harbo, H.F.; Gold, R.; Tintoré, M. Sex and gender issues in multiple sclerosis. *Ther. Adv. Neurol. Disord.* **2013**, *6*, 237–248. [CrossRef]
10. Yamoah, P.; Mensah, K.B.; Attakorah, J.; Padayachee, N.; Oosthuizen, F.; Bangalee, V. Adverse events following immunization associated with coronavirus disease 2019 (COVID-19) vaccines: A descriptive analysis from VigiAccess. *Hum. Vaccines Immunother.* **2022**, *18*, 2109365. [CrossRef]
11. Harris, T.; Nair, J.; Fediurek, J.; Deeks, S.L. Assessment of sex-specific differences in adverse events following immunization reporting in Ontario, 2012–15. *Vaccine* **2017**, *35*, 2600–2604. [CrossRef]
12. Zinzi, A.; Gaio, M.; Liguori, V.; Ruggiero, R.; Tesorone, M.; Rossi, F.; Rafaniello, C.; Capuano, A. Safety Monitoring of mRNA COVID-19 Vaccines in Children Aged 5 to 11 Years by Using EudraVigilance Pharmacovigilance Database: The CoVaxChild Study. *Vaccines* **2023**, *11*, 401. [CrossRef]
13. Baba, C.; Ozcelik, S.; Kaya, E.; Samedzada, U.; Ozdogar, A.T.; Cevik, S.; Dogan, Y.; Ozakbas, S. Three doses of COVID-19 vaccines in multiple sclerosis patients treated with disease-modifying therapies. *Mult. Scler. Relat. Disord.* **2022**, *68*, 104119. [CrossRef]
14. Dreyer-Alster, S.; Menascu, S.; Mandel, M.; Shirbint, E.; Magalashvili, D.; Dolev, M.; Flechter, S.; Givon, U.; Guber, D.; Stern, Y.; et al. COVID-19 vaccination in patients with multiple sclerosis: Safety and humoral efficacy of the third booster dose. *J. Neurol. Sci.* **2022**, *434*, 120155. [CrossRef]
15. Castaldo, M.; Waliszewska-Prosół, M.; Koutsokera, M.; Robotti, M.; Straburzyński, M.; Apostolakopoulou, L.; Capizzi, M.; Çibuku, O.; Ambat, F.D.F.; Frattale, I.; et al. Headache onset after vaccination against SARS-CoV-2: A systematic literature review and meta-analysis. *J. Headache Pain* **2022**, *23*, 41. [CrossRef]
16. Scavone, C.; Mascolo, A.; Rafaniello, C.; Sportiello, L.; Trama, U.; Zoccoli, A.; Bernardi, F.F.; Racagni, G.; Berrino, L.; Castaldo, G.; et al. Therapeutic strategies to fight COVID-19: Which is the status artis? *Br. J. Pharmacol.* **2021**, *179*, 2128–2148. [CrossRef]
17. Mascolo, A.; Scavone, C.; Rafaniello, C.; De Angelis, A.; Urbanek, K.; di Mauro, G.; Cappetta, D.; Berrino, L.; Rossi, F.; Capuano, A. The Role of Renin-Angiotensin-Aldosterone System in the Heart and Lung: Focus on COVID-19. *Front. Pharmacol.* **2021**, *12*, 667254. [CrossRef]
18. Pitzalis, M.; Idda, M.L.; Lodde, V.; Loizedda, A.; Lobina, M.; Zoledziewska, M.; Virdis, F.; Delogu, G.; Pirinu, F.; Marini, M.G.; et al. Effect of Different Disease-Modifying Therapies on Humoral Response to BNT162b2 Vaccine in Sardinian Multiple Sclerosis Patients. *Front. Immunol.* **2021**, *12*, 781843. [CrossRef]
19. Garjani, A.; Patel, S.; Bharkhada, D.; Rashid, W.; Coles, A.; Law, G.R.; Evangelou, N. Impact of mass vaccination on SARS-CoV-2 infections among multiple sclerosis patients taking immunomodulatory disease-modifying therapies in England. *Mult. Scler. Relat. Disord.* **2021**, *57*, 103458. [CrossRef]
20. Torres, P.; Sancho-Saldaña, A.; Gil Sánchez, A.; Peralta, S.; Solana, M.J.; Bakkioui, S.; González-Mingot, C.; Quibus, L.; Ruiz-Fernández, E.; Pedro-Murillo, E.S.; et al. A prospective study of cellular immune response to booster COVID-19 vaccination in multiple sclerosis patients treated with a broad spectrum of disease-modifying therapies. *J. Neurol.* **2023**, *270*, 2380–2391. [CrossRef]
21. König, M.; Torgauten, H.M.; Tran, T.T.; Holmøy, T.; Vaage, J.T.; Lund-Johansen, F.; Nygaard, G.O. Immunogenicity and Safety of a Third SARS-CoV-2 Vaccine Dose in Patients with Multiple Sclerosis and Weak Immune Response After COVID-19 Vaccination. *JAMA Neurol.* **2022**, *79*, 307–309. [CrossRef]
22. Achiron, A.; Mandel, M.; Gurevich, M.; Dreyer-Alster, S.; Magalashvili, D.; Sonis, P.; Dolev, M.; Menascu, S.; Harari, G.; Flechter, S.; et al. Immune response to the third COVID-19 vaccine dose is related to lymphocyte count in multiple sclerosis patients treated with fingolimod. *J. Neurol.* **2022**, *269*, 2286–2292. [CrossRef] [PubMed]
23. Madelon, N.; Heikkilä, N.; Royo, I.S.; Fontannaz, P.; Breville, G.; Lauper, K.; Goldstein, R.; Grifoni, A.; Sette, A.; Siegrist, C.-A.; et al. Omicron-Specific Cytotoxic T-Cell Responses After a Third Dose of mRNA COVID-19 Vaccine among Patients with Multiple Sclerosis Treated with Ocrelizumab. *JAMA Neurol.* **2022**, *79*, 399–404. [CrossRef] [PubMed]
24. Sessa, M.; Rafaniello, C.; Sportiello, L.; Mascolo, A.; Scavone, C.; Maccariello, A.; Iannaccone, T.; Fabbrozzi, M.; Berrino, L.; Rossi, F.; et al. Campania Region (Italy) spontaneous reporting system and preventability assessment through a case-by-case approach: A pilot study on psychotropic drugs. *Expert Opin. Drug Saf.* **2016**, *15*, 9–15. [CrossRef] [PubMed]

25. Sessa, M.; Sportiello, L.; Mascolo, A.; Scavone, C.; Gallipoli, S.; Di Mauro, G.; Cimmaruta, D.; Rafaniello, C.; Capuano, A. Campania Preventability Assessment Committee (Italy): A Focus on the Preventability of Non-steroidal Anti-inflammatory Drugs' Adverse Drug Reactions. *Front. Pharmacol.* **2017**, *8*, 305. [CrossRef]
26. Capuano, A.; Scavone, C.; Racagni, G.; Scaglione, F. NSAIDs in patients with viral infections, including COVID-19: Victims or perpetrators? *Pharmacol. Res.* **2020**, *157*, 104849. [CrossRef]

Disclaimer/Publisher's Note: The statements, opinions and data contained in all publications are solely those of the individual author(s) and contributor(s) and not of MDPI and/or the editor(s). MDPI and/or the editor(s) disclaim responsibility for any injury to people or property resulting from any ideas, methods, instructions or products referred to in the content.

MDPI
St. Alban-Anlage 66
4052 Basel
Switzerland
www.mdpi.com

Journal of Clinical Medicine Editorial Office
E-mail: jcm@mdpi.com
www.mdpi.com/journal/jcm

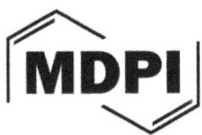

Disclaimer/Publisher's Note: The statements, opinions and data contained in all publications are solely those of the individual author(s) and contributor(s) and not of MDPI and/or the editor(s). MDPI and/or the editor(s) disclaim responsibility for any injury to people or property resulting from any ideas, methods, instructions or products referred to in the content.